T0262055

Critical Care MCQs

A Companion for Intensive Care Exams

Dr Steven Lobaz MBBS BMedSci FRCA FFICM

Consultant in Anaesthesia and Intensive Care Medicine
Barnsley Hospital NHS Foundation Trust, Barnsley, UK

Dr Mika Hamilton MBChB FRCA FFICM

Speciality Registrar (ST7) Anaesthesia and Intensive Care Medicine
The James Cook University Hospital, Middlesbrough, UK

Dr Alastair J Glossop BMedSci BMBS MRCP FRCA DICM FFICM

Consultant in Anaesthesia and Intensive Care Medicine
Sheffield Teaching Hospitals NHS Foundation Trust, Sheffield, UK

Dr Ajay Raithatha MBChB MRCP FRCA FFICM EDIC

Consultant in Anaesthesia and Intensive Care Medicine
Sheffield Teaching Hospitals NHS Foundation Trust, Sheffield, UK

i

tfm Publishing Limited, Castle Hill Barns, Harley, Shrewsbury, SY5 6LX, UK
Tel: +44 (0)1952 510061; Fax: +44 (0)1952 510192
E-mail: info@tfmpublishing.com
Web site: www.tfmpublishing.com

Editing, design & typesetting: Nikki Bramhill BSc Hons Dip Law
First edition: © 2015
Front cover images: © 2015 istockphoto; http://www.istockphoto.com
Paperback   ISBN: 978-1-903378-99-1
E-book editions: 2015
ePub   ISBN: 978-1-910079-15-7
Mobi   ISBN: 978-1-910079-16-4
Web pdf   ISBN: 978-1-910079-17-1

The entire contents of *Critical Care MCQs — A Companion for Intensive Care Exams* is copyright tfm Publishing Ltd. Apart from any fair dealing for the purposes of research or private study, or criticism or review, as permitted under the Copyright, Designs and Patents Act 1988, this publication may not be reproduced, stored in a retrieval system or transmitted in any form or by any means, electronic, digital, mechanical, photocopying, recording or otherwise, without the prior written permission of the publisher.

Neither the authors nor the publisher can accept responsibility for any injury or damage to persons or property occasioned through the implementation of any ideas or use of any product described herein. Neither can they accept any responsibility for errors, omissions or misrepresentations, howsoever caused.

Whilst every care is taken by the authors and the publisher to ensure that all information and data in this book are as accurate as possible at the time of going to press, it is recommended that readers seek independent verification of advice on drug or other product usage, surgical techniques and clinical processes prior to their use.

The authors and publisher gratefully acknowledge the permission granted to reproduce the copyright material where applicable in this book. Every effort has been made to trace copyright holders and to obtain their permission for the use of copyright material. The publisher apologizes for any errors or omissions and would be grateful if notified of any corrections that should be incorporated in future reprints or editions of this book.

Printed by Gutenberg Press Ltd., Gudja Road, Tarxien, PLA 19, Malta

Contents

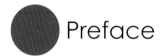 Preface

To many candidates the prospect of sitting an intensive care medicine exam can be daunting. The specialty is vast in its scope, one which is developing and evolving rapidly. However, with hard work and dedication, success can be achieved by the majority of candidates. We believe that this book, written by doctors who have collectively passed the UK FFICM and European Diploma examinations, is a perfect companion and guide to success in critical care exams. It encompasses both core syllabus topics and recent influential papers, and is an invaluable resource for preparation and success.

Good luck!

Dr Steven Lobaz MBBS BMedSci FRCA FFICM
Dr Mika Hamilton MBChB FRCA FFICM
Dr Alastair J Glossop BMedSci BMBS MRCP FRCA DICM FFICM
Dr Ajay Raithatha MBChB MRCP FRCA FFICM EDIC
January 2015

Acknowledgements

The authors would like to thank Dr Helen Ellis for her time and efforts in testing and critiquing the papers in this book. Her comments have proved invaluable during the final editorial process and we are very grateful for this.

We would also like to thank Nikki Bramhill at tfm publishing for helping to make this book a reality.

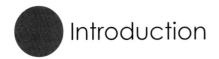 Introduction

Through five complete examination papers, each compromising 90 questions of 5 true or false stems, this book takes the reader through the core areas of intensive care medicine. Each paper is designed to cover a wide range of syllabus topics relevant to several major examination formats including: the UK Fellowship of the Faculty of Intensive Care Medicine (FFICM), the European Diploma in Intensive Care (EDIC), the Indian Diploma in Critical Care Medicine (IDCCM), the Diploma of the Irish Board of Intensive Care Medicine (DIBICM), the Australian and New Zealand Fellowship of the College of Intensive Care Medicine (CICM), and American board exams.

The questions are set at a level designed to test the knowledge of higher trainees in the specialty. A score of 72-74% (with a positive marking scoring system) is deemed the pass mark for each paper, which is comparable to the pass mark for the MCQ section of the FFICM examination.

Following each 90-question paper, an answer overview can be found. Each answer has the question title, summary of the true stems and a brief explanation and discussion attached. Relevant and up-to-date references are listed at the end of each answer.

A detailed list of further resources and recommendations relevant to critical care is provided at the end of the book, enabling readers to further their knowledge base and level of understanding.

Success in MCQ examinations requires a strong knowledge base but also good examination technique. We hope that this book will provide prospective candidates with the question practice and background reading required to be successful. We wish you the best of luck.

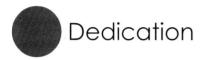 Dedication

I wish to dedicate this book to all the staff at the Royal Victoria Infirmary and Freeman Hospital, Newcastle-upon-Tyne, UK, in particular, Dr Kirk, Mr Hassan, Dr Smith and all staff involved in paediatric cardiology, surgery, anaesthesia and critical care. Without their efforts and expertise I would not have been given the most precious gift — the chance to be a father to my daughter Eva. Words cannot express my eternal gratitude. Thank you.

Dr Steven Lobaz MBBS BMedSci FRCA FFICM

"Believe in yourself! Have faith in your abilities!
Without a humble but reasonable confidence in your own
powers you cannot be successful or happy." **Norman Vincent Peale**

1 MCQ Paper 1: Questions

Question 1: In relation to the drug sugammadex:

a   It is recommended for immediate reversal of vecuronium.

b   It can effectively reverse cisatracurium.

c   16mg/kg is recommended intravenously for the immediate reversal of rocuronium.

d   It is an α-cyclodextrin that encapsulates aminosteroid neuromuscular blocking agents.

e   Sugammadex may be effective in treating rocuronium-induced anaphylaxis.

Question 2: For patients with coronary artery stents undergoing non-cardiac surgery:

a   Non-urgent surgery should be delayed in the immediate post-stent period.

b   Drug-eluting stents (DES) have reduced restenosis rates at 1 year, when compared to bare metal stents (BMS).

c   Bare metal stents (BMS) require 4-6 months of clopidogrel therapy.

d   Dual antiplatelet therapy is associated with an increased peri-operative mortality.

e   Biocompatible stents (e.g. Genous™ R-stent) require peri-operative bridging therapy.

Question 3: Regarding The Royal College of Anaesthetists' 4th National Audit Project (NAP4):

a   Airway complications in intensive care resulted in death or disability in less than 20% of cases.

b   End-tidal CO_2 monitoring (capnography) is not always necessary for intubation.

c   A difficult airway trolley is recommended for all intensive care units.

d   Regular audit of airway complications should occur.

e   Transfer of an intubated patient is deemed low risk for airway complications.

Question 4: In relation to a potential 'can't intubate, can't ventilate (CICV) scenario' in anaesthesia practice:

a   It is estimated to occur in 0.01 to 2.0 per 100,000 cases.

b   Jet ventilation is required for cricothyroidotomy with a cannula of >4mm diameter.

c   Over 90% of CICV situations are preventable.

d   Fixation error may lead to loss of situational awareness and poor decision making.

e   Cricothyroidotomy skills are retained for only a short period.

Question 5: In quinine sulphate overdose:

a   The QTc interval shortens.

b   Temporary deafness can occur.

c   Amiodarone is the anti-arrhythmic of choice for ventricular tachycardia (VT) with a pulse.

d   Quinine induces insulin release.

e   Continuous veno-venous haemofiltration (CVVH) will remove quinine.

Question 6: The pre-test heparin-induced thrombocytopenia (HIT) score:

a   Has four categories.

b   Has a maximum score of 4.

c   A score of 2 is given for a >50% fall in platelets.
d   A total score of 3 indicates a 20% pre-test probability of HIT.
e   A platelet fall in <4 days since heparin administration and no recent prior heparin exposure is given a zero score.

Question 7: Concerning bronchoscopy in critical care:

a   It is an essential diagnostic and therapeutic procedure.
b   One should wear full protective clothing during bronchoscopy.
c   Following bronchoscopy, the suction port should be immediately brushed through and the bronchoscope sent for decontamination.
d   It should be possible to visualise the first 2-7 divisions of each lobar bronchus.
e   During bronchial-alveolar lavage, 20-60ml 0.9% saline should be instilled prior to suctioning and specimen trap.

Question 8: In relation to the cerebral arterial circulation:

a   The basilar artery originates at the junction of the left and right vertebral arteries.
b   The basilar artery travels posterior to the brainstem.
c   The middle cerebral arteries supply the lateral aspect of the brain including the frontal, parietal, occipital, temporal and insular lobes.
d   70% of the arterial blood supply to the brain arises from the internal carotid arteries.
e   The posterior inferior cerebellar artery (PICA) is the largest of the cerebellar arteries arising from the vertebral artery.

Question 9: In acute graft versus host disease (AGVHD):

a   The skin, liver and gut are commonly involved.
b   Donor B lymphocytes attack host tissues.
c   Infliximab or mycophenolate mofetil are given as first-line treatment.
d   Calcineurin inhibitors are commonly used in the prophylaxis of AGVHD.
e   Transfusion-associated AGVHD has a mortality of less than 45%.

Question 10: Red cell transfusion and critical care:

a   The World Health Organisation (WHO) defines anaemia in men and women as a haemoglobin (Hb) <110g/L and <100g/L, respectively.

b   A transfusion trigger of 80g/L or below should be the default for critically ill patients.

c   The majority of blood transfusions given on intensive care are to treat major haemorrhage.

d   Transfusion to greater than Hb >80g/L assists weaning from mechanical ventilation.

e   A target of 100g/L should be maintained in patients with stable angina.

Question 11: Concerning heparin-induced thrombocytopenia (Type II HIT):

a   The platelet count typically falls by 30-50% within 5-10 days after initiation of heparin.

b   The incidence is 10x higher with unfractionated versus low-molecular-weight heparin (LMWH).

c   It is more common in male patients.

d   IgM antibodies to the heparin-PF4 antigen occurs on the surface of platelets.

e   Danaparoid has been used successfully to treat HIT-induced thrombosis.

Question 12: The larynx:

a   In adults extends from C3 to C6 in the midline.

b   The external branch of the superior laryngeal nerve innervates the cricothyroid muscle.

c   The superior laryngeal nerve is a branch of the vagus nerve.

d   Damage to the external branch of the superior laryngeal nerve results in a cadaveric vocal cord position.

e   Tracheostomy is performed through the cricothyroid membrane.

⬤ **Question 13: The following statements are true about electrocardiogram (ECG) monitoring:**

a   Standard calibration is 25mm/s and 1mV/cm.

b   Lead II is best for detecting arrhythmias.

c   CM5 lead is superior for detecting coronary ischaemia versus an individual limb lead.

d   A five-lead ECG has 60% sensitivity for detecting inferior or anterior ischaemia.

e   Normal axis is between 30 to 90°.

⬤ **Question 14: In relation to acute aortic dissection:**

a   The condition often presents with abrupt-onset sharp chest or back pain.

b   It is more common in females with a peak incidence between 50-70 years of age.

c   The European Society of Cardiology classifies the condition into Type A and Type B.

d   Adequate β-blockade should be established before initiation of vasodilator therapy in the medical management of acute aortic dissection.

e   Type A aortic dissection is managed medically.

⬤ **Question 15: Regarding defibrillation:**

a   Early defibrillation is paramount if indicated during cardiac arrest.

b   Transthoracic impedance is approximately 100 Ohms in adults.

c   Anteroposterior electrode placement is less effective than the sternal-apical position.

d   Biphasic defibrillators have a first shock efficacy of >86% for long duration ventricular fibrillation.

e   Biphasic defibrillators offer a survival advantage over monophasic devices.

Question 16: Considering intra-aortic balloon pump (IABP) use:

a   Myocardial oxygen supply is increased.
b   Carbon dioxide is used for balloon inflation.
c   Balloon inflation occurs in early systole.
d   Deflation occurs on the electrocardiogram R-wave peak.
e   The diameter of the balloon should not exceed 80-90% of the patient's descending aortic diameter.

Question 17: Indications for cardiac pacing include:

a   Permanent atrial fibrillation (AF) with atrioventricular (AV) block.
b   Symptomatic Mobitz Type I second-degree heart block.
c   Third-degree heart block.
d   Torsades de pointes.
e   Asystolic episodes.

Question 18: Considering the critical care management of acute liver failure (ALF):

a   N-acetylcysteine (NAC) is beneficial in non-paracetamol-induced ALF.
b   Intracranial pressure monitoring is advised in low-grade encephalopathy.
c   ALF is characterised by low cardiac output and often requires vasopressor support.
d   High positive end-expiratory pressures (PEEP) may exacerbate hepatic congestion.
e   Hepatocyte necrosis causes hyperglycaemia.

Question 19: Variceal bleeding:

a   Immediate mortality is estimated to be 2%.
b   Portal hypotension is the most common cause.
c   Terlipressin may be beneficial in reducing bleeding.
d   Broad-spectrum antibiotics should be given acutely.

e   A transjugular intrahepatic portosystemic shunt (TIPS) and liver transplantation may be considered in severe variceal bleeding.

Question 20: Regarding the Sengstaken-Blakemore tube (SBT):

a   80% of patients will rebleed once the balloon is deflated.
b   It is effective at controlling torrential bleeding from oesophago-gastric varices.
c   It has three lumens.
d   Insertion to the 55cm mark at the incisors indicates that the gastric balloon position is below the gastro-oesophageal junction.
e   The oesophageal balloon must be deflated every 6 hours.

Question 21: Regarding surgical resection of the oesophagus:

a   A lumbar epidural is likely to be beneficial.
b   A fibre-optic scope should be available to confirm correct double-lumen tube (DLT) placement.
c   Respiratory morbidity is high postoperatively.
d   Non-invasive ventilation in the early postoperative period is absolutely contraindicated.
e   Acute onset of fast atrial fibrillation at 3-7 days postoperatively may herald the development of an anastomotic leak.

Question 22: In relation to the classification of acute liver failure (ALF):

a   The O'Grady system classifies ALF into hyperacute, acute and subacute categories.
b   Is defined as 'acute' according to the O'Grady system, when jaundice to encephalopathy occurs in less than 1 month.
c   'Hyperacute' is when the onset of encephalopathy occurs less than 1 week after jaundice.
d   The Bernuau system classifies ALF as acute and subacute.
e   The Japanese system classifies ALF into fulminant and subfulminant categories.

Question 23: In relation to ethylene glycol (EG) poisoning:

a   It may present with an acute ascending motor and sensory neuropathy.

b   A normal anion gap acidosis is usually seen.

c   Alcohol dehydrogenase catabolises the metabolism of EG into metabolites including oxalate and glycolic acid.

d   Haemodialysis is not effective.

e   Fomepizole is a potent inducer of alcohol dehydrogenase and an effective treatment.

Question 24: The following statements concerning spontaneous bacterial peritonitis (SBP) in chronic liver disease are true:

a   The probability of survival at 2 years following one episode of SBP in cirrhosis is approximately 50%.

b   A neutrophil count of >150 neutrophils/mm^3 in ascites is diagnostic for SBP.

c   The administration of albumin may decrease the development of hepatorenal syndrome.

d   Ascitic culture is negative in up to 40% of cultures taken from patients with suspected SBP.

e   Routine antibiotic prophylaxis is not recommended in patients with cirrhosis and ascites, who have had one previous episode of SBP.

Question 25: Regarding alcoholic liver disease (ALD):

a   30% of cirrhotic patients develop hepatorenal syndrome (HRS) within 1 year of diagnosis.

b   One UK unit of alcohol contains 20-24g ethanol.

c   Patients may present with Wernicke's encephalopathy.

d   Ethanol metabolism causes accumulation of lipid in liver cells.

e   Infliximab (TNF-α inhibitor) is useful in preventing hepatorenal syndrome in severe ALD.

Question 26: Considering oxygen delivery (DO_2) in adults:

a DO_2 below 300ml/minute results in shock.

b   Clinical signs such as heart rate, blood pressure and urine output are useful signs of oxygen delivery in young adult patients.

c   At rest, the metabolic demands of an average person can be met by dissolved O_2 alone when breathing FiO_2 1.0 at 3 atmospheres.

d DO_2 is reliant on conduction, convection and diffusion.

e   Achieving supranormal values of DO_2 is beneficial in sepsis.

Question 27: Oesophageal Doppler:

a   Utilises the Doppler shift to measure blood velocity.

b   Velocity of blood (m/s) in the descending aorta can be calculated provided the aortic cross-sectional area is known.

c   It is assumed 70% of cardiac output is distributed caudally to the descending aorta.

d   Doppler probes must be removed after 1 week.

e   Is accurate when used with a working epidural.

Question 28: In relation to the PiCCO cardiac monitor, the following statements are true:

a   A central line is needed only.

b   Thermodilution is used to calibrate the pulse pressure algorithm.

c   Mean transit time (MTT) represents the time taken for all the thermal tracer to pass through the venous circulation, heart and lungs to the arterial circulation.

d   Pulmonary thermal volume (PTV) can be calculated from the downslope time (DST).

e   Global end-diastolic volume (GEDV) = (mean transit time x cardiac output) - pulmonary thermal volume.

Question 29: Derived variables from a pulmonary artery catheter:

a   A cardiac index of 2.1L/min/m^2 is normal.

b   Normal systemic vascular resistance index (SVRI) is 800-1200 dynes.sec/cm^5/m^2.

c   Pulmonary vascular resistance is normally <250 dynes.sec/cm^5.

d   Coronary artery perfusion pressure = systolic blood pressure - pulmonary artery occlusion pressure.

e   Stroke volume index (SVI) is normally 35-70ml/m^2/beat.

Question 30: Concerning liver transplantation for acute liver failure (ALF):

a   Most deaths after transplantation occur during the first 3 months postoperatively.

b   Risk of death is higher in recipients who received a graft from an identical ABO donor.

c   20% of liver transplants are performed in ALF patients.

d   Early postoperative impaired graft function is poorly tolerated.

e   After the first year following transplants, ALF patients have a better long-term survival than chronic liver failure patients.

Question 31: The lungs and bronchial tree:

a   The left lung has two fissures.

b   After 2.5cm the left main bronchus gives off the left upper lobe bronchus.

c   The left lower lobe bronchus is made up of five branches.

d   Lateral and posterior branches make up the right middle lobe bronchus.

e   The left main bronchus is shorter and wider than the right main bronchus.

Question 32: In relation to paracetamol (acetaminophen) overdose:

a   N-acetyl-p-benzo-quinone-imine (NAPQI) is produced by glucuronidation of paracetamol in the liver.
b   Plasma paracetamol levels on or above 100mg/L at 4 hours and 15mg/L at 15 hours after ingestion warrant treatment.
c   The toxicity nomogram is reliable in cases of staggered overdose.
d   Initial loading of N-acetylcysteine (NAC) 150mg/kg over 1 hour is recommended.
e   Hypersensitivity is a contraindication to NAC.

Question 33: Concerning recreational drug toxicity:

a   Dantrolene may be used for acute hyperpyrexia caused by ecstasy (MDMA).
b   Cocaine abuse should be considered in any young person presenting with acute chest pain.
c   Chlordiazepoxide may be effective for acute alcohol withdrawal.
d   Dilated pupils, hypotonia and hyporeflexia may occur in children following accidental ingestion of cannabis.
e   Mephedrone toxicity is associated with peripheral vasodilatation.

Question 34: In relation to the Glasgow Coma Scale (GCS):

a   It is incorporated in the Acute Physiology And Chronic Health Evaluation II (APACHE II) scoring system.
b   The FOUR score is inferior to the GCS as it cannot be carried out when the patient is intubated and ventilated.
c   A score of 8 or less is considered coma where airway reflexes may be inadequate.
d   May have prognostic significance after traumatic brain injury.
e   A patient who is opening eyes to pain, mumbles sounds and withdraws to a painful stimulus scores 9/15.

Question 35: Concerning cervical cord injury and critical care:

a   Fibre-optic intubation in patients with cervical cord injury has been proven to be a superior and safer technique, compared to orotracheal intubation with manual in-line stabilisation.

b   Maintaining patients in the semi-upright position optimises breathing.

c   The risk of deep vein thrombosis is increased three-fold.

d   In autonomic dysreflexia, hypertension typically occurs above the level of the lesion.

e   In non-penetrating spinal cord injury, administration of high-dose methylprednisolone within 8 hours of injury is a recommended treatment.

Question 36: Lumbar drain management:

a   A lumbar drain is an epidural catheter inserted into the subarachnoid space.

b   It may improve spinal cord perfusion following suprarenal aortic aneurysm repair.

c   The zero level should be at the level of the atria.

d   Drain height, maximum permitted drainage per hour and duration of drainage should be prescribed.

e   Excess cerebrospinal fluid (CSF) drainage is common and is associated with few minor complications.

Question 37: In relation to nerve conduction study patterns:

a   Motor conduction only is reduced in critical care polyneuropathy.

b   In motor neuron disease sensory nerve conduction is reduced.

c   Motor nerve conduction is reduced but increases with further repetition in myasthenia gravis.

d   Motor nerve conduction is slowed or blocked in Guillain-Barré syndrome.

e   Electromyography (EMG) shows fibrillations in motor neuron disease.

Question 38: In patients with brain herniation due to raised intracranial pressure (ICP):

a   Tentorial/uncal herniation causes pupillary dilatation and ptosis.

b   Tonsillar herniation occurs when the cerebellum herniates into the posterior fossa.

c   Compression of the midbrain may cause Cushing's syndrome.

d   Persistent ICP of <20mmHg is associated with a better outcome in traumatic brain injury.

e   Critically high ICP commonly causes hypotension and tachycardia.

Question 39: Concerning intracranial pressure (ICP) waveforms the following statements are true:

a   The normal ICP trace looks similar to an arterial trace in appearance.

b   P1 is caused by an arterial pressure percussion wave being transmitted from the choroid plexus to the ventricle.

c   P2 is the dichrotic wave due to aortic valve closure.

d   With high ICP, brain compliance reduces and the P1 component exceeds P2 with the wave becoming broader.

e   Plateau waves (Lundberg A waves) are always pathological.

Question 40: Pre-operative β-blockade use for non-cardiac surgery:

a   Should be started in patients with pre-existing ischaemic heart disease.

b   Is associated with increased mortality.

c   Is associated with a decrease in non-fatal myocardial infarction.

d   Is associated with increased stroke events.

e   Is based on robust clinical trial data.

Question 41: Mannitol 20%:

a   A 500ml bag contains 100g of mannitol.

b   Is alkalotic.

c   Mannitol solutions may crystallise at room temperature and should be discarded.

d   Exerts its effects by increasing diuresis.

e   0.25-1.0mg/kg should be given intravenously for significantly raised intracranial pressure.

Question 42: Pain management on critical care:

a   It is estimated that 45% of critical care patients remember experiencing pain during their stay.

b   The Behaviourial Pain Scale (BPS) is composed of four observational areas and is scored from 0 to a maximum of 8.

c   The Critical-care Pain Observation Tool (CPOT) is not suitable for intubated patients.

d   Uncontrolled pain has been linked to adverse patient consequences.

e   For non-neuropathic pain, intravenous opioids are considered for first-line management.

Question 43: In relation to prerequisites for brainstem death testing:

a   The aetiology of irreversible brain damage does not need to be known.

b   Testing should not be undertaken if thiopentone assay results are >5mg/L.

c   Core temperature should be greater than 35°C at the time of testing.

d   Sodium levels should be between 115 to 160mmol/L.

e   Phosphate should be greater than 0.5 but less than 3.0mmol/L.

Question 44: Echocardiography and critical care:

a   Ultrasound is sound with a frequency above 20MHz.
b   The speed of sound in tissue is 1570m/s.
c   Better resolution is observed with higher frequencies.
d   Severe aortic stenosis is classically defined as a valve area of 0.6-0.8cm^2.
e   A false-positive examination for infective endocarditis may occur in systemic lupus erythematosus (SLE).

Question 45: When considering transfer of critically ill patients:

a   A standard ambulance trolley is preferred for patient transfers.
b   Neurosurgical transfers are time-critical and need to be expedited regardless of stability.
c   Transfers for non-clinical reasons should only take place in exceptional circumstances and ideally only in daylight hours.
d   Departure checklists are a crucial aid and may prevent disaster.
e   Intra-hospital transfer does not increase complications in ventilated critically ill patients.

Question 46: In paediatric meningococcal disease:

a   Group B meningococcus is the most common cause in patients aged 3 months or older in the UK.
b   Classical signs are often absent in infants and may occur without a non-blanching rash.
c   Benzylpenicillin (intravenous or intramuscular) should be given pre-hospital without delay.
d   Intravenous ceftriaxone should be given immediately if meningococcal disease is suspected on arrival to hospital.
e   It is vital that lumbar puncture is performed without delay.

Question 47: Regarding paediatric airway emergencies:

a   Croup presents with high fever and dyspnoea.
b   Epiglottitis presents classically with drooling, dyspnoea, dysphagia and dysphonia.
c   Sevoflurane and topical anaesthesia is the airway technique of choice for removal of a foreign body with a Storz bronchoscope.
d   In the UK, the National Audit Project 4 (NAP4) showed that cricothyroidotomy was used in most cases where a child could not be intubated or ventilated.
e   A high-flow nasal cannula (HFNC) is well tolerated and beneficial in young infants with acute viral bronchiolitis.

Question 48: The following statements are true about human immunodeficiency virus (HIV) infection:

a   Fever is the most common presenting feature of seroconversion illness.
b   HIV DNA levels in the plasma correlate with serum CD4 count, rate of decline and progression to acquired immune deficiency syndrome (AIDS).
c   AIDS is defined by a CD4 level <200 cells/µl.
d   HIV infection frequently occurs after needle stick injuries.
e   Median survival in patients with HIV in the UK is 15 years.

Question 49: Regarding anti-retroviral therapy (ART) in human immunodeficiency virus (HIV):

a   Zidovudine (AZT) is a non-nucleoside reverse transcriptase inhibitor.
b   Fusion inhibitors block fusion of HIV with the cell membrane.
c   Lamivudine (3TC) can cause fatal lactic acidosis.
d   Initiating ART in the critical care unit is hazardous.
e   Nevirapine is currently effective against the HIV-2 subtype.

Question 50: Acute and chronic adverse effects of glucocorticoids include:

a   Distal muscle weakness.
b   Hypoglycaemia.

c   Peptic ulcer disease.
d   Osteonecrosis of the hip joint.
e   Adrenal insufficiency.

Question 51: Respiratory failure in a patient with rheumatoid arthritis on critical care may be caused by:

a   Bronchiolitis obliterans with organising pneumonia.
b   Methotrexate.
c   Gold salts.
d   Cricoarytenoid dysfunction.
e   Pleural and/or pericardial effusion.

Question 52: In relation to temperature regulation:

a   Temperature is sensed by A-δ fibres and C fibres.
b   Temperature elevation increases serum iron, which reduces bacterial growth.
c   An appropriate immediate dose of dantrolene for a 70kg male with suspected malignant hyperthermia is 100mg.
d   Asystole and ventricular fibrillation can occur below 28°C and 20°C, respectively.
e   Cerebral blood flow falls at an approximate rate of 7% per °C drop in temperature.

Question 53: The following statements are true about drowning:

a   Drowning is the second leading cause of unnatural death after road traffic accidents.
b   The diving response occurs due to cold water stimulation of the ophthalmic division of the trigeminal nerve.
c   It is unusual to find little or no fluid in the lungs of a drowning victim.
d   There are significant clinical differences evident between patients who have been submersed in salt water as compared to fresh water, affecting outcome.
e   Major electrolyte abnormalities secondary to aspiration of large fluid volumes are common after drowning.

Question 54: Pre-eclampsia:

a   Results from trophoblastic invasion of spiral arteries within the placenta.

b   Can result in foetal growth restriction.

c   Is more common in primiparous women.

d   Usually presents before 20 weeks' gestation.

e   Proteinuria with high blood pressure is required for diagnosis.

Question 55: Regarding eclampsia and HELLP syndrome:

a   Eclampsia is always preceded by symptoms of pre-eclampsia.

b   Eclampsia describes any seizures occurring during pregnancy.

c   HELLP syndrome is a combination of haemolysis, elevated liver enzymes and low platelets.

d   HELLP syndrome can occur without proteinuria or hypertension.

e   HELLP syndrome is a mild variant of pre-eclampsia.

Question 56: The following are International System of Units (SI) base units:

a   Kilogram.

b   Ampere.

c   Joule.

d   Mole.

e   Litre.

Question 57: In relation to haemoglobin, the following statements are true:

a   Adult haemoglobin contains two α and two β chains.

b   Haem is a porphyrin derivative containing iron in the ferric state.

c   Sickle cell anaemia is caused by the substitution of valine by glutamic acid in the β chains.

d   The Bohr effect describes an increased affinity for oxygen binding by haemoglobin in the presence of increased $PaCO_2$.

e   Porphyria is transmitted by autosomal dominant inheritance.

Question 58: During adult cardiopulmonary resuscitation, current UK resuscitation and related guidelines recommend that:

a   Adrenaline should be given before the third shock in a shockable rhythm.

b   Chest compressions should continue during charging of the defibrillator.

c   Hypotension is a reversible cause of a cardiac arrest.

d   There is no indication for the 'three-shock strategy'.

e   Following unsuccessful resuscitation, the patient should be observed for a minimum of 5 minutes before confirming death.

Question 59: During paediatric cardiopulmonary resuscitation of an 8-year-old child:

a   A compression/ventilation ratio of 15:2 is appropriate.

b   An adrenaline dose of 480µg would be appropriate.

c   A defibrillation energy level of 124J would be appropriate.

d   A bolus of 480ml of dextrose 5% would be appropriate for hypovolaemia.

e   Intraosseous access should be sited after 3 minutes, if attempts at gaining peripheral venous access are unsuccessful.

Question 60: During the resuscitation of a patient with major burns:

a   Early intubation is usually difficult if there is head and/or neck involvement.

b   Suxamethonium can be used safely for intubation.

c   The Parkland formula can be used to predict fluid requirement for the 24-hour period after presentation.

d   Early broad-spectrum antibiotics should be administered.

e   Patients who have sustained full-thickness burns will not require analgesia.

Question 61: Criteria for liver transplantation include:

a   An arterial pH of <7.35 despite adequate fluid resuscitation following paracetamol (acetaminophen)-induced acute liver failure.

b   Coexistent international normalised ratio (INR) >6.5 and creatinine >300µmol/L following paracetamol-induced acute liver failure.

c   An early arterial lactate concentration >3.5mmol/L.

d   Patients with end-stage hepatitis C cirrhosis.

e   Patients with fulminant Gilbert's disease.

Question 62: Pelvic trauma:

a   Patients presenting with an unstable pelvic fracture and shock have a mortality of up to 25%.

b   The pubic rami is the weakest point of the pelvic ring.

c   Springing of the pelvis should be performed in order to assess stability.

d   Early stabilisation can be achieved with a sheet or belt encircling the pelvis at the level of the iliac crests.

e   Patients with pelvic fractures must have a thoracic-abdominal-pelvic contrast CT prior to surgical intervention.

Question 63: In relation to clearing the cervical spine:

a   Up to 12% of major trauma patients have a cervical spine injury.

b   Prolonged immobilisation should be undertaken until the cervical spine is clinically cleared.

c   Spinal Cord Injury without Radiographic Abnormality (SCIWORA) is common in unconscious adult trauma patients.

d   Manual in-line stabilisation (MILS) during rapid sequence induction is best provided from in front of the patient.

e   The commonest mechanism of spinal cord injury in trauma is vertebral subluxation.

Question 64: The following conditions may cause a dominant R-wave in lead V1 on an electrocardiogram (ECG):

a   Pulmonary embolism.
b   Wolff-Parkinson-White Type B.
c   Inferior myocardial infarction.
d   Hypertrophic obstructive cardiomyopathy (HOCM).
e   Dressler's syndrome.

Question 65: In relation to medical statistics, the following can be considered correct:

a   The analysis of variance (ANOVA) test can be used with parametric data.
b   The standard error of the mean equals the standard deviation divided by the number of values.
c   The specificity is the number of true negatives divided by the total number with a negative test.
d   A pain score is an example of ordinal data.
e α error describes the probability of a positive finding from a study where the null hypothesis is correct.

Question 66: The following have been shown to improve mortality in acute respiratory distress syndrome (ARDS):

a   Inhaled β2-agonists.
b   Prone ventilation.
c   Treatment with intravenous glucocorticoids.
d   Use of high-frequency oscillatory ventilation (HFOV).
e   Ventilation at tidal volumes of 6ml per kg.

Question 67: The following are recognised strategies in the prevention of ventilator-associated pneumonia (VAP):

a   Daily sedation holds.

b   Head-up positioning of 30 to 45°.

c   Prone positioning.

d   Chlorhexidine mouthcare.

e   Daily ventilator tubing changes.

Question 68: Factors that influence inspired oxygen delivery (FiO$_2$) include:

a   Effective inspired oxygen concentration (EIOC) deteriorates as respiratory rate increases.

b   Increased inspired oxygen delivery is seen in patients with high tidal volumes.

c   The presence of a respiratory pause decreases inspired oxygen delivery.

d   Variable performance systems include the Venturi type masks.

e   Entrainment of environmental air increases delivered FiO$_2$.

Question 69: In relation to oxygen toxicity, the following statements are true:

a   The Paul Bert effect is seen with prolonged exposure to high inspired oxygen.

b   The Lorraine Smith effect can occur during diving at high pressures of >3 atmospheres.

c   Retinopathy of prematurity is solely due to high inspired oxygen.

d   Surfactant and maternal steroids have lowered the incidence of bronchopulmonary dysplasia in neonates.

e   Free oxygen radicals result in a progressive reduction in lung compliance associated with interstitial oedema and fibrosis.

Question 70: Indications for hyperbaric oxygen therapy include the following:

a   Acute blood loss.
b   Carbon monoxide poisoning.
c   Intracranial abscess.
d   Decompression sickness.
e   Clostridial myositis.

Question 71: Complications associated with ventilatory support include:

a   Laryngeal swelling.
b   Tracheal stenosis.
c   Pneumonia is the most common complication.
d   Hypertension.
e   Peak pressures >30cmH$_2$O are associated with barotrauma.

Question 72: Acid-base balance:

a   Plasma pH is equal to intracellular pH.
b   An increased strong ion difference indicates an alkalosis.
c   Acute renal failure will result in a reduced strong ion difference.
d   Respiratory compensation is triggered by an increased hydrogen ion concentration in cerebrospinal fluid.
e   Acidosis is defined as an increase in the hydrogen ion concentration of the blood, resulting in a fall in pH.

Question 73: The osmolar and anion gaps:

a   Methanol poisoning tends to present initially with an increased anion gap.
b   A normal serum osmolar gap is <10mOsm/kg.
c   The anion gap is increased by unmeasured anions.
d   The anion gap should be corrected for hypoalbuminaemia.
e   Paracetamol overdose can cause an elevated anion gap metabolic acidosis.

Question 74: Concerning the RIFLE classification system for acute renal failure (ARF):

a   There are separate criteria for creatinine and urine output.

b   When calculating the RIFLE classification, one should use the criteria that leads to the best possible classification stage.

c   Urine output of <0.5ml/kg/hr for 12 hours would meet criteria for RIFLE-R stage.

d   A serum creatinine ≥4mg/dL (350μmol/L) or an acute rise ≥0.5mg/dL (44μmol/L) would meet criteria for RIFLE-F stage.

e   In an ARF patient now requiring dialysis, who has not recovered renal function for >3 months, classification would be as RIFLE-E stage.

Question 75: In relation to arterial blood gas analysis:

a   The pH stat approach of blood gas measurement utilises temperature compensation.

b   Placing a blood gas syringe on ice will result in an increased $PaCO_2$.

c   Gas solubility increases as temperature falls.

d   Excessive heparin in the blood gas syringe will not affect the $PaCO_2$ result.

e   Leukocyte larceny causes a decreased PaO_2 value.

Question 76: In relation to sodium:

a   Sodium is the principal cation of the intracellular fluid.

b   Criteria for the diagnosis of the syndrome of inappropriate anti-diuretic hormone (SIADH) secretion includes finding a urinary sodium less than 20mmol/L.

c   One litre of 3% sodium chloride contains approximately 500mmol of sodium.

d   Hypernatraemia is always associated with hyperosmolality.

e   Normal serum osmolarity is 285-295mOsm/kg.

Question 77: Concerning critical care outreach services:

a   Critical care outreach services were largely introduced in the United Kingdom in the early 1990s.
b   The report "Comprehensive Critical Care" (Department of Health England, 2000) outlined outreach as an integral component.
c   Outreach services can avert admissions to critical care.
d   Outreach should aim to share skills with staff both on the wards and in the community.
e   Many outreach models utilise early warning scores (EWS) within the referral pathway.

Question 78: Concerning patients with acute renal failure (ARF):

a   Serum urea and creatinine can be considered as sensitive markers of glomerular filtration rate (GFR).
b   Laboratory examination of urine sediment showing occasional hyaline or finely granular casts is typical of acute tubular necrosis (ATN).
c   In pre-renal ARF, fractional excretion of sodium is typically <1%.
d   In a patient with ARF, findings of urine osmolality >500mOsm/kg and urine Na^+ <20mmol/L would be consistent with a pre-renal cause.
e   Anaemia is a typical finding.

Question 79: The following statements relating to thyroid physiology are true:

a   Thyrotropin releasing hormone (TRH) is produced in the paraventricular nucleus of the hypothalamus.
b   Thyroxine (T4) is converted to the more active tri-iodothyronine (T3) in the heart and pancreas by Type 1 deiodinases.
c   Thyroid stimulating hormone (TSH) receptors are part of the family of G-protein coupled receptors.
d   In plasma, approximately 75% of T4 and T3 is bound to hormone-binding proteins, with thyroxine binding globulin (TBG) being the major binding protein for both.
e   Only free T4 and free T3 are biologically active in tissues.

Question 80: Considering vasculitides:

a   Subglottic and tracheal stenosis are clinical manifestations of antineutrophil cytoplasmic antibody (ANCA)-associated vasculitis, and may be seen on chest X-ray.

b   Henoch-Schönlein purpura (HSP) is an ANCA-associated small vessel vasculitis.

c   Kawasaki disease presents in children with a short-lived fever.

d   Up to 50% of deaths from Churg-Strauss syndrome (CSS) occur due to cardiac complications.

e   Cryoglobulinemic vasculitis (CV) may present acutely with respiratory distress and acute kidney injury.

Question 81: Regarding the management of cardiac failure:

a   Enalapril decreases renal blood flow.

b   A left ventricular assist device (LVAD) will be ineffective in patients with biventricular failure.

c   The tip of an intra-aortic balloon pump should be situated distal to the origin of the left carotid artery.

d   Fluid overload is the most common complication following insertion of a ventricular assist device.

e   Low admission systolic blood pressure (<120mmHg) in a patient presenting with heart failure confers an increased risk of inpatient mortality.

Question 82: The following drugs may cause acute renal failure in the intensive care unit:

a   Radio-contrast agents.

b   Paracetamol (acetominophen).

c   Non-steroidal anti-inflammatory drugs.

d   Acyclovir.

e   Cyclosporin A.

Question 83: Considering the 2012 Surviving Sepsis guidelines:

a   Measurement of serum lactate and blood cultures prior to antibiotic administration should be undertaken within 6 hours of sepsis identification.

b   Corticosteroids should be administered in the treatment of sepsis.

c   A protocolised approach to blood glucose management should be undertaken targeting an upper blood glucose level of less than or equal to 110mg/dL (6.1mmol/L).

d   The use of procalcitonin levels is advised to guide antibiotic therapy.

e   A target tidal volume of 12ml/kg predicted body weight is recommended in sepsis-induced acute respiratory distress syndrome (ARDS).

Question 84: Concerning digoxin toxicity, the following statements are true:

a   Diltiazem can elevate the digoxin level.

b   In acute digoxin toxicity, hypokalaemia is common.

c   Yellow-green distortion is the commonest visual deficit seen in digoxin toxicity.

d   Downward sloping of the ST segment and inverted T-waves are electrocardiogram (ECG) findings indicative of digoxin toxicity.

e   A serum digoxin level greater than 10mg/mL in adults at steady state (i.e. 6-8 hours after acute ingestion or at baseline in chronic toxicity) is an indication for the therapeutic use of immunotherapy with digoxin Fab fragments (DigiBind®).

Question 85: Complications of the prone position include:

a   Quadriplegia.

b   Liver ischaemia.

c   Rhabdomyolysis.

d   Blindness.

e   Stroke.

Question 86: Regarding intensive care unit ventilation:

a Prolonging the expiratory time will increase the mean airway pressure.
b Increasing positive end-expiratory pressure (PEEP) may directly increase arterial oxygen tension.
c Decreased inspiratory time may cause gas trapping due to increased expiratory time.
d Morbid obesity may increase chest wall compliance.
e Auto-PEEP can be selected during controlled ventilation.

Question 87: Regarding cerebrospinal fluid (CSF):

a Formation is largely independent of intracranial pressure.
b Circulates from the lateral ventricles to the third ventricle via the aqueduct of Sylvius.
c Has a higher level of chloride and lower level of potassium than plasma.
d Has a lower specific gravity than plasma.
e Will display a low glucose relative to the plasma value in bacterial meningitis.

Question 88: Ventricular assist device (VAD) complications include:

a Right ventricular dysfunction is common after LVAD implantation.
b Haemorrhage.
c Air embolus.
d Haemolysis.
e Stroke.

Question 89: Therapeutic hypothermia after cardiac arrest:

a Directly decreases intracranial pressure.
b Promotes intracellular movement of calcium.
c May cause the appearance of delta waves on the electrocardiogram.

d   The aim is to achieve a core temperature of 32-34°C for 12-24 hours.

e   Should only be used in those whose initial rhythm was ventricular fibrillation (VF) or ventricular tachycardia (VT).

Question 90: Hepatitis E:

a   Along with hepatitis A, is globally responsible for the majority of acute liver failure cases.

b   Occurs in four groups with different clinical and epidemiologic features.

c   May masquerade as a drug-induced liver injury.

d   Genotypes 1 and 2 are associated with a higher mortality in pregnant women.

e   Autochthonous hepatitis E may be complicated by severe neurological complications.

Answer overview: Paper 1

Question:	a	b	c	d	e	Question:	a	b	c	d	e
1	F	F	T	F	T	46	T	T	T	T	F
2	T	T	F	F	F	47	F	T	T	F	T
3	F	F	T	T	F	48	T	F	T	F	F
4	F	F	T	T	T	49	F	T	T	T	F
5	F	T	F	T	F	50	F	F	T	T	T
6	T	F	T	F	T	51	T	T	T	T	T
7	T	T	T	F	T	52	T	F	F	F	T
8	T	F	T	T	T	53	T	T	T	F	F
9	T	F	F	T	F	54	F	T	T	F	F
10	F	F	F	F	F	55	F	F	T	T	F
11	T	T	F	F	T	56	T	T	F	T	F
12	T	T	T	F	F	57	T	F	F	F	T
13	T	T	T	F	F	58	F	T	F	F	T
14	T	F	F	T	F	59	T	F	T	F	F
15	T	F	F	T	F	60	F	T	F	F	F
16	T	F	F	T	T	61	F	F	T	T	F
17	T	T	T	T	T	62	F	T	F	F	F
18	T	F	F	T	F	63	T	F	F	F	T
19	F	F	T	T	T	64	T	F	F	T	F
20	F	T	T	T	F	65	T	F	F	T	T
21	F	T	T	F	T	66	F	T	F	F	T
22	T	T	T	F	F	67	T	T	F	T	F
23	T	F	T	F	F	68	T	T	F	F	F
24	T	F	T	T	F	69	F	F	F	T	T
25	F	F	T	T	F	70	T	T	T	T	T
26	T	F	T	F	F	71	T	T	T	F	F
27	T	F	T	F	F	72	F	T	T	F	F
28	F	T	F	T	T	73	F	T	T	T	T
29	F	F	T	F	T	74	T	F	F	T	T
30	T	F	F	T	T	75	T	F	T	F	T
31	F	F	T	F	F	76	F	F	T	T	F
32	F	T	F	T	F	77	F	T	T	T	T
33	T	T	T	T	F	78	F	F	T	T	F
34	T	F	T	T	F	79	T	F	T	F	T
35	F	F	T	F	F	80	T	F	F	T	T
36	T	T	F	T	F	81	F	F	F	F	T
37	F	F	F	T	F	82	T	T	T	T	T
38	T	F	F	T	F	83	F	F	F	T	F
39	T	T	F	F	T	84	T	F	T	F	F
40	F	T	T	T	F	85	T	T	T	T	T
41	T	F	F	F	F	86	F	T	F	F	F
42	F	F	F	T	T	87	T	F	T	T	T
43	F	T	F	T	T	88	T	T	T	T	T
44	F	F	T	T	T	89	T	F	F	T	F
45	F	F	T	T	F	90	T	F	T	T	T

1 MCQ Paper 1: Answers

Answer 1: In relation to the drug sugammadex: True c & e

F There are currently no data available regarding the use of sugammadex for the 'immediate reversal' of vecuronium. However, sugammadex is recommended for reversal of vecuronium once spontaneous T2 twitch has been achieved, using a dose of 4mg/kg to reverse 0.1mg/kg of vecuronium.

F Sugammadex is not effective against benzylisoquinolinium muscle relaxants (e.g. cisatracurium and mivacurium).

T Phase I-IV trials have shown sugammadex to be effective for rapid reversal of rocuronium-induced neuromuscular blockade (16mg/kg).

F Sugammadex is a member of the γ-cyclodextrin family, which encapsulates aminosteroid neuromuscular blocking agents (rocuronium, vecuronium, pancuronium).

T Debate still exists about whether sugammadex is effective in the management of rocuronium-induced anaphylaxis. Some case reports confer benefit.

1. http://wwwmedicinesorguk/EMC/medicine/21299/SPC/Bridion+1 00+mg+ml+solution+for+injection/2013.

2. Lobaz S, Clymer M, Sammut M. Safety and efficacy of sugammadex for neuromuscular blockade reversal. *Clin Med InsightsTher* 2014; 6: 1-14.

3. McDonnell N, Pavy T, Green L, Platt P. Sugammadex in the management of rocuronium-induced anaphylaxis. *Br J Anaesth* 2011; 106(2): 199-201.

Answer 2: For patients with coronary artery stents undergoing non-cardiac surgery: True a & b

T   There is an increased risk of stent thrombosis and myocardial infarction in the post-stenting period (4-6 weeks with BMS and up to 12 months with DES) in patients undergoing non-cardiac surgery.

T   First- and second-generation DES are antimitotic and designed to decrease new tissue formation in the luminal surface and thus reduce the incidence of stent restenosis. DES have a reduced incidence of in-stent restenosis compared to BMS (0-3% vs 5-10%, respectively at 1 year), but an increased late stent thrombosis rate (DES 0.6% per year). This is due to less complete endothelisation, warranting the need for a longer period of dual antiplatelet therapy with DES.

F   BMS require 4-6 weeks of clopidogrel and aspirin (dual antiplatelet therapy) followed by aspirin for life. If surgery is required in the first 4 weeks post-insertion, then bridging therapy with tirofiban or heparin is recommended if aspirin therapy cannot be maintained. If surgery is required for more than 4 weeks post-insertion of a BMS, clopidogrel should be stopped but aspirin therapy continued.

F   There is an increased risk of surgical bleeding (up to 50%) for patients on dual antiplatelet therapy undergoing surgery, although there does not appear to be an associated increased mortality risk.

F   There is some evidence that bridging therapy in the peri-operative period with tirofiban and/or heparin allows clopidogrel to be stopped for surgery and may reduce complications of stent thrombosis and bleeding in both BMS and DES patients. Biocompatible stents (e.g. the Genous™ R-stent) require only 10 days of clopidogrel followed by lifelong aspirin. Bridging therapy for biocompatible stents is not deemed necessary.

1.   Moore C, Leslie S. Coronary artery stents: management in patients undergoing non-cardiac surgery. Johnston I, Harrop-Griffiths W, Gemmell L, Eds. In: *AAGBI Core Topics in Anaesthesia* 2012; 2: 17-27.

2.   Bolsin S, Hiew C, Birdsey G, *et al.* Coronary artery stents and surgery; the basis of sound perioperative management. *Health* 2013; 5(10): 1730-6.

3.   Chassot PG, Delabays A, Spahn DR. Perioperative antiplatelet therapy: the case for continuing therapy in patients at risk of myocardial infarction. *Br J Anaesth* 2007; 99: 316-28.

Answer 3: Regarding The Royal College of Anaesthetists 4th National Audit Project (NAP4): True c & d

F   Only 20% of the total cases reported to the NAP4 involved intensive care unit (ICU) patients. However, when airway complications did occur within the ICU, they were more likely to be associated with a much higher incidence of death or severe disability (61%), when compared to the anaesthesia or emergency department.

F   Capnography is paramount for monitoring anyone with an endotracheal tube or tracheostomy. It may prevent significant harm by indicating oesophageal intubation or displacement of a tracheostomy or endotracheal tube and is recommended by The Royal College of Anaesthetists as a standard of care in the UK.

T   A dedicated difficult airway trolley is recommended for all intensive care units. All staff should be familiar with items on the trolley.

T   Regular audit and education is important to improve staff awareness and patient care when dealing with any intubated/tracheostomised patient.

F   All staff undertaking any routine movement/turns or transfer of intubated patients, need to be alert to the potential risk of airway displacement and have an established management plan if this were to occur.

1.   RCOA/DAS. 4th National Audit Project, 2011. Major complications of airway management in the UK. The Royal College of Anaesthetists and the Difficult Airway Society. http://www.rcoa.ac.uk/nap4.

Answer 4: In relation to a potential 'can't intubate, can't ventilate (CICV) scenario' in anaesthesia practice: True c, d & e

F   The CICV or can't intubate, can't oxygenate (CICO) scenario is an inability to secure the patient's airway with an endotracheal tube and an inability to ventilate a patient's lungs by conventional non-invasive means. This is a rare complication, estimated to occur in 0.01 to 2.0 per 10,000 cases.

F   Cannula cricothyroidotomy requires jet ventilation to ventilate a patient's lungs when a narrow-bore cannula (e.g. 2mm diameter) is used. A dedicated wide-bore proprietary cannula (>4mm) fits a standard 15mm connector and does not require jet ventilation.

T   Data from the United States suggest that >90% of CICV situations are preventable with adequate pre-operative airway assessment and preparation.

T   The fixation in trying to 'achieve endotracheal intubation at all costs', and the persistence in trying an airway method that has already failed, results in significant human error, loss of situational awareness and poor decision making.

T   Skills in any cricothyroidotomy technique are retained for a short period of time only. It is recommended that chosen techniques should be practised every 3-6 months for optimal performance and skill retention.

1.   Popat M. The unanticipated difficult airway: the can't intubate, can't ventilate scenario. Johnston I, Harrop-Griffiths W, Gemmell L, Eds. In: *AAGBI Core Topics in Anaesthesia* 2012; 4: 44-55.

2.   The Difficult Airway Society (DAS). http://www.das.uk.com/files/cvci-Jul04-A4.pdf.

Answer 5: In quinine sulphate overdose: True b & d

F   Quinine prolongs the QTc interval, with a subsequent risk of ventricular tachycardia (VT) and acute arrhythmias developing.

T   Quinine sulphate overdose can also cause blindness.

F   Quinine sulphate overdose may precipitate ventricular fibrillation (VF) that is resistant to cardioversion with amiodarone.

T   Quinine sulphate overdose induces insulin release and often causes hypoglycaemia.

F   Continuous veno-venous haemofiltration (CVVH) does not remove quinine.

1.   Worthley LI. Clinical Toxicology: Part II. Diagnosis and management of uncommon poisonings. *Crit Care Resusc* 2002; 4(3): 216-30.

Answer 6: The pre-test heparin-induced thrombocytopenia (HIT) score: True a, c & e

T   There are four categories used when calculating the HIT score (sometimes referred to as the 'four Ts'): Thrombocytopenia, Timing of platelet fall, Thrombosis and exclusion of other potential causes of Thrombocytopenia.

F   The maximum score is 8.

T   Thrombocytopenia with a >50% fall or nadir greater than or equal to 20 x 10^9/L is given 2 points.

F   A score of 0-3 confers low probability (<5% HIT), a score of 4-5 intermediate (10-30%) and a score of 6-8 high pre-test probability for HIT (20-80%).

T   A platelet fall <4 days since heparin exposure and/or with no recent previous heparin exposure is given a score of zero.

1.   Doane M. Heparin-induced thrombocytopenia (Part 1). Anaesthesia Tutorial of the Week 243, 2011. www.aagbi.org/education/educational-resources/tutorial-week.

Answer 7: Concerning bronchoscopy in critical care: True a-c & e

T   Bronchoscopy is an essential diagnostic and therapeutic procedure in the ICU.

T   One should wear full protective clothing during bronchoscopy, e.g. mask, eye protection and gown, as airway secretions may cause significant healthcare worker contamination.

T   The suction port should be immediately brushed through and the scope sent for decontamination once bronchoscopy is complete.

F   The first 2-5 divisions should be possible to visualise during bronchoscopy.

T   20-60ml 0.9% saline should be instilled prior to suctioning and specimen trap when undertaking bronchial-alveolar lavage.

1.   Waldmann C, Soni N, Rhodes A. *Oxford Desk Reference Critical Care.* Oxford, UK: Oxford University Press, 2008.

Answer 8: In relation to the cerebral arterial circulation: True a & c-e

T   This is true. The basilar artery does originate at the junction between the left and right vertebral arteries.

F   The basilar artery travels <u>anterior</u> to the brainstem.

T   The lateral aspects of the brain including the frontal, parietal, occipital, temporal and insular lobes are supplied by the middle cerebral arteries.

T   Anterior and middle cerebral arteries arise from the internal carotid arteries and supply 70% of the arterial blood supply to the brain.

T   The posterior inferior cerebellar artery (PICA) arises from the vertebral artery and is the largest of the cerebellar arteries.

1.   Smith T, Pinnock C, Lin T. *Fundamentals of Anaesthesia*, 3rd ed. Cambridge, UK: Cambridge University Press, 2009.

2.   Moss E. The cerebral circulation. *Br J Anaesth CEPD reviews* 2001; 1(3): 63-71.

Answer 9: In acute graft versus host disease (AGVHD): True a & d

T   AGVHD is a complication of allogeneic haematopoietic stem cell transplantation (HSCT) and commonly involves the skin, liver and gut. Typically, a maculopapular rash usually starts on palms and soles, but may start on any part of the skin before spreading. In severe forms, toxic epidermal necrolysis may occur. Diarrhoea can be copious. Jaundice and cholestasis often herald liver involvement.

F   AGVHD is due to T-cells from the donor blood, bone marrow and stem cells attacking the tissues of the host.

F   Steroids form the first-line therapy for AGVHD but may be only effective in <50% of patients. Second-line therapy for AGVHD includes: extracorporeal photopheresis, Il-2 receptor antibodies, T-cell immunosuppression (cyclosporine, tacrolimus), anti-TNF antibodies (infliximab, etanercept), mTOR inhibitors (sirolimus) and mycophenolate mofetil (MMF).

T   Calcineurin inhibitors (ciclosporin/tacrolimus) are commonly used for AGVHD prophylaxis.

F   Transfusion-associated graft versus host disease (TA-GVHD) is associated with an almost 100% mortality.

1.   http://www.bcshguidelines.com/documents/bjh_9129_Rev_EV.pdf.

2.   Clevenger B, Kelleher A. Hazards of blood transfusion in adults and children. *Contin Educ Anaesth Crit Care Pain* 2014; 14(3): 112-8.

Answer 10: Red cell transfusion and critical care: All False

F   The WHO defines anaemia as <130g/L in men and <120g/L in women. Severe anaemia is defined as <80g/L.

F   A transfusion threshold of 70g/L or below is recommended by the British Committee for Standards in Haematology (BCSH), with a target range 70-90g/L. This is based on evidence suggesting that a liberal approach to blood transfusion correction has no benefit over a more restrictive transfusion policy. Patients with traumatic brain injury, subarachnoid haemorrhage or ischaemic stroke may benefit from Hb >90g/L. The TRISS study found that there was no difference in outcome between septic patients in the ICU with a low (7g/dL) versus high (9g/dL) transfusion trigger. A transfusion trigger of 7g/dL in septic patients is safe and results in fewer transfusions.

F   Studies suggest only 20% of transfusions on critical care are used to treat haemorrhage with the majority being given for anaemia. About 60% of patients admitted to intensive care are anaemic on admission.

F   Although a contentious issue, red cell transfusion should not be used routinely as a strategy to assist weaning from mechanical ventilation when the Hb is >70g/L.

F   In patients suffering from an acute coronary syndrome (ACS), the BCSH recommends maintaining Hb >80g/L. In critically ill patients with stable angina, Hb should be maintained >70g/L.

1.   Retter A, Wyncoll D, Pearse R, *et al*. Guidelines on the management of anaemia and red cell transfusion in adult critically ill patients. *Br J Haematol* 2013; 160: 445-64.

2.   Hébert PC, Wells G, Blajchman MA, *et al;* Transfusion Requirements in Critical Care Investigators, Canadian Critical Care Trials Group. A multicenter, randomised, controlled clinical trial of transfusion requirements in critical care. *N Engl J Med* 1999; 340(6): 409-17.

3.   Carson JL, Terrin ML, Noveck H, *et al;* FOCUS Investigators. Liberal or restrictive transfusion in high-risk patients after hip surgery. *N Engl J Med* 2011; 365: 2453-62.

4.   Holst LB, Haase N, Wetterslev J, *et al;* TRISS Trial Group. Lower versus higher threshold for transfusion in septic shock. *N Engl J Med* 2014; 371(5): 1381-91.

● Answer 11: Concerning heparin-induced thrombocytopenia (Type II HIT): True a, b & e

T   Type II (immune) HIT is rare. The platelet count typically falls by 30-50% within 5-10 days after starting heparin therapy.

T   The incidence of HIT occurs more frequently (10x) with unfractionated heparin compared to low-molecular-weight heparins (LMWH).

F   HIT is more common in female patients.

F   A complex can be formed between a heparin antigen and platelet factor 4 (PF4). This complex is immunogenic. The patient develops an immune response, where typically IgG antibodies form against the heparin-platelet factor 4 complex on the surface of platelets. Once IgG attaches to the platelets they then become activated resulting in a consumptive coagulopathy and HIT development.

T   Heparin/LMWH should be stopped immediately on diagnosing HIT. Providing there is not extensive bleeding, non-heparin anticoagulation is required for at least 14 days to treat and prevent thrombosis, either using direct thrombin inhibitors (e.g. argatroban, lepirudin) or Factor Xa inhibitors (e.g. danaparoid, fondaparinux).

1.   Doane M. Heparin-induced thrombocytopenia (Part 1). Anaesthesia Tutorial of the Week 243, 2011. www.aagbi.org/education/educational-resources/tutorial-week.

● Answer 12: The larynx: True a-c

T   The larynx extends from C3 to C6.

T   Damage may occur during surgery, such as thyroidectomy, causing loss of cord tension and hoarseness.

T   It is a branch of the vagus nerve and passes deep to the internal and external carotid arteries before dividing into external and internal branches.

F   The recurrent laryngeal nerve is also a branch from the vagus nerve and provides motor innervation to all intrinsic muscles of the larynx (except cricothyroid) and sensory innervation below the vocal cords. Bilateral palsy results in total loss of vocal cord function and severe stridor and dyspnoea — the (cadaveric) midline vocal cord position.

F   Cricothyroidotomy is performed in an emergency situation through the cricothyroid ligament. Tracheostomy is performed between the 1st to 4th tracheal rings.

1.   Erdmann AG. *Concise Anatomy for Anaesthesia.* Cambridge, UK: Cambridge University Press, 2002.

Answer 13: The following statements are true about electrocardiogram (ECG) monitoring: True a-c

T   Standard ECG calibration is 25mm/s and 1mV/cm.

T   Lead II is considered the best lead for detecting arrhythmias, as it monitors the axis of left ventricular depolarisation.

T   The CM5 lead is superior for detecting coronary ischaemia versus an individual limb lead. The right arm lead is placed on the manubrium and the left leg electrode is placed in the standard V5 position. Lead II is selected on the monitor.

F   A five-lead ECG has a 90% sensitivity for detecting inferior or anterior ischaemia when leads II, V4 and V5 are selected continuously.

F   The normal ECG axis is -30° (minus) to +90°. Left axis deviation is present if the mean axis lies between -30° and -90°, and right axis deviation is present if the mean axis is +90° to 180°.

1.   Waldmann C, Soni N, Rhodes, A. *Oxford Desk Reference Critical Care.* Oxford, UK: Oxford University Press, 2008.

2.   www.fammed.wisc.edu/medstudent/pcc/ecg/axis.htm.

Answer 14: In relation to acute aortic dissection: True a & d

T   Aortic dissection is a tearing of layers within the aortic wall, either of the intima or from intramural haemorrhage and haematoma in the media causing intimal perforation. Other signs include syncope and abdominal pain.

F   Acute aortic dissection is more common in males with a peak incidence at 50-70 years of age.

F   The Stanford Classification system has two types of dissection; Type A (involving the ascending aorta) and Type B (involving the descending aorta, distal to the left subclavian artery). The European Society of Cardiology classification is made up of five classes (1 to 5). The DeBakey classification describes three types of dissection (Types I, II and III).

T   Blood pressure titration to a systolic 100-120mmHg is recommended. β-blockers should be the first-line agents used (esmolol, metoprolol, labetalol) unless contraindicated, in which case calcium channel blockers (verapamil, diltiazem) should be utilised. Patients should be adequately β-blocked before the use of vasodilators (sodium nitroprusside, glyceryl trinitrate or hydralazine) to prevent reflex tachycardia, an increased force of ventricular contraction and greater aortic wall stress, which may potentially worsen aortic dissection.

F   Acute Type A aortic dissection is a surgical emergency. Most Type B dissections are managed medically initially but up to a third will eventually require surgery.

1.   Hebballi R, Swanevelder J. Diagnosis and management of aortic dissection. Contin Educ Anaesth Crit Care Pain 2009; 9(1): 14-8.
2.   Parsons PE, Wiener-Kronish JP. Critical Care Secrets, 5th ed. Missouri, USA: Elsevier Mosby, 2013.

Answer 15: Regarding defibrillation: True a & d

T   According to the Resuscitation Council UK, the chain of survival during cardiac arrest includes: early recognition and call for help, early cardiopulmonary resuscitation, early defibrillation and post-resuscitation care.

F   Transthoracic impedance in an adult is approximately 70-80 Ohms.

F   Anteroposterior electrode placement is more effective in atrial fibrillation than sternal-apical positioning, during synchronised DC cardioversion/defibrillation.

T   Biphasic defibrillators have a first shock efficacy of 86-98% for long duration ventricular fibrillation/ventricular tachycardia, compared to 54-91% with monophasic devices.

F No survival benefit has been demonstrated with biphasic defibrillators compared to monophasic defibrillators.

1. Resuscitation Council (UK). Advanced life support, 6th ed. London, UK: Resuscitation Council (UK), 2011. www.resus.org.uk.
2. Waldmann C, Soni N, Rhodes, A. *Oxford Desk Reference Critical Care*. Oxford, UK: Oxford University Press, 2008.

Answer 16: Considering intra-aortic balloon pump (IABP) use: True a, d & e

T With IABP use, blood is displaced proximally augmenting diastolic pressure and increasing coronary perfusion and myocardial oxygen supply.

F Helium is used to inflate the balloon as its low density and rapid diffusion coefficient allows rapid inflation and deflation. There is also less risk of a gas embolus with helium, if the balloon were to rupture or leak.

F The IABP inflates at the onset of diastole (middle of the T-wave on the electrocardiogram [ECG] and dichrotic notch on the arterial trace), thus augmenting coronary blood supply with proximal displacement of blood.

T IABP deflation occurs at the onset of systole, immediately before the opening of the aortic valve (this corresponds with the peak of the R-wave on the ECG or a point just before systolic upstroke on the arterial line).

T The diameter of the IABP balloon should not exceed 80-90% of a patient's descending aortic diameter, so as not to fully occlude the aorta.

1. Alaour B, English W. Intra-aortic balloon pump counterpulsation. Anaesthesia Tutorial of the Week 220, 2011. www.aagbi.org/education/educational-resources/tutorial-week.
2. Krishna M, Zacharowski K. Principles of intra-aortic balloon pump counterpulsation. *Contin Educ Anaesth Crit Care Pain* 2009; 9(1): 24-8.

Answer 17: Indications for cardiac pacing include: All True

T   Permanent atrial fibrillation (AF) with atrioventricular (AV) block is a Class I indication for cardiac pacing according to the European Society of Cardiology (ESC) 2013 guidelines.

T   Mobitz Type I second-degree heart block is an indication for pacing if symptomatic.

T   Third-degree heart block is an indication for pacing.

T   Overdrive pacing for prevention or treatment of torsade de pointes is sometimes used.

T   Asystolic episodes are an indication for pacing.

1.   The Taskforce on Cardiac Pacing and Resynchronization therapy of the European Society of Cardiology (ESC). ESC guidelines on cardiac pacing and cardiac resynchronisation therapy. *Eur Heart J* 2013; 34: 2281-329.

2.   Waldmann C, Soni N, Rhodes A. *Oxford Desk Reference Critical Care*. Oxford, UK: Oxford University Press, 2008.

Answer 18: Considering the critical care management of acute liver failure (ALF): True a & d

T   N-acetylcysteine (NAC) is proven to be effective for both paracetamol-induced ALF and in patients with non-paracetamol-induced ALF showing early hepatic encephalopathy (Grade I/II). NAC may increase non-transplant survival.

F   Intracranial pressure (ICP) monitoring is recommended in ALF patients with high-grade encephalopathy, in centres where there is ICP monitoring expertise and in patients awaiting acute liver transplantation. ICP monitoring is not without risk, as bleeding has been reported to occur in 4-20% of cases, resulting in death in up to 5% of cases.

F   ALF is characterised by a hyperdynamic state with high output cardiac failure, low mean arterial pressure (MAP) and low systemic vascular resistance (SVR) often seen. Increased nitric oxide (NO) production and cyclic guanosine monophosphate (cGMP) may contribute to the haemodynamic disturbances seen. Fluid resuscitation and the use of vasopressors may be required.

T   In treating respiratory failure in ALF, the lowest level of PEEP that achieves adequate oxygenation should be targeted. High levels of PEEP may exacerbate hepatic congestion and cerebral oedema.

F   Hepatocyte necrosis causes glycogen depletion, defective glycogenolysis and gluconeogenesis, predisposing to hypoglycaemia.

1.   Wang DW, Yin YM, Yao YM. Advances in the management of acute liver failure. *World J Gastroenterol* 2013; 19(41): 7069-77.

Answer 19: Variceal bleeding: True c-e

F   Regardless of medical/surgical and endscopic management, acute variceal bleeding still carries an immediate mortality of 8%, with an associated 20% risk of death after 6 weeks.

F   Portal hypertension is associated with a portal pressure gradient of greater than 5mmHg. At gradients greater than 10mmHg, blood flow through the hepatic portal system is redirected from the liver into areas with lower venous pressures. Collateral circulation thus develops in the lower oesophagus, abdominal wall, stomach, and rectum. The small blood vessels in these areas become distended and thin-walled, appearing as varicosities.

T   Terlipressin reduces flow to splanchnic vessels and reduces venous blood flow to the upper gastrointestinal (GI) tract and thus may be effective in reducing variceal bleeding.

T   Broad-spectrum antibiotics have been demonstrated to reduce the risk of variceal rebleeding and mortality from sepsis in cirrhosis.

T   A TIPS procedure and even liver transplantation may need to be considered for severe variceal bleeding, warranting referral to tertiary centres for consideration.

1.   Waldmann C, Soni N, Rhodes A. *Oxford Desk Reference Critical Care.* Oxford, UK: Oxford University Press, 2008.

2.   Arguedas M. "The critically ill liver patient: the variceal bleeder". *Semin Gastrointest Dis* 2003; 14(1): 34-8.

Answer 20: Regarding the Sengstaken-Blakemore tube (SBT): True b-d

F   Up to 50% of patients will rebleed following SBT deflation.

T   A SBT is effective at controlling torrential bleeding from gastro-oesophageal varices.

T   A SBT has three lumens: one each for oesophageal balloon inflation, gastric aspiration and gastric balloon inflation.

T   A position of the SBT 55cm at the incisors indicates a position well below the gastro-oesophageal junction.

F   The oesophageal balloon of the SBT should be deflated every 4 hours for 15 minutes to reduce potential mucosal damage.

1.   Waldmann C, Soni N, Rhodes A. *Oxford Desk Reference Critical Care.* Oxford, UK: Oxford University Press, 2008.

Answer 21: Regarding surgical resection of the oesophagus: True b, c & e

F   A thoracic epidural will aid effective postoperative analgesia, improving mobility and cough. It should be considered in all patients if not contraindicated.

T   There is a significant morbidity/mortality associated following double-lumen endotracheal tube displacement and/or incorrect positioning. Respiratory failure post-oesophagectomy is common and may affect up to 25% of patients. There should be a low threshold for using a fibre-optic scope to confirm initial DLT placement and subsequent intra-operative tube position checks.

T   Respiratory morbidity following oesophagectomy is common with respiratory complications occurring in approximately 25% of patients. These patients may require critical care re-admission and early intervention with potential re-intubation. Cardiovascular complications (12%) and anastomotic leak (16%) may also complicate the postoperative period.

F   The use of non-invasive positive pressure ventilation (NPPV) for respiratory failure in the immediate postoperative period following oseophagectomy is controversial, but not absolutely contraindicated. High inspiratory (IPAP) and expiratory (EPAP,

CPAP) pressures may hypothetically cause anastomotic distension and subsequent leak. However, there is increasing evidence that these concerns may be overstated and that NPPV use for postoperative respiratory failure may decrease re-intubation need and acute respiratory distress syndrome (ARDS), without increasing the risk of anastomotic leakage. Although, gastric distension is unlikely below inspiratory pressures of $25cmH_2O$, the use of nasogastric drainage is advocated by many, as this would reduce the risk of distension. Further studies are warranted.

T Anastomotic leak may occur typically between 3-7 days and may present with non-specific signs such as pyrexia, general malaise, respiratory infection and cardiac arrhythmias (often atrial fibrillation is seen).

1. Rucklidge M, Sanders D, Martin A. Anaesthesia for minimally invasive oesophagectomy. *Contin Educ Anaesth Crit Care Pain* 2010; 10(2): 43-7.

2. Sherry KM, Smith FG. Anaesthesia for oesophagectomy. *Contin Educ Anaesth Crit Care Pain* 2003; 3(3): 87-90

3. Michelet P, D'Journo XB, Seinaye F, *et al.* Non-invasive ventilation for the treatment of postoperative respiratory failure after oesophagectomy. *Br J Surg* 2009; 96: 54-60.

Answer 22: In relation to the classification of acute liver failure (ALF): True a-c

T The O'Grady system classifies ALF as follows: hyperacute (<1 week), acute (<1 month) and subacute (<3 months), depending on the time of jaundice to encephalopathy.

T The O'Grady system classifies ALF as 'acute' when jaundice to encephalopathy occurs after 7 days and up to 1 month.

T The O'Grady system classifies ALF as 'hyperacute' when jaundice to encephalopathy occurs within less than 1 week.

F The Bernuau system classifies ALF into fulminant (1-2 weeks from jaundice to encephalopathy) and subfulminant (2 weeks+ from jaundice to encephalopathy).

F The Japanese system classifies ALF into 'fulminant' (which is split up into subclasses: acute 0-9 days and subacute 9 days-8 weeks) and 'late-onset' (period is 8-24 weeks from jaundice to encephalopathy).

1.   Bernal W, Wendon J. Acute liver failure. *New Engl J Med* 2014; 369: 2525-34.

Answer 23: In relation to ethylene glycol (EG) poisoning: True a & c

T   EG poisoning presents in three phases depending on timing: initially (30-60 minutes) after ingestion acute intoxication occurs. This may also result in excitatory symptoms, cerebral oedema, convulsions and coma. The second phase occurs at 12-18 hours with predominantly cardiovascular effects including dysrhythmias and cardiac failure. Profound metabolic acidosis often causes death during this phase. Phase three occurs at 2-3 days with predominantly renal failure and acute tubular necrosis due to calcium deposition. Finally, a delayed neurologic phase can occur 5-20 days post-ingestion, presenting with neurological effects including profound limb weakness, cranial nerve palsies and sensory disturbance.

F   EG causes an increased anion gap acidosis. Other causes of a raised anion gap acidosis include: lactate, toxins (ethanol, ethylene glycol, methanol, paraldehyde, aspirin, cyanide, iron, isoniazid), and ketoacidosis (diabetes, alcohol). Causes of a normal anion gap acidosis include: gastrointestinal losses (diarrhoea), renal loss of bicarbonate (proximal renal tubular acidosis), renal failure and hyperchloraemic acidosis.

T   The enzyme alcohol dehydrogenase catabolises the metabolism of EG into toxic metabolites including: glycoaldehyde, glycolate (35%), formate, oxalate (2.3%), glycine, hippuric acid, and benzoic acid. Oxalate may combine with ionised calcium resulting in hypocalcaemia and renal failure due to crystal deposition. EG toxic metabolites are responsible for the profoundly high anion gap acidosis and associated toxic signs and symptoms.

F   Renal replacement therapy is a very effective treatment for EG poisoning, as it corrects acid-base status and eliminates EG and some of the harmful metabolites.

F   Fomepizole is a potent inhibitor of alcohol dehydrogenase preventing the production of toxic metabolites of EG. It is given as a loading dose 15mg/kg and then 10mg/kg every 12 hours for the next 48 hours. After which, the dose is increased to 15mg/kg 12-hourly. It is continued until plasma EG levels are less than 20mg/dL.

1. Glossop AJ, Bryden DC. Case report: an unusual presentation of ethylene glycol poisoning. *J Intensive Care Soc* 2009; 10(2): 118-21.

Answer 24: The following statements concerning spontaneous bacterial peritonitis (SBP) in chronic liver disease are true: True a, c & d

T   Following one episode of SBP in cirrhosis, the probability of survival at 2 years is 50%.

F   A neutrophil count greater than 250/mm^3 is diagnostic for SBP. SBP accounts for about 20% of acute on chronic liver failure cases.

T   The administration of albumin in SBP may decrease the frequency of development of hepatorenal syndrome in patients with chronic liver disease.

T   Ascitic culture is negative in 40% of SBP cases despite signs and symptoms indicative of SBP. The most common pathogens are *Escherichia coli*, *Streptococcal* and *Enterococcal* species. Patients who are culture-negative, but have a neutrophil count >250/mm^3, should still be treated for SBP. Broad-spectrum antibiotics should be started immediately following a diagnosis of SBP.

F   It is recommended that cirrhotic patients with ascites, who have had one previous episode of SBP, receive lifelong prophylactic antibiotics.

1. EASL. EASL clinical practice guidelines on the management of ascites, spontaneous bacterial peritonitis, and hepatorenal syndrome in cirrhosis. *J Hepatol* 2010; 53: 397-417.

2. Jackson P, Gleeson D. Alcoholic liver disease. *Contin Educ Anaesth Crit Care Pain* 2010; 10(3): 66-71.

3. Lee J, Kwang-Hyub H, Sang H. Ascites and spontaneous bacterial peritonitis: an Asian perspective. *J Gasteroenterol Hepatol* 2009; 24(9): 1494-503.

4. Segarra-Newnham M, Henneman A. Antibiotic prophylaxis for prevention of spontaneous bacterial peritonitis in patients without gastrointestinal bleeding. *Ann Pharmacother* 2010; 44(12): 1946-54.

Answer 25: Regarding alcoholic liver disease (ALD): True c & d

F   Patients with advanced cirrhosis and ascites, which may be caused by alcohol, are at a high risk of developing hepatorenal syndrome (HRS). 18% develop HRS within 1 year, with up to 39% developing HRS by 5 years.

F   One UK unit of alcohol contains 10-12g ethanol. A typical pint of beer contains 2 units, a bottle of normal strength beer 1.5 units, a glass of wine 1-3 units depending on size. Ethanol intake in excess of 40g per day in men and 10-20g per day in women is associated with an increased relative risk of developing liver disease.

T   Patients with alcoholic liver disease may present with Wernicke's encephalopathy (nystagmus, opthalmoplegia, ataxia and confusion) secondary to thiamine deficiency.

T   ALD is divided into three histological types, which may all coexist in the same patient. Ethanol metabolites cause accumulation of lipid in liver cells (steatosis). 90-100% occur in heavy drinkers and resolves within a few months of alcohol cessation. Ethanol metabolism can also generate oxygen species and neo-antigens which cause inflammation — alcoholic hepatitis. This inflammatory response may be mild or lead to full blown multi-organ failure. Prolonged hepatocellular damage results in liver fibrosis and hepatocyte destruction. This causes hepatic function decline, portal hypertension due to disruption in liver blood flow and ultimately cirrhosis. 8-20% of heavy drinkers will develop cirrhosis.

F   Serum levels of tumour necrosis factor-α (TNF-α) are raised in ALD and alcoholic hepatitis in particular. In severe alcoholic hepatitis, steroids are recommended demonstrating a short-term survival benefit. The side effects of steroids, risk of GI bleeding and potential increased risk of sepsis preclude the use of steroids in some patients. Inhibition of TNF-α with monoclonal antibodies, e.g. infliximab and etanercept, was found to increase mortality in alcoholic hepatitis. However, pentoxifylline, an oral anti-TNF-α agent (via phosphodiesterase inhibition), has been associated with a reduced hepatorenal syndrome risk and may be considered in severe alcoholic hepatitis in patients who cannot receive steroids.

1. Kiser TH. Hepatorenal syndrome. *Int J Clin Med* 2014; 5: 102-10.
2. Jackson P, Gleeson D. Alcoholic liver disease. *Contin Educ Anaesth Crit Care Pain* 2010; 10(3): 66-71.
3. Parker R, Armstrong MJ, Corbett C, *et al.* Systematic review: pentoxifylline for the treatment of severe alcoholic hepatitis. *Aliment Pharmacol Ther* 2013; 37(9): 845-54.
4. http://www.medscape.com/viewarticle/782533.
5. Flood S, Bodenham A, Jackson P. Mortality of patients with alcoholic liver disease admitted to critical care: a systematic review. *J Intensive Care Soc* 2012; 13(2): 130-5.

Answer 26: Considering oxygen delivery (DO_2) in adults: True a & c

T When oxygen delivery falls below 300ml/minute, it fails to match oxygen uptake and shock ensues.

F Younger patients compensate for shock well and may have relatively normal vital signs despite profound shock.

T The metabolic demands of an average person can be met by dissolved O_2 alone when breathing FiO_2 1.0 at 3 atmospheres at rest.

F DO_2 is reliant on convection from the environment and diffusion into the blood.

F Achieving supranormal values of DO_2 in sepsis have not been demonstrated to be beneficial in septic patients, with attempts often proving detrimental.

1. Waldmann C, Soni N, Rhodes A. *Oxford Desk Reference Critical Care.* Oxford, UK: Oxford University Press, 2008.

Answer 27: Oesophageal Doppler: True a & c

T The Doppler frequency is $f_d=2f_0 v\cos\theta/c$ where v is velocity of blood flow, θ is the angle between the ultrasound beam and blood flow, c is ultrasound velocity in that medium, f_0 is the transmitting frequency. Rearranged blood velocity may be calculated.

F Velocity of blood flow in the descending aorta is measured using a flexible ultrasound probe and the Doppler principle. The shift in reflected ultrasound wave frequency, from moving red cells, is proportional to the velocity of blood flow. The velocity of blood flow in cm/s or stroke distance (calculated from the area under the trace curve), is combined with the cross-sectional area of the descending aorta (using a nomogram based on age, weight and height) to estimate stroke volume (SV). Cardiac output (Q) is then estimated by applying Q = SV x heart rate.

T   A number of assumptions are made with oesophageal Doppler. It is assumed that cardiac output or aortic blood flow is distributed caudally to the descending aorta and rostrally to the great vessels and coronary arteries in a constant ratio of 70:30, respectively. Other assumptions are that a flat velocity profile exists within the aorta, the estimated cross-sectional area is close to the mean systolic diameter, there is negligible diastolic blood flow and the velocity of blood flow in the aorta is measured accurately.

F   Oesophageal Doppler probes have been used for up to 14 days without complications.

F   Oesophageal Doppler may be potentially inaccurate in the presence of a working epidural due to the vasodilation and reduction in systemic vascular resistance caused by epidural drug administration.

1.   Waldmann C, Soni N, Rhodes A. *Oxford Desk Reference Critical Care.* Oxford, UK: Oxford University Press, 2008.

Answer 28: In relation to the PiCCO cardiac monitor, the following statements are true: True b, d & e

F   The PiCCO requires a central line and specialised (usually femoral) arterial catheter.

T   Thermodilution is used to calibrate the pulse pressure algorithm in PiCCO.

F   The mean transit time (MTT) is the time taken for half the tracer to pass through the venous circulation, heart and lungs to the arterial circulation.

T   The downslope time (DST) represents the time it takes for thermal tracer to be eluted from the largest chamber in the circuit, which is the pulmonary blood volume and extravascular lung water or termed the pulmonary thermal volume (PTV).

T Global end-diastolic volume (GEDV) can be calculated using the following equations:

MTT x cardiac output (CO) = intrathoracic thermal volume (ITTV).

ITTV - PTV = GEDV.

1. http://www.pulsion.com/fileadmin/pulsion_share/Products/PiCCO/Philips_PiCCO_Application_Note.pdf.

Answer 29: Derived variables from a pulmonary artery catheter: True c & e

F This is low.
Cardiac index (CI) = cardiac output/body surface area.
The normal range is between 2.8-4.2L/min/m^2.

F Normal systemic vascular resistance index (SVRI) is between 1760-2600 dynes.sec/cm^5/m^2.
SVRI = 80 x (mean arterial pressure [MAP]) - central venous pressure (CVP)/CI.
Normal systemic vascular resistance (SVR) is 800-1200 dynes.sec/cm^5.

T Normal pulmonary vascular resistance (PVR) is <250 dynes.sec/cm^5.
PVR = 80 x (mean pulmonary artery pressure [MPAP]) - pulmonary artery occlusion pressure (PAOP)/cardiac output (CO).

F Left ventricle coronary perfusion pressure (LVCPP) = diastolic blood pressure (DBP) - pulmonary artery occlusion pressure (PAOP).
Normal range is 60-80mmHg.

T Normal stroke volume index (SVI) is 35-47ml/m^2/beat.
SVI = cardiac index (CI)/heart rate x 1000.

1. Bersten AD, Soni N. *Oh's Intensive Care Manual*, 6th ed. Butterworth Heinemann Elsevier, 2009.

2. Edwards (2014). Normal haemodynamic parameters. http://ht.edwards.com/scin/edwards/sitecollectionimages/products/mininvasive/ar10523-normal_card_1lr.pdf.

Answer 30: Concerning liver transplantation for acute liver failure (ALF): True a, d & e

T Survival rates following liver transplantation for ALF are 79% at 1 year and 72% at 5 years. Most deaths occur within the first 3 postoperative months.

F Risk of death following liver transplantation for ALF is higher among older recipients and in those receiving older or partial grafts. It is also higher in recipients who received a donor graft from donors without an identical ABO blood group.

F Less than 10% of liver transplants are performed in ALF patients. Peri-operative management of transplantation for ALF is challenging with survival rates consistently lower than those seen following elective liver transplantation for chronic liver disease.

T Early postoperative impaired graft function is poorly tolerated and predisposes to intracranial hypertension and sepsis.

T The initial mortality following liver transplantation in ALF is higher than in chronic liver failure patients. After the first year, however, this trend reverses and ALF patients have better long-term survival.

1. Bernal W, Wendon J. Acute liver failure. *New Engl J Med* 2014; 369: 2525-34.

2. Wang DW, Yin YM, Yao YM. Advances in the management of acute liver failure. *World J Gastroenterol* 2013; 19(41): 7069-77.

Answer 31: The lungs and bronchial tree: True c

F There is only one fissure in the left lung — an oblique fissure separating upper and lower lobes. The right lung is made up of two fissures — the oblique and horizontal fissures.

F After 2.5cm the right main bronchus gives off the right upper lobe bronchus.

T The right lower lobe bronchus is also made up of superior, medial, anterior, lateral and posterior basal branches.

F Lateral and medial branches make up the right middle lobe bronchus.

F The left main bronchus is longer and narrower, about 5cm in adults. The right main bronchus is wider and easier to enter.

1. Erdmann AG. *Concise Anatomy for Anaesthesia.* Cambridge, UK: Cambridge University Press, 2002.

Answer 32: In relation to paracetamol (acetaminophen) overdose: True b & d

F   Paracetamol is broken down into metabolites in the liver. Most metabolites are produced by glucuronidation and sulphation to non-toxic conjugates. However, a small percentage are oxidised by cytochrome P450 to form the highly toxic metabolite NAPQI. Normally, NAPQI is detoxified by conjugation with glutathione to form cysteine and mercapturic acid, which is then renally excreted. In overdose, insufficient glutathione results in excess NAPQI causing hepatic damage and necrosis.

T   Ingestion of paracetamol levels <75mg/kg is unlikely to cause serious harm. Plasma paracetamol levels on or above 100mg/L at 4 hours and 15mg/L at 15 hours warrant immediate treatment with NAC.

F   The nomogram should not be used in staggered overdose, as it is unreliable. N-acetylcysteine should be started without delay in this situation.

T   The initial (1st) infusion of NAC is recommended by the Medicines and Healthcare Products Regulatory Agency (MHRA), to be 150mg/kg over 1 hour. The 2nd infusion of 50mg/kg is then given over the next 4 hours and the 3rd infusion of 100mg/kg over the next 16 hours. If ingestion occurred within 8 hours of starting NAC, the patient will usually be fit following 21 hours of antidote. However, the international normalised ratio (INR), plasma creatinine, venous pH or bicarbonate and alanine aminotransferase (ALT) should be checked before treatment cessation. Further treatment of 100mg/kg over a further 16 hours is warranted if abnormalities in laboratory bloods are identified (e.g. doubled ALT, ALT 2x upper limit of normal, INR >1.3). Further bloods are required at 8-16 hours to assess progress.

F   Hypersensitivity is not a contraindication to NAC. The benefits of acetylcysteine outweigh the risks of hypersensitivity in such cases, and patients should receive treatment. Hypersensitivity often presents with rash and may present within the first hour of treatment. Chlorphenamine (Piriton) may reduce symptoms.

1.   Sharma C, Mehta V. Paracetamol: mechanisms and updates *Contin Educ Anaesth Crit Care Pain* 2014; 14(4): 153-8.
2.   http://www.mhra.gov.uk/Safetyinformation/DrugSafetyUpdate/CON185624.
3.   www.toxbase.org.

Answer 33: Concerning recreational drug toxicity: True a-d

T   Dantrolene in combination with resuscitation and other cooling measures may be used for MDMA toxicity. MDMA can precipitate serotonin syndrome. The classic triad of symptoms include: 1) neuromuscular excitability (tremor, stiffness, hyperpyrexia, clonus, myoclonus); 2) autonomic disturbance (mydriasis, tachycardia, hypertension, flushing, hyperthermia); 3) mental changes (headache, poor concentration, agitation, coma).

T   The effects of cocaine are predominantly sympathomimetic, tachypnoea, tachycardia, hypertension, chest pain, myocardial ischaemia, vasospasm, vascular infarction or dissection, agitation, paranoia, anxiety, psychosis, stroke, seizures and coma.

T   Acute alcohol withdrawal may result in delirium tremens and death. Chlordiazepoxide is often used to attenuate alcohol withdrawal. Lorazepam and clonidine are sometimes used in critical care to attenuate alcohol withdrawal.

T   Dilated pupils, hypotonia and hyporeflexia may occur in children following accidental ingestion of cannabis.

F   Mephedrone (4-methylmethcathinone) toxicity is relatively unknown. It has been responsible for a number of deaths globally. Toxicity includes: peripheral vasoconstriction, tachycardia, anxiety, excessive sweating, palpitations, agitation, hypertension, convulsions, coma, chest pain, and raised creatine phosphokinase (CpK).

1.   Nicholson Roberts T, Thompson JP. Illegal substances in anaesthetic and intensive care patients. *Contin Educ Anaesth Crit Care Pain* 2013; 13(1): 42-6.
2.   http://www.evidence.nhs.uk/formulary/bnf/current/4-central-nervous-system/410-drugs-used-in-substance-dependence/4101-alcohol-dependence.
3.   www.toxbase.org.

Answer 34: In relation to the Glasgow Coma Scale (GCS): True a, c & d

T	The GCS is incorporated into the Acute Physiology And Chronic Health Evaluation II (APACHE II) scoring system. It is also incorporated into other critical care scoring systems such as the Sequential Organ Failure Score (SOFA) and Multi-organ Dysfunction Score (MODS).

F	Full assessment of coma with the GCS cannot be done when the patient is intubated and ventilated. The FOUR score (Full Outline of Responsiveness score) replaces the verbal scoring of the GCS with observation of brainstem reflexes and is becoming more commonly used. It scores each component: eye response, motor response, brainstem reflexes and respiration from 0-4.

T	A score of 8/15 or below is deemed significant coma, where airway reflexes may be obtunded requiring invasive ventilation for airway protection and control.

T	The GCS pre-intubation following traumatic brain injury has prognostic significance. For example, in one study by Timmons *et al*, GCS motor score was found to be a strong predictor of 2-week mortality in this group of patients.

F	This patient scores 8/15: eyes opening to pain = E2 out of 4, mumbles sounds = V2 out of 5, withdraws to painful stimuli = M4 out of 6. The breakdown of the GCS is as follows: E: 4 = spontaneous eye opening, 3 = eyes open to voice, 2 = eyes open to pain, 1 = no eye opening. M: 6 = obeys commands, 5 = localises pain, 4 = withdraws to painful stimuli or flexion, 3 = abnormal flexion (decorticate response), 2 = extension to pain (de-cerebrate response), 1 = no movement. V: 5 = orientated normal speech, 4 = confused speech, 3 = inappropriate words, 2 = inappropriate sounds, 1 = no speech/sounds.

1.	Bouch DC, Thompson JP. Severity scoring systems in the critically ill. *Contin Educ Anaesth Crit Care Pain* 2008; 8(5): 181-5.

2.	Patel S, Hirsch N. Coma. *Contin Educ Anaesth Crit Care Pain* 2013; 14(5): 220-3.

3.	Timmons SD, Bee T, Webb S, *et al*. Using the abbreviated injury severity and Glasgow Coma Scale scores to predict 2-week mortality after traumatic brain injury. *J Trauma* 2011; 71(5): 1172-8.

Answer 35: Concerning cervical cord injury and critical care: True c

F   Fibre-optic intubation has not been proven to be superior or safer to standard laryngoscopy and orotracheal intubation, with manual in-line stabilisation, in cervical cord injury.

F   Maintaining patients with cervical spinal cord injury in the supine position may optimise/improve breathing function when compared to the semi-upright position. Abdominal contents are pushed higher into the chest, improving apposition with the ribcage. The diaphragmatic curvature radius is reduced, restoring the fulcrum lost with higher abdominal compliance, improving breathing efficiency.

T   Loss of mobility and vasodilatation with venous pooling, in spinal cord injury, results in a higher (up to three-fold) increased risk of deep vein thrombosis and subsequent complications.

F   Autonomic dysreflexia develops in individuals with a spinal cord injury level at or above T6. Potentially life-threatening hypertension can occur below the level of the lesion causing seizures, retinal haemorrhages, pulmonary oedema, renal failure, stroke, myocardial infarction and death (due to strong peripheral sympathetic responses due to stimuli below the level of the lesion). Pupillary constriction and nasal congestion with bradycardia, sweating and flushing is typically seen above the level of the lesion due to descending inhibitory response as far down as the lesion (unopposed parasympathetic responses).

F   The National Acute Spinal Cord Injury Studies (NASCIS) II and III, and a Cochrane systematic review of all randomised clinical trials (Bracken MB, 2002) verified significant improvement in motor function and sensation in patients with complete or incomplete spinal cord injury who were treated within 8 hours with high doses of methylprednisolone (30mg/kg initial bolus over 15 minutes, followed 45 minutes after this bolus with an infusion 5.4mg/kg/hr for 23 hours). However, following these studies, the methodology of NASCIS II and III was revisited with the validity of these results brought into question. An increased incidence of severe sepsis and severe pneumonia was noted in NASCIS III in those treated with steroids. Due to this controversy, administration of steroids remains at the preference of the institution and physician.

1. McGill J. Airway management in trauma: an update. *Emerg Med Clin N Am* 2007; 25: 603-22.
2. Denton M, McKinlay J. Cervical cord injury and critical care. *Contin Educ Anaesth Crit Care Pain* 2009; 9(3): 82-6.
3. Stephenson RO, Berliner J, Meier RH, *et al*. Autonomic dysreflexia in spinal cord injury. Medscape reference, 2013. http://emedicine.medscape.com/article/322809-overview.
4. Chin LS, Wyler AR. Spinal cord injuries treatment and management. Medscape reference, 2012. http://emedicine.medscape.com/article/793582-treatment.

Answer 36: Lumbar drain management: True a, b & d

T   A lumbar drain is an epidural catheter inserted into the subarachnoid space to drain cerebrospinal fluid (CSF) from around the spinal cord.

T   Suprarenal aortic aneurysm (thoracic) patients are at particular risk of spinal cord ischaemia and paraplegia development. Lumbar drains may be used in selected patients in an attempt to improve perfusion to the spinal cord and offset any oedema effects caused by ischaemia. This may reduce paraplegia complications.

F   The zero level should be at the level of the drain insertion site (i.e. lumbar level).

T   The variable height reservoir can be raised or lowered to achieve the prescribed drain height. Drain height is typically 10-20cmH$_2$O. When CSF pressure exceeds the drain height set, CSF will drain into the variable height reservoir and drainage bag. The maximum permitted amount of drainage per hour (typically 20-30ml) is set. The duration of drainage (typically 48 hours post-op) is also prescribed. CSF should be sent for culture, cell count, protein and glucose at least every 48 hours or more frequently depending on the clinical condition.

F   Excessive CSF drainage is associated with a number of rare but serious complications including: tension pneumocephalus (due to a siphoning effect [via catheter] of air), raised intracranial pressure and herniation, subdural haemorrhage, intradural haematoma and infection.

1. American Association of Neuroscience Nurses (AANN). *Care of the patient with a lumbar drain*, 2nd ed. AANN Reference Series for Clinical Practice, 2007.
2. http://www.aann.org/pdf/cpg/aannlumbardrain.pdf.

Answer 37: In relation to nerve conduction study patterns: True d

F   Both motor and sensory conduction is reduced in critical care polyneuropathy.

F   Motor conduction shows reduced amplitude, with sensory conduction being normal in motor neuron disease.

F   Motor conduction is reduced and falls further with repetition in myasthenia gravis. Sensation is normal. On electromyography (EMG) there is increased jitter on single fibre testing.

T   In Guillain-Barré syndrome, motor nerve conduction is slowed or blocked. Sensory conduction is also reduced or absent. EMG may show denervation later.

F   EMG fibrillations are seen in critical care polyneuropathy. Widespread denervation is seen in motor neuron disease on EMG.

1. Waldmann C, Soni N, Rhodes A. *Oxford Desk Reference Critical Care*. Oxford, UK: Oxford University Press, 2008.

Answer 38: In patients with brain herniation due to raised intracranial pressure (ICP): a & d

T   Tentorial/uncal herniation causes pupillary dilatation and ptosis. Although trans-tentorial herniation can occur when the brain moves up or down across the tentorium, descending herniation is much more common.

F   Tonsillar herniation occurs when the cerebellum herniates through the foramen magnum into the spinal canal. This causes compression of the midbrain with blood pressure and heart rate changes. Flaccid paralysis is also usually seen.

F   Compression of the midbrain during tonsillar herniation may cause a Cushing's response (severe hypertension and bradycardia) in about one third of cases.

T   Persistently high ICP over 20-25mmHg is associated with worse outcomes in traumatic brain injury.

F   Cushing's response is more commonly seen, classically evident as hypertension and bradycardia.

1.   Waldmann C, Soni N, Rhodes A. *Oxford Desk Reference Critical Care.* Oxford, UK: Oxford University Press, 2008

2.   Brant WE, Helms CA. *Fundamentals of Diagnostic Radiology.* Philadelphia, USA: Lippincott, Williams & Wilkins, 2007: 69.

Answer 39: Concerning intracranial pressure (ICP) waveforms (Figure 1.1) the following statements are true: True a, b & e

T   The normal ICP trace looks similar to an arterial trace.

T   P1 is caused by the percussion wave caused by the arterial pressure being transmitted from the choroid plexus to the ventricle.

F   P3 is the dichrotic wave due to aortic valve closure. P2 is the tidal wave due to brain compliance.

F   With high ICP, P2 exceeds P1 and the wave becomes broader.

T   Lundberg A waves or plateau waves are slow vasogenic waves seen in patients with critical perfusion. They are always pathological and indicate reduced cerebral compliance. B waves occur 0.5-2/minute and can be seen in normal individuals. C waves are of little importance.

1.   Marion DW, Darby J, Yonas H. Acute regional blood flow changes caused by severe head injuries. *J Neurosurg* 1991; 74: 407-14.

2.   Clemens P. Traumatic brain injury: outcome and pathophysiology, 2007. http://www.frca.co.uk/article.aspx?articleid=100915.

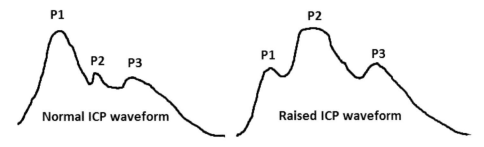

Figure 1.1. ICP waveforms.

Answer 40: Pre-operative β-blockade use for non-cardiac surgery: True b, c & d

F   The POISE trial confirmed a decrease in non-fatal myocardial infarction when β-blockers were given pre-operatively in patients with ischaemic heart disease for non-cardiac surgery, but found that all-cause mortality increased with increased bradycardic, hypotensive and stroke events.

T   The Dutch Echocardiographic Cardiac Risk Evaluation Applying Stress Echocardiography (DECREASE) series of studies suggested benefit with pre-operative β-blockade. These trials were discredited due to serious flaws. A recent meta-analysis by Bouri et al in 2013 found that pre-operative β-blockade in non-cardiac surgery significantly increased all-cause 30-day mortality by 27% (p=0.04). β-blockers reduced non-fatal myocardial infarction, but were associated with increased hypotensive and stroke events, leaving a net increase in deaths. The Bouri meta-analysis questions the validity of current guidelines, based on the DECREASE trials (Poldermans et al), by the European Society of Cardiology (ESC), which recommends the use of pre-operative β-blockade. The true answer whether to use pre-operative β-blockade or not remains currently a matter of debate, but use may harm patients overall.

T   In the POISE trial, myocardial infarction (MI) was reduced occurring in 4.2% vs. 5.7% (metoprolol vs. placebo, respectively), p=0.0017.

T   In the POISE trial, β-blockers increased stroke rates, occurring in 1% vs. 0.5% of patients (metoprolol vs. placebo, respectively), p=0.0053.

F   The evidence for the use of β-blockers peri-operatively for non-cardiac surgery was not based on robust data, due to discredited studies (DECREASE series).

1.   POISE Study Group, Devereaux PJ, Yang H, Yusuf S. Effects of extended-release metoprolol succinate in patients undergoing non-cardiac surgery (POISE Trial): a randomised controlled trial. *Lancet* 2008; 371: 1839-47.

2.   Bouri S, Shun-Shin MJ, Cole GD, *et al.* Meta-analysis of secure randomised controlled trials of β-blockade to prevent perioperative death in non-cardiac surgery. *Heart* 2014; 100(6): 456-64.

Answer 41: Mannitol 20%: True a

T   20% mannitol = 200mg/ml, therefore 200mg x 500ml = 100,000mg = 100g.

F   Mannitol solutions are acidotic (pH 6.3).

F   Mannitol may crystallise at room temperature but can be made soluble again by warming the solution prior to use.

F   Mannitol exerts its effects via multiple mechanisms. Plasma expansion reduces blood viscosity and this in turn improves regional cerebral microvascular flow and oxygenation. Cardiac output is also increased due to increased intravascular volume, increasing cerebral blood flow, resulting in compensatory vasoconstriction reducing cerebral oedema. An osmotic gradient is established between plasma and brain cells, drawing water from the cerebral extracellular space into the vasculature, reducing cerebral oedema. An intact blood brain barrier is required for these actions to work. Peak effect is 30-45 minutes and lasts for around 6 hours. Mannitol effectively reduces ICP while the serum osmolality is <320mOsm/L.

F   The current recommendations from the Brain Trauma Foundation and the European Brain Injury Consortium identify level II and III evidence for the use of mannitol in reducing intracranial pressure following traumatic brain injury. 0.25g-1.0g/kg is recommended over 20 minutes. This is repeated 1-2 times after 4-8 hours. Higher doses

>2g/kg convey no further benefit and are associated with a greater incidence of side effects. For a 70kg patient administration would thus involve: 0.5g/kg-1.0g/kg = 35-70g dose = 20% mannitol solution = 200mg/ml =175-350ml to be given.

1.   Shawkat H, Westwood MM, Mortimer A. Mannitol: a review of its clinical uses. *Contin Educ Anaesth Crit Care Pain* 2012; 12(2): 82-5.

2.   Haddad SH, Arabi YM. Critical care management of severe traumatic brain injury in adults. *Scand J Trauma, Resusc Emerg Med* 2012; 20: 12. http://www.sjtrem.com/content/20/1/12.

Answer 42: Pain management on critical care: True d & e

F   It is estimated that >70% of critical care patients remember experiencing pain during their critical care stay.

F   The BPS is composed of three observational areas (facial expression, upper limb movements and compliance with mechanical ventilation). Each is scored from 1 to 4, with higher numbers indicating discomfort. The BPS score ranges from 3 (no pain) to 12 (most pain). It has been studied and validated in both deeply sedated and moderately sedated patients.

F   The CPOT assesses four areas (facial expression, movements, muscle tension and ventilator compliance). Each area is scored from 0-2, with total scores ranging from 0 (no pain) to 8 (most pain). It is validated in both intubated and non-intubated critical care patients. CPOT has superior reliability and validity when used in non-verbal critically ill adults. Chronic pain or delirium may make ascertaining a pain level difficult with CPOT.

T   Uncontrolled pain is common in critically ill patients. Uncontrolled pain is associated with many adverse physiological and psychological consequences and may cause increased overall morbidity and death. Consequences include: arrhythmias, immune system alteration, increased catecholamine and cortisol release, depression, anxiety and post-traumatic stress disorder.

T   Intravenous opioids (e.g. alfentanil) are considered first line for the treatment of non-neuropathic pain on the critical care unit. Enteral gabapentin or carbamazepine in addition to opioids may be considered for neuropathic pain management.

1.   Stites M. Observational pain scales in critically ill adults. *Crit Care Nurs* 2013; 33(3): 68-79.

2.   Barr J, Puntillo K, Ely EW, *et al.* Clinical practice guidelines for the management of pain, agitation, and delirium in adult patients in the intensive care unit. *Crit Care Med* 2013; 41(1): 263-306.

Answer 43: In relation to prerequisites for brainstem death testing: True b, d & e

F   There should be no doubt that the patient's condition is caused by irreversible brain damage. In some patients the final diagnosis is never fully established despite extensive investigation. Brainstem death testing should be only done after a period of observation and further investigation that there is no possibility of a reversible or treatable condition.

T   Prior to brainstem death testing, it is imperative to exclude the possibility of coma due to residual sedatives, analgesics or muscle relaxants. If there is doubt that residual thiopentone remains, then assays can be undertaken. As such, brainstem death testing should not be done if thiopentone levels are >5mg/L.

F   Core temperature should be greater than 34°C at the time of testing. Brainstem reflexes are usually lost at temperatures of less than 28°C.

T   In relation to plasma sodium levels, low values <115mmol/L and high values >160mmol/L are associated with coma and contraindicate brainstem death testing.

T   Significant weakness is unlikely with serum phosphate or magnesium between 0.5-3.0mmol/L.

1.   Academy of Medical Royal Colleges. A code of practice for the diagnosis and confirmation of death, 2010. http://www.aomrc.org.uk/publications/statements/doc_details/42-a-code-of-practice-for-the-diagnosis-and-confirmation-of-death.html.

Answer 44: Echocardiography and critical care: True c-e

F   Ultrasound is sound with frequencies above 20kHz. Echo machines use frequencies of 2-10MHz.

F   The speed of sound is: 1540m/s in soft tissue, 1570m/s in blood and 330m/s in air.

T   Better resolution is seen with higher frequencies, but at the expense of shorter wavelengths and reduced image depth. Longer wavelengths and lower frequencies are useful for imaging at depth due to better penetration.

T   Echo can be used to assess valvular dysfunction, stenotic and regurgitant lesions amongst other pathologies. Echo can provide a bedside diagnosis in the unstable critical care patient with massive pulmonary embolus. Severe aortic stenosis classically is defined as a valve area of 0.6-0.8cm^2 and a mean pressure gradient of >40-50mmHg.

T   Lesions that resemble vegetations such as papillary fibroma, rupture or redundant chordae, non-specific valve thickening, calcification, SLE or cardiac thrombus can give false-positive findings for infective endocarditis. Echo features of infective endocarditis include: an oscillating intracardiac mass on a valve or supporting structure, intracardiac abscess, new dehiscence of a prosthetic valve or new valvular regurgitation.

1.   Waldmann C, Soni N, Rhodes A. *Oxford Desk Reference Critical Care*. Oxford, UK: Oxford University Press, 2008.

Answer 45: When considering transfer of critically ill patients: True c & d

F   A standard ambulance trolley is not suitable for the transfer of critically ill patients. Ideally, a critical care trolley should be able to carry all equipment including O_2 supply and ventilator, syringe drivers, suction pump and back-up batteries. These items should be secure and placed below the patient. The trolley should be secured and fixed within the ambulance and able to withstand up to 10G forces in all directions.

F   Neurosurgical transfers are time-critical, but the risks of delay must be balanced against the risks of transferring an unstable or ill-prepared patient and/or transfer team.

T   Transfers for non-clinical reasons should only take place in exceptional circumstances and ideally only in daylight hours.

T   Departure checklists, such as those produced by the Association of Anaesthetists of Great Britain and Ireland (AAGBI), should be mandatory prior to transfer. They allow a quick final check of personnel, equipment, patient, logistics, contact numbers, location, sedation and drugs, notes and investigations. They may prove crucial in ensuring an uneventful transfer and prevent disaster. Clear documentation should be done throughout transfer and is a legal requirement.

F   The OUTCOMEREA study group found that intra-hospital transfers of ventilated critically ill patients was associated with increased complications such as pneumothorax, atelectasis, ventilator-associated pneumonia, hypoglycaemia and hyperglycaemia, and hypernatraemia. Intra-hospital transfer was also associated with an increased length of stay in ventilated patients, but had no significant impact on mortality.

1.   Dinsmore J. Traumatic brain injury: an evidence-based review of management. *Contin Educ Anaesth Crit Care Pain* 2013; 13(6): 189-95.

2.   http://www.aagbi.org/sites/default/files/interhospital09.pdf.

3.   OUTCOMEREA Study Group. Safety of intrahospital transport in ventilated critically ill patients: a multicenter cohort study. *Crit Care Med* 2013; 41: 1919-28.

Answer 46: In paediatric meningococcal disease: True a-d

T   Due to vaccination programmes for *Haemophilus influenzae* Type b, serogroup C meningococcus and pneumococcal disease, the epidemiology of bacterial meningitis has changed in the last 20 years. Serogroup B meningococcus is the most common cause of meningitis and meningococcal disease in children aged 3 months or older. There is currently no vaccine for serogroup B meningococcus.

T   Symptoms and signs of meningitis and meningococcal disease are often non-specific. Classical signs of meningitis are often absent in infants. Patients commonly present with fever, vomiting, respiratory symptoms, irritability and sometimes seizures.

T   Benzylpenicillin is recommended by the National Institute for Health and Care Excellence (NICE), UK, to be given pre-hospital as soon as the diagnosis of meningococcal infection is suspected, providing there is no history of anaphylaxis to penicillin. Administration of antibiotics should not delay urgent transfer to hospital.

T   Intravenous cetriaxone or cefotaxime (indicated if co-administering with calcium-containing infusions, the baby is premature, has hypoalbuminaemia or is acidotic) should be given immediately to any child suspected of having meningococcal disease.

F   Ideally, lumbar puncture should be performed in suspected meningococcal disease. However, there are numerous contraindications, which may prevent lumbar puncture being safely undertaken. In such circumstances it is reasonable to avoid lumbar puncture. It is vital that administration of antibiotics is not delayed. Contraindications to lumbar puncture include: signs of raised intracranial pressure (reduced consciousness, focal neurological signs, unequal, dilated or poorly reactive pupils), shock, extensive or spreading purpura, post-convulsions (unless stabilised), coagulation abnormalities, local skin infection, or in the presence of respiratory insufficiency.

1.   National Institute for Health and Clinical Excellence (NICE). Bacterial meningitis and meningococcal septicaemia. Management of bacterial meningitis and meningococcal septicaemia in children and young people younger than 16 years. NICE Clinical Guideline 102, 2010. London, UK: NICE, 2010. http://www.nice.org.uk.

2.   http://www.nice.org.uk/nicemedia/live/13027/49341/49341.pdf.

Answer 47: Regarding paediatric airway emergencies: True b, c & e

F   A child with croup has a distinctive barking cough and stridor may be heard. Bacterial tracheitis may present in a similar way to croup, but often the patient fails to respond to croup management and is systemically septic with a high fever and a toxic appearance. Bacterial tracheitis can be life-threatening and is often caused by *Staphylococcus aureus* or *Haemophilus influenzae* Type B. Findings at tracheobronchoscopy include mucopurulent exudates, ulceration and sloughing of tracheal mucosa. Airway protection and broad-spectrum antibiotics (ceftriaxone intravenously for 14 days) is important for management.

T Acute epiglottitis is a life-threatening emergency. It is most commonly due to *Haemophilus influenzae* Type B. Acute epiglottitis presents with severe throat pain, fever, irritability and respiratory distress, which progresses rapidly. Key features include the 4Ds: drooling, dyspnoea, dysphagia and dysphonia. Airway management is important with close observation being mandatory. In the event of airway deterioration, prompt intubation may be required. In an arrested patient, an emergency needle cricothyroidotomy may be needed. Antibiotics (co-amoxiclav or cefuroxime) are recommended. If invasive ventilation is needed, then the patient should be kept intubated until an audible leak around the endotracheal tube is heard. Patients with croup (laryngotracheobronchitis) commonly present between ages 6 months to 4 years. Croup is most commonly caused by the parainfluenza virus. Classic symptoms include a barking cough, stridor, hoarse voice and respiratory distress. Croup is generally short-lived. Management involves the use of systemic and inhaled steroids and nebulized adrenaline.

T Sevoflurane and topical anaesthesia is the airway technique of choice for removal of a foreign body with a Storz bronchoscope. Maintenance of spontaneous breathing is of paramount importance. Intravenous induction and muscle relaxation should only be used if the anaesthetist is confident that no air trapping will occur (ball-gas effect) with associated barotrauma risk.

F The NAP4 found, that in the UK, formal surgical tracheostomy was used in most cases of failed intubation and ventilation in children.

T A high-flow nasal cannula (HFNC) with a flow rate equal to or above 2L/kg/min is well tolerated and beneficial in young infants, with acute respiratory syncytial virus (RSV) bronchiolitis.

1.   Cheng HC, Dai ZK, Wu JR, Chen IC. Pediatric upper airway emergencies. Taiwan Society of Pediatric Pulmonology, 2012.

2.   Roberts S, Thornington RE. Paediatric bronchoscopy. *Contin Educ Anaesth Crit Care Pain* 2005; 5(2): 41-4.

3.   Prasad Y. The difficult paediatric airway. Anaesthesia Tutorial of the Week 250, 2012. www.aagbi.org/education/educational-resources/tutorial-week.

4.   Milesi C, Baleine J, Matecki S, *et al.* Is treatment with high flow nasal cannula effective in acute viral bronchiolitis? A physiologic study. *Int Care Med* 2013; 39(6): 1088-94.

Answer 48: The following statements are true about human immunodeficiency virus (HIV) infection: True a & c

T   Fever is seen in over 75% of patients with primary HIV infection (seroconversion illness). Other symptoms include fatigue, headache, rash and lymphadenopathy.

F   High HIV RNA levels (viral load) correlates with the rate of decline of T-helper cells (CD4 count) and progression to acquired immunodeficiency syndrome (AIDS).

T   AIDS is defined by the finding of one of the AIDS-defining conditions in a patient with HIV, or by the finding of a CD4 count of <200 cells/µl.

F   HIV transmission occurs in about 0.3% cases of needle stick injuries where a HIV-positive patient was involved, and thus can be considered a rare event.

F   Median survival in HIV patients treated with anti-retroviral therapy in the UK is about 30 years, and is likely to increase.

1.   Hare CB. Clinical overview of HIV disease, 2006. HIV Insite. UCSF. http://hivinsite.ucsf.edu/InSite?page=kb.

2.   Bersten AD, Soni N. *Oh's Intensive Care Manual*, 6th ed. Butterworth Heinemann Elsevier Publishing, 2009.

Answer 49: Regarding anti-retroviral therapy (ART) in human immunodeficiency virus (HIV): True b-d

F   Zidovudine is a nucleoside analogue reverse transcriptase inhibitor.

T   This is true, fusion inhibitors block fusion of HIV with the cell membrane. Enfuvirtide (T20) is an example of such a drug.

T   Life-threatening lactic acidosis with hepatomegaly and steatosis is associated with nucleoside reverse transcriptase inhibitors (NRTI), e.g. zidovudine (AZT), lamivudine (3TC), stavudine (d4T). Withdrawal of the inciting NRTI drug is important therapy.

T   Anti-retroviral therapy initiation in the critical care unit is often hazardous due to unpredictable absorption, lack of parenteral formulations and hypersensitivity reactions. Guidance should be sought from your local infectious diseases team.

F   The non-nucleoside reverse transcriptase inhibitors (NNRts) (e.g. efavirenz, nevirapine) are effective against the HIV-1 subtype only and not HIV-2.

1.   Bersten AD, Soni N. *Oh's Intensive Care Manual*, 6th ed. Butterworth Heinemann Elsevier Publishing, 2009.
2.   Chow DC, Day LJ, Souza SA, Shikuma CM. Metabolic complications of HIV therapy. *IAPAC Mon* 2006; 12(9): 302-17.
3.   http://hivinsite.ucsf.edu/InSite?page=kb.
4.   Crothers, K. Huang, L. Critical care of patients with HIV, 2006. HIV Insite. UCSF. http://hivinsite.ucsf.edu/InSite?page=kb.
5.   The British National Formulary (BNF) 66. Joint Formulary Committee 66 (September 2013). BMJ Publishing Group Ltd and Royal Pharmaceutical Society. http://www.bnf.org/bnf/index.htm.

Answer 50: Acute and chronic adverse effects of glucocorticoids include: True c-e

F   Proximal muscle weakness is more commonly seen in patients receiving long-term steroids (steroid-induced myopathy).

F   Hyperglycaemia is a common side effect of steroid use, and patients receiving steroids should have blood glucose levels closely monitored.

T   Peptic ulcer disease and gastrointestinal haemorrhage is associated with steroid use. Caution should be exercised in patients with a prior history of such conditions, when prescribing steroids.

T   Avascular osteonecrosis of large joints (e.g. knees and hips) may occur with chronic steroid use.

T   There is a risk of adrenal insufficiency, particularly in patients with chronic steroid use and sudden cessation of therapy. Guidelines for steroid supplementation in patients on long-term steroids or with repeated short-term courses should be closely followed, for patients admitted to critical care and also in the peri-operative period. Other adverse features of glucocorticoid therapy include: infection (atypical), hypertension, emotional instability, insomnia, psychosis, fluid retention, impaired wound healing, pancreatitis, increased coronary and cerebrovascular events and osteoporosis.

1.   Parsons PE, Wiener-Kronish JP. *Critical Care Secrets*, 5th ed. Missouri, USA: Elsevier Mosby, 2013.

Answer 51: Respiratory failure in a patient with rheumatoid arthritis on critical care may be caused by: All True

T   There is a wide differential for shortness of breath/respiratory failure in a patient with rheumatoid arthritis presenting to critical care. Parenchymal involvement such as that seen in interstitial lung disease and bronchiolitis obliterans may be a cause. Other causes include typical and atypical pneumonia, rheumatoid nodules, pulmonary oedema and heart failure.

T   Drug-related lung toxicity can be caused by methotrexate, leflunomide, tumour necrosis factor (TNF) inhibitors, gold, penicillamine and other disease-modifying agents (DMARDs) in patients taking such medications for rheumatoid arthritis management.

T   Gold salts may cause drug-related lung toxicity.

T   Rheumatoid disease involving the airway may manifest with upper airway obstruction, sleep apnoea, Caplan syndrome (rheumatoid pneumoconiosis manifesting as intrapulmonary nodules) and cricoarytenoid dysfunction.

T   Pleural and pericardial effusions are commonly associated with rheumatoid arthritis and may cause respiratory failure if of significant size.

1.   Parsons PE, Wiener-Kronish JP. *Critical Care Secrets*, 5th ed. Missouri, USA: Elsevier Mosby, 2013.

Answer 52: In relation to temperature regulation: True a & e

T   Temperature is sensed by A-δ fibres and C fibres.

F   Temperature elevation reduces serum iron, which can subsequently reduce bacterial growth.

F   The initial immediate dose of dantrolene in suspected cases of malignant hyperthermia is 2.5mg/kg, followed by additional boluses of 1mg/kg as required up to a maximum dose of 10mg/kg. Therefore, this patient should initially receive a dose of 175mg.

F   Ventricular fibrillation can occur below a temperature of 28°C and asystole below a temperature of 20°C.

T   Cerebral blood flow falls at an approximate rate of 7% per °C drop in temperature. This is postulated to be due to reduced cardiac output and increased blood viscosity.

1.   Bersten AD, Soni N. *Oh's Intensive Care Manual*, 6th ed. Butterworth Heinemann Elsevier, 2009.

2.   Association of Anaesthetists of Great Britain and Ireland. Malignant hyperthermia crisis AAGBI safety guideline. http://www.aagbi.org/sites/default/files/mh_guideline_for_website.pdf.

Answer 53: The following statements are true about drowning: True a-c

T   Drowning is the second leading cause of unnatural death after road traffic accidents in the UK.

T   Drowning is characterised by apnoea, generalised vasoconstriction and bradycardia, resulting in a shunt of blood to the heart and brain.

T   It was initially postulated that laryngeal spasm occurred in approximately 15% of drowning victims, resulting in dry drowning. It is now thought that death without pulmonary aspiration rarely occurs.

F   Submersion in salt water as compared to fresh water is not thought to make a significant clinical difference in outcome.

F   Major electrolyte abnormalities secondary to aspiration of large fluid volumes in patients with drowning are rare, unless drowning occurs in extremely electrolyte-rich liquids.

1.   Carter E, Sinclair R. Drowning. *Contin Educ Anaesth Crit Care Pain* 2011; 11(6): 210-3.

2.   Bersten AD, Soni N. *Oh's Intensive Care Manual*, 6th ed. Butterworth Heinemann Elsevier, 2009.

Answer 54: Pre-eclampsia: True b & c

F   The pathophysiology is highly variable, but it is thought that failure of trophoblastic invasion of spiral arteries within the placenta is involved.

T   Foetal growth restriction occurs in pre-eclampsia secondary to hypoperfusion and hypoxaemia of the placenta.

T   Pre-eclampsia is more common in primiparous women and is also more common in first pregnancies with a particular partner.

F   Pre-eclampsia is rare before 20 weeks' gestation, but the prognosis is poorer the earlier the condition presents.

F   To diagnose pre-eclampsia, the patient will have a persistently high systolic (>140mmHg) and/or diastolic blood pressure (>90mmHg) after 20 weeks' gestation and one or more of the following: proteinuria, low platelet count, impaired liver function, renal impairment, pulmonary oedema, new-onset headaches and visual disturbances. Proteinuria is not required to diagnose pre-eclampsia.

1.   Yentis SM, Hirsch NP, Smith GB. *Anaesthesia and Intensive Care A-Z. An Encyclopaedia of Principles and Practice*, 3rd ed. Edinburgh, UK: Elsevier Butterworth Heinemann, 2004.

2.   Turner JA. Diagnosis and management of pre-eclampsia - an update. *Int J Women's Health* 2010; 2: 327-37.

3.   The American College of Obstetricians and Gynaecologists. Hypertension in Pregnancy, 2013. http://www.acog.org/Resources_And_Publications/Task_Force _and_Work_Group_Reports/Hypertension_in_Pregnancy.

Answer 55: Regarding eclampsia and HELLP syndrome: True c & d

F   Eclampsia can occur without symptoms of pre-eclampsia.

F   The term eclampsia is used to describe grand mal seizures occurring during pregnancy, which do not have another identifiable cause.

T   HELLP syndrome is generally considered to be a variant of pre-eclampsia. Both conditions usually occur during the later stages of pregnancy, or sometimes after childbirth. HELLP syndrome is a combination of haemolysis, elevated liver enzymes and low platelets.

T   HELLP syndrome can occur without proteinuria or hypertension, but the majority of patients will have pre-eclamptic symptoms.

F   HELLP syndrome is a severe form of disease, which occurs in approximately 20% of cases of severe pre-eclampsia. HELLP syndrome may require delivery of the foetus.

1.   Turner JA. Diagnosis and management of preeclampsia - an update. *Int J Women's Health* 2010; 2: 327-37.

Answer 56: The following are International System of Units (SI) base units: True a, b & d

T   There are seven base units in the SI system from which all other units are derived. These base units are the metre, kilogram, second, ampere, kelvin, candela and mole.

T   The ampere is a fundamental unit, with 6.241×10^{18} electrons (or one coulomb) per second constituting one ampere.

F   The joule is a derived unit. It is equal to the energy expended in applying a force of one newton through a distance of one metre or in passing an electric current of one ampere through a resistance of one ohm for one second.

T   The mole is a fundamental unit. It is defined as the amount of any substance that contains as many elementary entities or atoms as there are atoms in 12 grams of pure carbon-12. This corresponds to the Avogadro constant, which has a value of 6.0221413×10^{23} atoms or constituent particles per mole of a given substance.

F   The litre is a non-SI metric system unit of volume equal to 1 cubic decimetre (dm^3), 1000 cubic centimetres (cm^3) or 1/1000 cubic metre.

1.   Davis PD, Kenny GNC. *Basic Physics and Measurement in Anaesthesia*, 5th ed. Edinburgh, UK: Butterworth Heinemann, 2003.

2.   International Bureau of Weights and Measures. *The International System of Units (SI)*, 8th ed, 2006: 120.

Answer 57: In relation to haemoglobin, the following statements are true: True a & e

T   Adult haemoglobin contains two α and two β chains. Foetal haemoglobin contains two α and two γ chains.

F   The iron in haem is in the ferrous state. Oxidation of iron to the ferric state forms methaemoglobin.

F   Glutamic acid is replaced by valine at the sixth amino acid position.

F   The Bohr effect describes the physiological state where hemoglobin's oxygen binding affinity is inversely related both to acidity and to the concentration of carbon dioxide. Affinity is reduced by increasing values of $PaCO_2$, acidity, temperature and 2,3-diphosphoglycerate (2,3-DPG).

T   Porphyria is transmitted by autosomal dominant inheritance.

1.   Smith T, Pinnock C, Lin T. *Fundamentals of Anaesthesia*, 3rd ed. Cambridge, UK: Cambridge University Press, 2009.

Answer 58: During adult cardiopulmonary resuscitation, current UK resuscitation and related guidelines recommend that: True b & e

F   Intravenous adrenaline 1mg should be given after the third shock in a shockable rhythm, as per guidance from the Resuscitation Council (UK).

T   The Advanced Life Support guidelines state that every 5-second increase in the pre-shock pause, almost halves the chance of successful defibrillation.

F   Hypovolaemia is a reversible cause of cardiac arrest, in addition to hypoxia, hypothermia, tension pneumothorax, cardiac tamponade, toxins, thrombosis and electrolyte/metabolic disturbances.

F   The 'three-shock strategy' is appropriate in patients who have had a witnessed or monitored ventricular fibrillation (VF) or ventricular tachycardia (VT) arrest, in the cardiac catheter laboratory or early after cardiac surgery.

T   The 5-minute time period for observation following failed resuscitation before confirmation of death, was recommended by the Academy of Medical Royal Colleges in the 2008 publication "A code of practice for the diagnosis and confirmation of death".

1.   Resuscitation Council (UK). Advanced life support, 6th ed. London, UK: Resuscitation Council (UK), 2011. www.resus.org.uk.
2.   Academy of Medical Royal Colleges. A code of practice for the diagnosis and confirmation of death. London, UK: Academy of Medical Royal Colleges, 2008.

Answer 59: During paediatric cardiopulmonary resuscitation of an 8-year-old child: True a & c

T   A compression/ventilation ratio of 15:2 is appropriate in an 8-year-old child.

F   Weight (kg) can be estimated from the formulae:

$<$1yr = (age x 0.5)+ 4, age in months
1-5yr = (age x 2)+ 8, age in years
6-12yr = (age x 3)+ 7, age in year

So this child would be expected to weigh approximately 31kg. An adrenaline dose of 10μg/kg as per European Paediatric Life Support guidelines would be 310μg.

T   Energy (J) = weight (kg) x 4. Thus, 31kg x 4 = 124J; therefore, a defibrillation energy level of 124-130J depending on defibrillator settings (always round up) would be appropriate, during paediatric cardiopulmonary resuscitation of an 8-year-old child in pulseless ventricular tachycardia (VT) or ventricular fibrillation (VF).

F   Glucose solutions are not recommended for volume expansion.

F   Intraosseous access should be sited after three unsuccessful attempts at gaining peripheral venous access or 90 seconds, in time duration, of attempts.

1.   Resuscitation Council (UK). European paediatric life support (EPLS), 3rd ed. London, UK: Resuscitation Council (UK). www.resus.org.uk.

Answer 60: During the resuscitation of a patient with major burns: True b

F   Airway swelling does not generally occur at an early stage; however, appropriate preparation for a potentially difficult airway should always be made.

T   Suxamethonium is safe to use in the first 24 hours after a burn, but can cause hyperkalaemia after this time due to the generation of extra-junctional acetylcholine receptors.

F   The Parkland formula can be used to predict fluid requirement for the 24 hours from time of burn injury, and uses the formula:

Fluid volume requirements = total body surface area (TBSA) burned (%) x Wt (Kg) x 4ml.

Half of requirements should be given in the first 8 hours, then the remaining half over the next 16 hours. Fluid replacement subsequent to this will be determined by clinical state, urine output and overall fluid losses.

F   Infection is a significant cause of mortality in major burns, but there is no conclusive evidence to support early prophylactic antibiotics.

F   Full-thickness burns are painless due to nerve destruction, but a mixed picture of full- and partial-thickness burns is common.

1.   Bishop S, Maguire S. Anaesthesia and intensive care for major burns. *Contin Educ Anaesth Crit Care Pain* 2012; 12(3): 118-22.

2.   Kasten KR, Makley AT, Kagan RJ. Update on the critical care management of severe burns. *J Intensive Care Med* 2011; 26(4): 223-36.

Answer 61: Criteria for liver transplantation include: True c & d

F   An arterial pH <7.3 despite volume resuscitation is included in the King's College Criteria for emergency liver transplantation.

F   In addition, Grade III or IV encephalopathy needs to be present with a coexistent INR >6.5 and creatinine >300μmol/L following acetaminophen-induced acute liver failure, to meet the King's College Criteria for emergency liver transplantation.

T   An early arterial lactate concentration >3.5mmol/L (median 4 hours) or a lactate concentration >3.0mmol/L following a median of 12 hours of fluid resuscitation forms part of the Modified King's College Criteria.

T   Patients with end-stage hepatitis C cirrhosis would be appropriate candidates for liver transplantation. Patients with uncontrolled drug dependency and persistent alcohol misuse, however, may not be eligible for transplantation dependent on local policy.

F   Fulminant Gilbert's disease does not meet the criteria for transplantation. A fulminant clinical course of Wilson's disease may necessitate transplantation.

1.   Bernal W, Wendon J. Liver transplantation in adults with acute liver failure. *J Hepatol* 2004; 40: 192-7.

2.   Bernal W, Donaldson N, Wyncoll D, Wendon J. Blood lactate as an early predictor of outcome in paracetamol-induced acute liver failure: a cohort study. *Lancet* 2002; 359(9306): 558-63.

3.   Devlin J, O'Grady J. Indications for referral and assessment in adult liver transplantation: a clinical guideline, 2000. http://www.bsg.org.uk/images/stories /docs/clinical/guidelines/liver/adult_liver.pdf.

Answer 62: Pelvic trauma: True b

F   The mortality from pelvic trauma may approach 50% in patients with an unstable pelvic fracture and shock.

T   The pubic rami is the weakest point of the pelvic ring.

F   Springing of the pelvis can exacerbate bleeding and thus should not be part of routine practice in patients with acute pelvic trauma.

F   Early stabilisation can be achieved with a sheet or belt. This should encircle the hips at the level of the greater trochanters.

F   Not all patients with pelvic fractures must have a thoracic-abdominal-pelvic contrast CT prior to surgical intervention. Some patients will be too unstable for CT to be performed.

1.   Waldmann C, Soni N, Rhodes A. *Oxford Desk Reference Critical Care.* Oxford, UK: Oxford University Press, 2008.

Answer 63: In relation to clearing the cervical spine: True a & e

T   Up to 12% of major trauma patients have a cervical spine injury. In addition, up to 14% of these may be unstable.

F   Prolonged immobilisation increases the risk of pressure ulcers, hospital-acquired pneumonia, venous thromboembolism and causes difficulty with airway management and central venous access. Prompt clearance of the cervical spine should be undertaken in liaison with radiological and spinal surgical guidance in accordance with locally established protocols.

F   SCIWORA occurs mainly in children, and is thought to occur in 10-20% of all paediatric spinal cord injuries, although figures vary. It has been rarely reported in the adult population.

F   Traditional teaching would state that MILS should be undertaken from the back rather than the front of the patient. This is because MILS from the front in theory could interfere with cricoid pressure and impair access to the cricothyroid space, should a surgical airway be necessary. In reality, it is a matter of personal preference and whichever method is deemed the safest at the time should be used.

T   The commonest mechanism of spinal cord injury in trauma is vertebral subluxation.

1.   Cranshaw J, Nolan J. Airway management after major trauma. *Contin Educ Anaesth Crit Care Pain* 2006; 6(3): 124-7.

2.   Scott TE, Coates PJB, Davies SR, Gay DAT. Clearing the spine in the unconscious trauma patient: an update. *J Intensive Care Soc* 2012; 13(3): 227-31.

3.   Bonner S, Smith C. Initial management of acute spinal cord injury. *Contin Educ Anaesth Crit Care Pain* 2013: 13(6): 224-31.

Answer 64: The following conditions may cause a dominant R-wave in lead V1 on an electrocardiogram (ECG): True a & d

T   Acute pulmonary embolism may cause acute right heart strain and thus a dominant R-wave may be seen in lead V1.

F   Wolff-Parkinson-White Type A causes a dominant R-wave in lead V1.

F   Posterior myocardial infarction may cause a dominant R-wave in lead V1.

T   HOCM may cause a dominant R-wave in lead V1.

F   Dressler's syndrome is an autoimmune pericarditis that occurs typically 4-6 weeks post-myocardial infarction. Global ST segment elevation and T-wave inversion may be seen. The ECG can also show low QRS amplitude, in patients with a large pericardial effusion.

1. Longmore M, Wilkinson I, Baldwin A, Wallin E. *Oxford Handbook of Clinical Medicine*. Oxford, UK: Oxford University Press, 2010.

Answer 65: In relation to medical statistics, the following can be considered correct: True a, d & e

T The analysis of variance (ANOVA) test can be used with parametric data if there are more than two groups being analysed.

F The standard error of the mean equals the standard deviation divided by the square root of the number of values, and is an indication of how well the mean of a sample represents the true population mean.

F The specificity is the negative predictive value. Specificity is the number of true negatives divided by the total without the condition.

T A pain score is an example of ordinal data.

T α error describes the probability of a positive finding from a study being wrong. This is known as a type I error or false positive. β error is a type II error or false negative, and describes the chance of not picking up a difference where one exists.

1. McCluskey A, Lalkhen AG. Statistics I-V. *Contin Educ Anaesth Crit Care Pain* 2007-2008; I 7(3): 95-9, II 7(4): 127-30, III 7(5): 167-70, IV 7(6): 208-12, V 8(4): 143-6.
2. Hanna-Juma S. Statistics in anaesthesia (Part 1). Anaesthesia Tutorial of the Week 302, 2014. www.aagbi.org/education/educational-resources/tutorial-week.

Answer 66: The following have been shown to improve mortality in acute respiratory distress syndrome (ARDS): True b & e

F The BALTI-2 trial suggested β-2 agonists may increase mortality in ARDS.

T The PROSEVA study demonstrated a mortality benefit in patients with ARDS. A total of 237 patients were assigned to the prone group, and 229 patients were assigned to the supine group. 28-day mortality was 16.0% in the prone group and 32.8% in the supine group (p<0.001).

F   The use of steroids in ARDS is controversial; methylprednisolone given at least 7 days after the onset of ARDS has been suggested to reduce time spent on mechanical ventilation, but has not shown conclusively to reduce mortality.

F   HFOV does not improve mortality in ARDS, and has been demonstrated to increase mortality compared to current best practice.

T   As initially described in the ARDSNET study, low tidal volume ventilation (6-7ml/kg) reduces mortality in ARDS. This is now considered a standard of practice in patients with ARDS.

1.   Smith FG, Perkins GD, Gates S, *et al*, for the BALTI-2 study investigators. Effect of intravenous β-2 agonist treatment on clinical outcomes in acute respiratory distress syndrome (BALTI-2): a multicentre, randomised controlled trial. *Lancet* 2012; 379: 21-7.

2.   Guerin C, Reignier J, Richard JC, *et al*. Prone positioning in severe acute respiratory distress syndrome. *New Engl J Med* 2013; 368(2): 159-68.

3.   The National Heart, Lung and Blood Institute Acute Respiratory Distress Syndrome (ARDS) Clinical Trials Network. Efficacy and safety of corticosteroids for persistent acute respiratory distress syndrome. The National Heart, Lung and Blood Institute Acute Respiratory Distress Syndrome (ARDS) Clinical Trials Network. *N Engl J Med* 2006; 354: 1671-84.

4.   Ferguson ND, Cook DJ, Guyatt GH, *et al*, for the OSCILLATE Trial Investigators and the Canadian Critical Care Trials Group. High-frequency oscillation in early acute respiratory distress syndrome. *New Engl J Med* 2013; 368(9): 795-805.

5.   Young D, Lamb SE, Shah S, *et al*. High-frequency oscillation for acute respiratory distress syndrome. *New Engl J Med* 2013; 368: 806-13.

6.   The Acute Respiratory Distress Syndrome Network. Ventilation with lower tidal volumes as compared with traditional tidal volumes for acute lung injury and the acute respiratory distress syndrome. *New Engl J Med* 2000; 342(18): 1301-8.

Answer 67: The following are recognised strategies in the prevention of ventilator-associated pneumonia (VAP): True a, b & d

T   Daily sedation holds have been demonstrated to reduce patient time spent on the ventilator, and thus reduce the incidence of VAP.

T   Head-up positioning of 30 to 45° reduces micro-aspiration, and thus the incidence of VAP.

F   Prone positioning improves mortality in severe ARDS, but its impact on VAP rates *per se* is as yet unclear.

T   Chlorhexidine mouthcare has been demonstrated to reduce the incidence of VAP.

F   Daily changes of ventilator tubing may increase the VAP risk due to cross-contamination from excess handling of equipment.

1.   Hunter JD. Ventilator-associated pneumonia. *Br Med J* 2012; 344: e3325.

2.   Guerin C, Reignier J, Richard JC, *et al.* Prone positioning in severe acute respiratory distress syndrome. *New Engl J Med* 2013; 368(2): 159-68.

Answer 68: Factors that influence inspired oxygen delivery (FiO_2) include: True a & b

T   Effective inspired O_2 concentration (EIOC) deteriorates as respiratory rate increases. This is a patient factor.

T   Increased inspired oxygen delivery is seen in patients with high tidal volumes. This is a patient factor.

F   The presence of a respiratory pause increases the FiO_2 reservoir available to the patient.

F   Venturi type masks are fixed performance systems and deliver a set concentration of oxygen independent of patient effort. They utilise the Bernoulli principle.

F   Entrainment of air usually dilutes oxygen flow reducing FiO_2 delivered.

1.   Waldmann C, Soni N, Rhodes A. *Oxford Desk Reference Critical Care.* Oxford, UK: Oxford University Press, 2008.

Answer 69: In relation to oxygen toxicity, the following statements are true: True d & e

F   The Paul Bert effect is central nervous system toxicity due to oxygen delivered at high pressure of >3 atmospheres.

F   The Lorraine Smith effect is the pulmonary condition of lung toxicity due to prolonged exposure to high inspired oxygen at high pressures.

F   Retinopathy of prematurity continues to be seen despite controlled oxygen therapy, suggesting a multi-factorial cause.

T   Surfactant and maternal steroids have lowered the incidence of bronchopulmonary dysplasia in neonates.

T   Free oxygen radicals result in a progressive reduction in lung compliance associated with interstitial oedema and fibrosis.

1.   Waldmann C, Soni N, Rhodes A. *Oxford Desk Reference Critical Care.* Oxford, UK: Oxford University Press, 2008.

2.   Acott C. "Oxygen toxicity: A brief history of oxygen in diving". *South Pacific Underwater Medicine Society Journal* 1999; 29(3): 150-5.

Answer 70: Indications for hyperbaric oxygen therapy include the following: All True

All conditions listed are indications for hyperbaric oxygen therapy including acute blood loss, carbon monoxide poisoning, intracranial abscess, decompression sickness and clostridial myositis.

1.   Waldmann C, Soni N, Rhodes A. *Oxford Desk Reference Critical Care.* Oxford, UK: Oxford University Press, 2008.

Answer 71: Complications associated with ventilatory support include: True a-c

T   Laryngeal swelling is a recognised complication of respiratory support.

T   Tracheal stenosis is a recognised complication of respiratory support.

T   VAP is a recognised complication of respiratory support.

F   Hypotension following positive pressure ventilation is more frequently seen, due to hypovolaemia and reduced venous return.

F   Peak pressures >45cmH$_2$O and plateau pressures >35cmH$_2$O are associated with barotrauma. More recently, studies have suggested downward revision of these targets.

1.   Waldmann C, Soni N, Rhodes A. *Oxford Desk Reference Critical Care.* Oxford, UK: Oxford University Press, 2008.

Answer 72: Acid-base balance: True b & c

F   Plasma pH exceeds intracellular pH by approximately 0.6 pH units.

T   A strong ion difference dictates the buffer base concentration.

T   In acute renal failure there will be an accumulation of strong ions reducing extracellular strong ion difference.

F   Central chemoreceptors are stimulated by an increased concentration of hydrogen ions. However, the compensatory response is triggered by peripheral chemoreceptors at the aortic and carotid bodies.

F   The correct term for an increase in the hydrogen ion concentration of the blood is acidaemia. Acidosis and alkalosis refer to the processes that lower or raise the pH, respectively.

1.   Bersten AD, Soni N. *Oh's Intensive Care Manual*, 6th ed. Butterworth Heinemann Elsevier, 2009.

2.   Yentis SM, Hirsch NP, Smith GB. *Anaesthesia and Intensive Care A-Z. An Encyclopaedia of Principles and Practice*, 3rd ed. Edinburgh, UK: Elsevier Butterworth Heinemann, 2004.

3.   Parsons PE, Wiener-Kronish JP. *Critical Care Secrets*, 5th ed. Missouri, USA: Elsevier Mosby, 2013.

Answer 73: The osmolar and anion gaps: True b-e

F   Methanol poisoning causes an increased serum <u>osmolar gap initially</u> due to toxic alcohol. This increases serum osmolality, which subsequently reduces as the toxic alcohol is metabolised. The anion gap then rises later as acid products of metabolism accumulate.

T   A normal serum osmolar gap is <10mOsm/kg.

T   The anion gap is increased by unmeasured anions. Such anions include: lactate, phosphates and sulphates.

T   The anion gap is the difference in the measured cations (positively charged ions) and the measured anions (negatively charged ions): this equals $([Na^+] + [K^+]) - ([Cl^-] + [HCO_3^-])$. A classic pneumonic to remember the causes of a raised anion gap acidosis is MUDPILERS (methanol, uremia, diabetic ketoacidosis, propylene glycol, isoniazid, lactic acidosis, ethylene glycol, rhabdomyolysis and salicylates). The anion gap can be corrected for hypoalbuminaemia, where the corrected anion gap = observed anion gap + 25% (normal albumin - observed albumin).

T   Paracetamol overdose can cause an elevated anion gap metabolic acidosis. This is due to the accumulation of 5-oxoproline.

1.   Parsons PE, Wiener-Kronish JP. *Critical Care Secrets*, 5th ed. Missouri, USA: Elsevier Mosby, 2013.

2.   Gabow PA, Kaehny WD, Fennessey PV, *et al.* Diagnostic importance of an increased serum anion gap. *New Engl J Med* 1980; 303(15): 854-8.

Answer 74: Concerning the RIFLE classification system for acute renal failure (ARF)(Table 1.1): True a, d & e

T   There are separate criteria for creatinine and urine output.
F   The criteria on calculation which leads to the worst possible classification should be used.
F   This is the urine output criteria for RIFLE-I.

Table 1.1. RIFLE classification.

RIFLE grade of renal dysfunction	Glomerular filtration rate (GFR)	Serum creatinine	Urine output (ml/kg/hr)
Risk	Decrease >25%	Increase x 1.5	<0.5 for 6 hr
Injury	Decrease >50%	Increase x 2.0	<0.5 for 12 hr
Failure	Decrease >75%	Increase x 3.0 or rise in serum creatinine >4mg/dL (350μmol/L) and acute rise >0.5mg/dL (44μmol/L) within 48 hr	<0.3 for 24 hr or anuria for 12 hr
Loss	Persistent loss of kidney function >4 wk		
End-stage renal disease	Dialysis dependent >3 months		

T   A serum creatinine ≥4mg/dL (350μmol/L) or an acute rise ≥0.5mg/dL (44μmol/L) would meet criteria for RIFLE-F stage.

T   In a patient with ARF, now requiring dialysis who has not recovered renal function for >3 months, classification would be as RIFLE-E stage.

1.   KDIGO. Kidney Disease Improving Global Outcomes (KDIGO): KDIGO Clinical Practice Guideline for Acute Kidney Injury. Kidney International. *Kidney Int* Supplements 2012; 2: 2.

2.   Bellomo R, Ronco C, Kellum JA, *et al*. Acute renal failure - definition, outcome measures, animal models, fluid therapy and information technology needs: the Second International Consensus Conference of the Acute Dialysis Quality Initiative (ADQI) Group. *Crit Care* 2004; 8(4): R204-12.

3.   Lin CY, Chen YC. Acute kidney injury classification: AKIN and RIFLE criteria in critical patients. *World J Crit Care Med* 2012; 1(2): 40-5.

Answer 75: In relation to arterial blood gas analysis: True a, c & e

T   Blood gas analysers can convert pH and gas tensions to values corresponding to the patient core temperature. The alpha stat approach is to act on values as measured at 37°C.

F   The solubility coefficient increases when placing a blood gas syringe on ice, resulting in a fall in measured $PaCO_2$ values.

T   Gas solubility increases as temperature falls; this will result in a lower $PaCO_2$ and an alkaline pH.

F   Heparin will equilibrate with $PaCO_2$ of room air, with an excess causing a reduction in $PaCO_2$ value.

T   Extreme leukocytosis, for example, in patients with leukaemia, may be seen and is termed 'leukocyte larceny'. White blood cells metabolize plasma oxygen in arterial blood gas samples, which may result in a falsely low PaO_2 result due to continued metabolic activity of white blood cells in the sample, resulting in pseudo-hypoxaemia.

1.   Bersten AD, Soni N. *Oh's Intensive Care Manual*, 6th ed. Butterworth Heinemann Elsevier, 2009.

2.   Muzic DS, Chaney MA. What's new with alpha-stat vs pH-stat? Society of Cardiovascular Anesthesiologists. Drug and Innovation Review, 2006. http://ether.stanford.edu/library/cardiac_anesthesia/Cardiac%20Surgery%20and%20 20CPB/Alpha-stat%20and%20ph-stat.pdf.

3.   Sacchetti A, Grynn J, Pope A, Vasso S. Leukocyte larceny: spurious hypoxemia confirmed with pulse oximetry. *J Emerg Med* 1990; 8(5): 567-9.

Answer 76: In relation to sodium: True c & d

F   Sodium is the principal cation of the extracellular fluid. Potassium is the principal intracellular cation.

F   Urinary sodium is greater than 20mmol/L in SIADH.

T   One litre of 3% sodium chloride contains 513mmol of sodium.

T   Hypernatraemia is caused by excess sodium and/or loss of water.

F   Osmolarity is defined as the number of osmoles of solute per litre of solution (osmol/L or Osm/L). Osmolality is defined as the number of osmoles of solute per kilogram of solvent (osmol/kg or Osm/kg).

1.   Bersten AD, Soni N. *Oh's Intensive Care Manual*, 6th ed. Butterworth Heinemann Elsevier, 2009.

2.   Spasovski G, Vanholder R, Allolio B, *et al*. Clinical practice guideline on diagnosis and treatment of hyponatraemia. *Intensive Care Med* 2014; 40: 320-31.

Answer 77: Concerning critical care outreach services: True b-e

F   Outreach was largely introduced in the year 2000 following publication of the Audit Commission's (1999) "Critical to Success" report.

T   One of the four key areas identified for organisation of services by the Department of Health England (DoH) was outreach.

T   Outreach services can avert admissions to critical care by identifying deteriorating patients and helping to prevent admission.

T   Outreach should aim to share skills with staff both on the wards and in the community, to improve training and skill mix. Outreach can also gather information to assess the experiences of patients and/or relatives in order to direct future improvements.

T   Early Warning Scores (EWS) are integral to outreach models.

1.   Ball C, Kirkby M, Williams S. Effect of the critical care outreach team on patient survival to discharge from hospital and readmission to critical care: non-randomised population based study. *Br Med J* 2003; 327:1014-6.

2.   Department of Health. Comprehensive critical care: a review of adult critical care services. London, UK: Department of Health, 2000: 15.

3.   McArthur-Rouse F. Critical care outreach services and early warning scoring systems: a review of the literature. *J Adv Nursing* 2001; 36: 696-704.

4.   Marsh S, Pittard A. Outreach: 'the past, present and future'. *Contin Educ Anaesth Crit Care Pain* 2012; 12(2): 78-85.

Answer 78: Concerning patients with acute renal failure (ARF): True c-d

F   Serum urea and creatinine are relatively insensitive markers of GFR. They are heavily influenced by factors such as: age, gender, nutritional status and muscle mass.

F   The finding of occasional hyaline or finely granular casts on examination of urine sediment would be typical of pre-renal azotaemia. Renal tubular epithelial cells and granular casts in urine sediment would be more suggestive of ATN.

T   This is the ratio of the clearance of sodium to the clearance of creatinine.

FENa = ([urine Na$^+$ x plasma Cr]/[plasma Na$^+$ x urine Cr]) x 100.

<1% suggests pre-renal azotaemia, >2% suggests parenchymal renal disease or urinary obstruction.

T   Renal causes will tend to have a urine osmolality <400mOsm/kg and urine Na$^+$ >40mmol/L.

F   Anaemia is a characteristic finding in chronic renal failure.

1.   Schrier RW, Wang W, Poole B, Mitra A. Acute renal failure: definitions, diagnosis, pathogenesis, and therapy. *J Clin Invest* 2004; 114(1): 5-14.

2.   Provan D. *Oxford Handbook of Clinical and Laboratory Investigation*. Oxford, UK: Oxford University Press, 2005.

Answer 79: The following statements relating to thyroid physiology are true: True a, c & e

T   Thyrotropin releasing hormone (TRH) is a tri-peptide hormone, produced in the medial neurones of the paraventricular nucleus of the hypothalamus. TRH stimulates the release of thyroxine stimulating hormone (TSH) and prolactin from the anterior pituitary gland.

F   80% of T3 comes from T4 5'-monodeiodination with 20% of T3 coming from thyroidal secretion. Type 1 5'deiodinase is primarily found in the liver and kidney. An alternative 3'monodeiodination removes an inner iodine ring and forms the inactive reverse T3 (rT3).

T   TSH receptors are part of the family of G-protein coupled receptors with the classic 'serpentine' 7 transmembrane segments. Upon binding of the ligand, there is activation of adenylate cyclase with a resultant increase in the intracellular concentration of cyclic adenosine monophosphate (cAMP). Stimulation of the TSH receptor via this cAMP second messenger system regulates the transcription of genes central to thyroid hormone synthesis.

F   Approximately 99.97% of plasma T4 and 99.7% of T3 are non-covalently bound to proteins. Thyroid binding globulin (TBG) is the pre-dominant binding protein (TBG has approximately 10 times the affinity for T4 versus T3), transthyretin carries some T4 and albumin carries small amounts of T3 and T4.

T   Only free T4 and free T3 are biologically active in tissues and are regulated by negative feedback loops. Conditions altering TBG levels such as pregnancy, chronic liver failure and acute hepatitis affect total T4 and T3, but do not alter free T4 and T3 levels. For example, pregnancy raises total T4 and chronic liver disease lowers total T4, thus free T4 should be measured.

1.   Kumar P, Clark M. *Kumar and Clark's Clinical Medicine*, 7th ed. Edinburgh, UK: Saunders Elsevier, 2009.

2.   De Lloyd A, Bursell J, Gregory JW, *et al*. TSH receptor activation and body composition. *J Endocrinol* 2010; 204: 13-20.

Answer 80: Considering vasculitides: True a, d & e

T   ANCA-associated vasculitides include granulomatosis with polyangiitis (known as Wegener's granulomatosis), microscopic polyangiitis and eosinophilic granulomatosis with polyangiitis (formerly Churg-Strauss syndrome). Clinical features include alveolar haemorrhage, flu-like symptoms, stenotic lesions (which if tracheal may be visible on chest X-ray), haemoptysis, haematuria, renal failure and polyarthralgia.

F   Henoch-Schönlein purpura (HSP) is an acute immunoglobulin A (IgA)-mediated disorder and is non-ANCA-associated. It is characterised by generalised vasculitis predominantly involving the skin, GI tract, kidneys, joints and, rarely, the lungs and central nervous system.

F   Kawasaki disease is an acute febrile vasculitis syndrome of early childhood. The prognosis is generally good but a small percentage may die from coronary artery aneurysm. The acronym 'febrile' may be used to summarise the main clinical features: prolonged fever (>5 days), enanthem, bulbar conjunctivitis, rash, internal organ involvement, lymphadenopathy and extremity changes.

T   Churg-Strauss syndrome (CSS) is characterised by a triad of asthma, eosinophilia and vasculitis. Roughly half of the mortality associated with CSS is attributed to cardiac complications such as cardiomyopathy, myocarditis, coronary arteritis, conduction delays and sudden death.

T   Cryoglobulinemic vasculitis (CV) may present acutely with respiratory distress and acute kidney injury. CV is a small-vessel systemic vasculitis that results in deposition of cryoglobulins on vessel walls and subsequent activation of the complement system. The classic triad is purpura, weakness and arthalgia with other broad systemic manifestations involving the respiratory and renal system, GI tract and central nervous system.

1.   Berden A, Goceroglu A, Jayne D, et al. Diagnosis and management of ANCA-associated vasculitis. Br Med J 2012; 344: e26.

2.   Scheinfield NS, Jones EL, Langman CB, et al. Henoch-Schönlein purpura. Medscape reference, 2013. http://emedicine.medscape.com/article/984105-overview.

3.   Frankel SK, Schwarz MI. The pulmonary vasculitides. Am J Respir Crit Care Med 2012; 186: 216-24.

4.   Zaidan M, Mariotte E, Galicier L, *et al.* Vasculitic emergencies in the intensive care unit: a special focus on cryoglobulinemic vasculitis. *Ann Intensive Care* 2012; 2: 31.

Answer 81: Regarding the management of cardiac failure: True e

F   Enalapril increases renal blood flow although glomerular filtration rate remains unaltered.

F   By improving left ventricular function, forward flow is improved with a LVAD which can result in subsequent improved right ventricular function.

F   It should be situated with its tip 2-3cm distal to the origin of the left subclavian artery.

F   Bleeding is the most common complication following insertion of a LVAD. Other complications include driveline infection, thromboembolic events, ventricular and atrial arrhythmias, renal failure and respiratory failure (usually due to fluid overload).

T   Patients presenting with low systolic blood pressure and heart failure are less likely to have preserved systolic function and have a three to four times increased in-hospital and discharge mortality compared to those patients presenting with higher systolic pressures.

1.   Sasada M, Smith S. *Drugs in Anaesthesia and Intensive Care*, 3rd ed. Oxford, UK: Oxford Universiy Press, 2003.

2.   Harris P, Kuppurao L. Ventricular assist devices. *Contin Educ Anaesth Crit Care Pain* 2012; 12(3): 145-51.

3.   Krishna M, Zacharowski K. Prinicples of intra-aortic balloon pump counterpulsation. *Contin Educ Anaesth Crit Care Pain* 2009; 9(1): 24-8.

4.   Bersten AD, Soni N. *Oh's Intensive Care Manual*, 6th ed. Butterworth Heinemann Elsevier, 2009.

Answer 82: The following drugs may cause acute renal failure in the intensive care unit: All True

T   Radio-contrast agents are well recognised in causing acute renal failure in patients admitted to the intensive care unit.

T   At therapeutic dosages, acetaminophen can be nephrotoxic in glutathione-depleted patients (chronic alcohol ingestion, starvation, or fasting) or in those taking drugs stimulating the P-450 microsomal oxidase enzymes (e.g. anticonvulsants). Acute renal failure due to acetaminophen manifests as acute tubular necrosis (ATN).

T   Non-steroidal anti-inflammatory drugs are well recognised in causing acute renal failure in patients admitted to the intensive care unit.

T   Acyclovir is a well-recognised cause of acute renal failure in patients admitted to the intensive care unit.

T   Cyclosporin A may cause acute renal failure.

1.   Bersten AD, Soni N. *Oh's Intensive Care Manual*, 6th ed. Butterworth Heinemann Elsevier, 2009.

Answer 83: Considering the 2012 Surviving Sepsis guidelines: True d

F   The Surviving Sepsis Campaign recommends two care bundles: the first to be completed within 3 hours (measure lactate level, obtain blood cultures prior to antibiotic administration, administer broad-spectrum antibiotics and administer 30ml/kg crystalloid for hypotension or lactate >4mmol/L) and second to be completed within 6 hours (vasopressors for refractory hypotension targeting a mean arterial blood pressure >65mmHg, measurement of central venous pressure and central venous oxygen saturations $ScvO_2$, re-measure lactate if initially elevated).

F   Corticosteroids should only be given in sepsis complicated by septic shock refractory to fluid resuscitation and vasopressor therapy. If septic shock is not correctable with fluids and vasopressors, IV hydrocortisone is given 50mg qds (200mg/day).

F   A protocolised approach to blood glucose management on the ICU should be undertaken with an upper blood glucose value of less than or equal to 180mg/dL. The NICE-Sugar trial demonstrated no benefit with glucose management to an upper limit less than or equal to 110mg/dL.

T   The use of low procalcitonin levels or similar biomarkers (such as C-reactive protein [CRP]) to assist the clinician in the discontinuation of empiric antibiotics in patients initially presenting with sepsis, but with no ongoing evidence of infection, is recommended.

F   A target tidal volume of 6ml/kg predicted body weight is recommended in sepsis-induced ARDS.

1.   Dellinger RP, Levy MM, Rhodes A, *et al.* Surviving Sepsis Campaign: international guidelines for management of severe sepsis and septic shock: 2012. *Crit Care Med* 2013; 41: 580-637.

2.   Angus DC, van der Poll T. Severe sepsis and septic shock. *New Engl J Med* 2013; 369: 840-51.

Answer 84: Concerning digoxin toxicity, the following statements are true: True a & c

T   Verapamil, erythromycin, diltiazem and tetracycline are all drugs that can elevate the digoxin level.

F   Hyperkalaemia is often seen in acute toxicity secondary to inactivation of the Na^+/K^+-ATPase pump. Initial potassium values may correlate with prognosis in acute digoxin toxicity.

T   Clinically, yellow-green discoloration is the commonest visual deficit of digoxin toxicity.

F   Baseline ECG findings in a patient taking digoxin are downward sloping of the ST segment and inverted T-waves and are thus not indicative of toxicity. ECG findings in digoxin toxicity can show almost any dysrhythmia.

F   Indications for DigiBind® in acute digoxin toxicity are: cardiac arrest due to digoxin, life-threatening dysrhythmia, K^+ >5mmol/L, >10mg digoxin ingested (adult) or >12ng/ml serum level (note units: nanogram). DigiBind® contains 38mg of digoxin-specific Fab fragments. It is reconstituted with water. The number of vials required is calculated by: number of vials = (serum digoxin concentration (ng/L) x weight (kg)/100. Each vial will bind about 0.5mg of digoxin and is given over 30 minutes or as a bolus in cardiac arrest.

1.   Thacker D, Sharma J. Digoxin toxicity. *Clin Pediatr* (Phila) 2007; 46(3): 276-9.

2.   Nickson C. Digibind. 2007. www.lifeinthefastlane.com.

Answer 85: Complications of the prone position include: All True

T   There are case reports of cervical cord injury due to impaired blood supply due to neck positioning whilst proned.

T   Turning prone reduces the cardiac index and can obstruct or reduce venous return through inferior vena cavae (IVC) compression. This can cause liver ischaemia, visceral ischaemia and/or pancreatitis.

T   Rhabdomyolysis has been reported secondary to limb compartment syndrome associated with the prone position.

T   Complications of the prone position are numerous. Debate still exists whether the prone position itself causes postoperative visual loss or not. There is an association with spinal surgery, the prone position and blindness. This is often caused by ischaemic optic neuropathy and central retinal artery occlusion. An extensive number of eye injuries and complications from a large number of mechanisms have also occurred during the prone position.

T   Carotid or vertebral artery compression has resulted in stroke following proning, particularly in patients who already have a degree of arterial stenosis.

1.   Edgcombe H, Carter K, Yarrow S. Anaesthesia in the prone position. *Br J Anaesth* 2008; 100(2): 165-83.

Answer 86: Regarding intensive care unit ventilation: True b

F   The mean airway pressure is increased by prolonging the ventilator inspiratory time. This may increase arterial oxygen tension but it may also reduce venous return.

T   Increasing PEEP may directly increase arterial O_2 tension.

F   Increased inspiratory time may cause gas trapping due to decreased expiratory time.

F   Generally, morbid obesity reduces chest wall compliance.

F   Auto-PEEP or intrinsic PEEP due to inadequate patient expiration may impair ventilator triggering.

1. Waldmann C, Soni N, Rhodes A. *Oxford Desk Reference Critical Care.* Oxford, UK: Oxford University Press, 2008.

Answer 87: Regarding cerebrospinal fluid (CSF): True a, c-e

T   CSF formation is largely independent of intracranial pressure. Removal of CSF increases with increasing intracranial pressure.

F   CSF passes from the lateral ventricles to the third ventricle via the foramen of Munro, then to the fourth ventricle via the aqueduct of Sylvius.

T   CSF has a higher level of chloride and lower level of potassium than plasma.

T   The specific gravity of plasma is 1.010 and of CSF is 1.004-1.007.

T   Bacterial meningitis is suggested by turbid or purulent CSF fluid, a raised white cell count, raised protein and low glucose.

1. Smith T, Pinnock C, Lin T. *Fundamentals of Anaesthesia*, 3rd ed. Cambridge, UK; Cambridge University Press, 2009.

Answer 88: Ventricular assist device (VAD) complications include: All True

VAD complications include: device malfunction, bleeding, right heart failure, myocardial infarction, cardiac arrhythmias, pericardial drainage, hypertension, arterial non-CNS thrombosis, haemolysis, air embolus, infection, neurologic dysfunction and stroke, renal and hepatic dysfunction, respiratory failure and psychiatric episodes. Bleeding and infection are the most frequent complications.

1. Harris P, Kuppurao L. Ventricular assist devices. *Contin Educ Anaesth Crit Care Pain* 2012; 12(3): 145-51.

2. Krishnamani R, DeNofrio D, Konstam MA. Emerging ventricular assist devices for long-term cardiac support. *Nat Rev Cardiol* 2010; 7: 71-6.

Answer 89: Therapeutic hypothermia after cardiac arrest: True a & d

T   Therapeutic hypothermia promotes cerebral vasoconstriction which reduces intracranial pressure.

F   Therapeutic hypothermia is thought to limit reperfusion injury through many mechanisms, one of which is reducing calcium flux.

F   Hypothermia may cause Osborne or J-waves, which are positive deflections at the end of the QRS complex. Delta waves are seen in Wolff-Parkinson-White syndrome.

T   A target temperature of 32-34°C for therapeutic hypothermia following return of spontaneous circulation after cardiac arrest was the initial recommendation made by the International Liaison Committee on Resuscitation. However, a recent trial of therapeutic hypothermia after cardiac arrest has controversially found no evidence of benefit with a target temperature of 32-34°C compared to 36°C. At present, the role of therapeutic hypothermia in critical care is unclear, with most still using a target temperature of 32-34°C for at least 24 hours post-cardiac arrest. Further trials are warranted.

F   The International Liaison Committee on Resuscitation recommended that therapeutic hypothermia be used when the initial rhythm was ventricular fibrillation, but that "such cooling may also be beneficial for other rhythms". The results of the recent TTM trial have cast doubt on these recommendations, with further investigation warranted.

1.   Luscombe M, Andrzejowski JC. Clinical applications of induced hypothermia. *Contin Educ Anaesth Crit Care Pain* 2006; 6(1): 23-7.

2.   Nichani R, McGrath B, Owen T, *et al*. Cooling practices and outcome following therapeutic hypothermia for cardiac arrest. *J Intensive Care Soc* 2012; 13(2): 102-6.

3.   Yentis SM, Hirsch NP, Smith GB. *Anaesthesia and Intensive Care A-Z. An Encyclopaedia of Principles and Practice*, 3rd ed. Edinburgh, UK: Elsevier Butterworth Heinemann, 2004.

4.   Nielsen N, Wetterslev J, Cronberg T, *et al*. Targeted temperature management at 33°C versus 36°C after cardiac arrest. *New Engl J Med* 2013; 369(23): 2197-206.

Answer 90: Hepatitis E: True a, c-e

T   Acute hepatitis E infection accounts for a large proportion of acute liver disease in developing countries.

F   Hepatitis E occurs in two major groups. Genotypes 1 and 2 are human viruses associated with water-borne and faecal-oral transmission. Genotypes 3 and 4 are swine viruses common in domestic and wild pigs and infect humans as accidental hosts (zoonoses).

T   Hepatitis E may masquerade as a drug-induced liver injury in 3-13% of cases.

T   Hepatitis E is a single stranded RNA virus. Genotypes 1 and 2 (epidemic) is associated with few extrahepatic complications and carries a higher mortality in pregnant women. Fulminant hepatitis in pregnancy is more common with genotype 1 infection.

T   Autochthonous hepatitis E is caused by genotypes 3 and 4, which often presents with a mild subclinical infection. Up to 21% of adults in the United States have anti-HEV antibody, but few with a history of acute hepatitis. Autochthonous hepatitis E is spread via food (pork) and has higher disease rates in older men. It has a large spectrum of serious complications including acute on chronic liver failure, neurologic disorders (polyradiculopathy, Guillain-Barré syndrome, Bell's palsy, peripheral neuropathy, ataxia, mental confusion), which may overshadow the liver injury. Chronic infection can occur in immunocompromised patients. Hepatitis E (genotypes 1 and 4) has been prevented by vaccination (approved only in China currently).

1.   Bernal W, Wendon J. Acute liver failure. *New Engl J Med* 2014; 369: 2525-34.

2.   Hoofnagle JH, Nelson KE, Purcell RH. Hepatitis E. *New Engl J Med* 2012; 367: 1237-44.

3.   Leise MD, Poterucha JJ, Talwalkar JA. Drug-induced liver injury. *Mayo Clin Proc* 2014; 89(1): 95-106.

2 MCQ Paper 2: Questions

Question 1: Cricothyroidotomy (surgical or cannula):
a   The oesophagus may be damaged.
b   There is a low incidence of complications (<7% cases).
c   Narrow-bore cannula cricothyroidotomy is suitable if complete upper airway occlusion has occurred.
d   Surgical cricothyroidotomy has a high success rate in an unanticipated difficult airway.
e   The technique should be abandoned if bleeding occurs.

Question 2: The minimum standard for monitoring during general anaesthesia includes:
a   Capnography.
b   Oxygen analyser with audible alarm.
c   Electrocardiography.
d   Tidal volume and airway pressures.
e   Pulse oximetry.

Question 3: Management of tracheostomy and laryngectomy emergencies:
a   If the patient is making spontaneous breathing efforts, hand ventilation using a Mapleson C circuit should be used initially to assess the tracheostomy patency.
b   High-flow oxygen should be applied to the face and tracheostomy.
c   A suction catheter should be used to assess tracheostomy patency.
d   A laryngeal mask over the stoma site is inappropriate for ventilation.
e   A size 7.0 cuffed endotracheal tube should be used to intubate the stoma.

Question 4: Cerebrospinal fluid (CSF):

a   Is produced in the arachnoid villi in the lateral ventricles.
b   Is produced at a rate of about 576ml per day.
c   In the lumbar region, CSF pressure is normally 6-10cm H_2O in the lateral position.
d   Is approximately 35ml in volume around the spinal cord.
e   Intracranial pressure varies normally with CSF volume changes.

Question 5: Central venous pressure (CVC) catheter position on chest X-ray:

a   The tip should be in the superior vena cava (SVC) or at the junction of the SVC and right atrium.
b   The tip should ideally be outside the pericardial reflection.
c   The tip should be at or above the carina.
d   Subclavian vein catheters must not be allowed to lie with their tip abutting the wall of the SVC.
e   The true intravenous position cannot be inferred from a plain chest X-ray.

Question 6: Pleural aspiration and chest drain management:

a   Smaller chest drains are preferable for bronchopleural fistulas (BPF).
b   The use of thoracic ultrasound in radiology to mark the effusion site, prior to aspiration or a Seldinger chest drain insertion on the unit, is recommended.
c   The neurovascular bundle runs along the superior border of the rib.
d   The 'safe triangle' is defined by the anterior border of latissimus dorsi, lateral border of pectoralis major, base superior to the horizontal level of the nipple and apex below the axilla.
e   A 2-3cm incision above the upper edge of the rib, which is the inferior border of the relevant rib space, is recommended for thoracostomy.

Question 7: In neutropenic sepsis:

a   Intensive care management is often required.
b   Is diagnosed when the neutrophil count is <1.0 x 10^9 per litre.

c   Is an anticipated consequence of chemotherapy and radiotherapy.
d   Fluoroquinolone should be given to all chemotherapy patients as prophylaxis.
e   Piperacillin with tazobactam and gentamicin should be given as the initial empirical antibiotics.

Question 8: Left ventricular assist devices (LVAD):
a   Take blood from the right atrium and injects into the pulmonary artery.
b   Result in reduced left ventricular (LV) preload and increased cardiac output.
c   Are indicated in cardiac failure refractory to maximal medical therapy as a bridge to transplant.
d   LVAD implantation versus medical therapy in patients ineligible for heart transplant results in worse survival.
e   Pulsatile and non-pulsatile flow devices are available.

Question 9: Disseminated intravascular coagulation (DIC):
a   Thrombocythaemia and elevated fibrin degradation products support the diagnosis.
b   May be chronic with little overt clinical effects.
c   Removal of the precipitating cause and blood component therapy is key to management.
d   Results in a prolonged bleeding time.
e   On thromboelastography (TEG) trace, Type I DIC may initially present with a prolonged R-time.

Question 10: Regarding temperature management following cardiac arrest:
a   Mild hypothermia/normothermia (36°C) improves neurological outcome.
b   32-34°C is the recommended target temperature.
c   Fever may adversely affect neurological outcome.
d   The TTM trial showed a target temperature of 33°C to be associated with increased patient harm.
e   Prognostication after out-of-hospital cardiac arrest is not affected by cooling.

Question 11: Therapeutic hypothermia (<36°C):

a   Shivering increases O_2 consumption by 40-100%.
b   Can cause insulin resistance.
c   Cooling decreases metabolism by 30% per 1°C below 37°C.
d   Risk of ventricular tachycardia (VT) arises at temperatures of <32°C.
e   Myocardial contractility decreases in most patients.

Question 12: Tumour lysis syndrome:

a   Is mostly associated with acute leukaemia and high-grade lymphoma.
b   Can occur spontaneously.
c   May present with life threatening hyperkalaemia.
d   Forced alkaline diuresis is advocated.
e   Rasburicase oxidises the compound allantoin to the more water-soluble uric acid.

Question 13: Arterial pressure monitoring:

a   The ulnar artery is the dominant blood supply to the hand.
b   Allen's test should never be performed.
c   Systolic blood pressure measurement in the dorsalis pedis artery will be 10-20mmHg lower than in the central circulation.
d   During spontaneous breathing of a normovolaemic patient, intrathoracic pressure and lung volumes produce cyclical variations in blood pressure.
e   Mean arterial pressure (MAP) is calculated by: (systolic BP - diastolic BP) + 1/3 diastolic pressure.

Question 14: Adult congenital heart disease (CHD):

a   90% of children with CHD amenable to treatment survive to adulthood.
b   Atrial septal defects are the most common defect.
c   Arrhythmias are a common complication.
d   Pulmonary hypertension occurs as a result of left to right shunts.
e   A Mustard-Senning repair of transposition of the great arteries is associated with right ventricular failure and arrhythmias in adult life.

Question 15: Upper gastrointestinal (GI) endoscopy:

a   Gastroduodenal erosions are the most common cause of acute upper GI haemorrhage.
b   The Rockall score predicts re-intervention and mortality pre-endoscopy.
c   The modified Glasgow score predicts bleeding risk and the need for endoscopy.
d   Endoscopic adrenaline injection alone is the treatment of choice for non-variceal bleeding or ulcers.
e   High-dose proton pump inhibitors are recommended post-endoscopy if bleeding is present.

Question 16: Electrical bioimpedance cardiac output monitoring:

a   Performs well in critically ill patients.
b   Is invasive.
c   Measures variations in electrical impedance caused by vascular blood flow.
d   Can estimate changes in cardiac output with electrodes placed on the thorax.
e   May be conducted with electrodes placed on the limbs.

Question 17: Severe acute pancreatitis:

a   Aggressive fluid therapy may offer little benefit after the first 12-24 hours of treatment.
b   Broad-spectrum antibiotics should be started prophylactically.
c   A contrast-enhanced CT scan is warranted in all patients within 48 hours of diagnosis.
d   Early enteral nutrition is recommended.
e   In stable patients with infected necrosis, surgical endoscopic intervention should be undertaken within the first week.

Question 18: Preload status:

a   Transmural pressure is proportional to cardiac chamber dilatation.
b   Cardiac transmural pressure is the difference between intravascular and extravascular pressure.
c   Central venous pressure measurement is a good preload index.
d   Global end-diastolic volume index (GEDVI) represents blood in the heart chambers only and is normally 650-800ml/m².
e   Intrathoracic blood volume index (ITBVI) is measured directly.

Question 19: Uncommon liver disorders:

a   Reye's syndrome represents an abrupt failure of mitochondria.
b   HELLP (haemolysis, elevated liver enzymes, low platelets) syndrome is always associated with pre-eclampsia.
c   α1-antitrypsin deficiency is the main genetic cause of liver disease in children.
d   Serum copper is low in Wilson's disease.
e   Budd-Chiari syndrome occurs when the portal vein is obstructed by thrombosis or tumour.

Question 20: Selective oral decontamination (SOD) and selective digestive decontamination (SDD):

a   SDD has been found to reduce respiratory tract infections and overall mortality in a number of meta-analyses.
b   SDD patients are given intravenous co-amoxiclav (Augmentin®) in addition to oral decontamination for 4 days.
c   Oral chlorhexidine gluconate is recommended by some for oral disinfection.
d   Is recommended by the Surviving Sepsis Campaign guideline (2012) in an attempt to reduce ventilator-associated pneumonia (VAP).
e   Use is associated with increased bacterial resistance.

Question 21: Hepatitis B (HBV):

a   Is a single-stranded RNA virus.

b   Most patients develop persistent infection.

c   Ongoing viraemia should be presumed in any patient who tests positive for hepatitis B surface antigen (HBsAg).

d   Lamivudine is immunomodulatory and blocks HBV replication.

e   Hepatocellular carcinoma is uncommon in chronic HBV infection.

Question 22: Transjugular intrahepatic portosystemic shunt (TIPS):

a   Is the percutaneous formation of a tract between the hepatic vein and intrahepatic portal vein.

b   Is indicated in severe encephalopathy.

c   A portosystemic gradient of less than 12mmHg is deemed a success following TIPS.

d   Shunt stenosis is uncommon.

e   Hepatic encephalopathy is unlikely following TIPS insertion.

Question 23: Hepatitis C (HCV) therapy:

a   Acute liver failure due to hepatitis C infection is uncommon.

b   Pegylated interferon-alfa inhibits viral replication and forms the mainstay of HCV therapy.

c   Ribavirin is a cyclophilin A inhibitor.

d   The enzyme NS3/4A cleaves HCV polyprotein and is the target of boceprevir.

e   Anaemia is a common complication of protease inhibitors used in triple therapy regimens.

Question 24: Regarding lithium dilution cardiac output (LiDCO) monitoring:

a   Measures cardiac output via lithium transpulmonary dilution.
b   A dose of 0.3ml of lithium is injected using central or peripheral venous access.
c   A sensor is connected using a specialised arterial line.
d   Continuous cardiac output can be measured and is proven reliable in critical care patients.
e   Allows analysis of pulse pressure and stroke volume variation.

Question 25: Nasogastric (NG) and nasojejunal (NJ) feeding tubes:

a   Enteral nutrition is associated with a reduced risk of bacterial and toxin translocation.
b   Gastric residual volumes of 200ml increases the risk of reflux/aspiration and feeding should be stopped.
c   NJ feeding is indicated post-gastro-oesophageal surgery.
d   NG tubes should not be passed further than 65cm.
e   NJ tubes are easily placed.

Question 26: Intra-abdominal hypertension:

a   Normal intra-abdominal pressure (IAP) is 12-15mmHg in critically ill patients.
b   Is classified into four grades of severity according to the World Society of Abdominal Compartment Syndrome (WSACS).
c   Intravesical pressure measurement is zeroed at the iliac crest in the mid-axillary line.
d   Abdominal perfusion pressure should be maintained below 50mmHg.
e   Acute abdominal compartment syndrome can still occur following surgical decompression and a postoperative 'open abdomen'.

Question 27: Caffeine:
a   Energy drinks (e.g. Red Bull™) contain about 80mg/250ml caffeine.
b   Tremors and hyporeflexia may occur.
c   Peak plasma concentration occurs 5-90 minutes after ingestion.
d   A fatal dose >150-200mg/kg (5-10g) is described in the literature.
e   Diazepam (0.1-0.3mg/kg) may be considered for agitation and hypertension.

Question 28: Detection of fluid responsiveness:
a   Clinical assessment is good value for detecting fluid responsiveness.
b   Static markers of preload (central venous pressure and pulmonary artery occlusion pressure) predict fluid responsiveness reliably.
c   Variation in arterial pulse pressure can predict fluid responsiveness in ventilated patients.
d   Arterial pulse pressure variation cannot be used to assess fluid response in spontaneously breathing patients.
e   Passive leg raising may aid prediction of fluid response in spontaneously breathing patients.

Question 29: Radiation poisoning and exposure:
a   Sievert (Sv) is defined as the absorption of 1J of ionising radiation by 1kg of matter.
b   Nausea, vomiting and fatigue with low appetite may occur following exposure at a dose of 0.5-1.5 Grays (Gy).
c   Wearing a lead apron reduces the exposure dose to 0mSv.
d   Skin burns may occur at 0.5Gy.
e   CT of the chest and abdomen is associated with an approximate 1 in 200,000 lifetime cancer risk.

Question 30: In relation to brain tissue oxygenation and microdialysis:

a   Brain tissue oxygen maintained >25mmHg is associated with better outcomes.
b   Microdialysis catheters are placed into the cerebrospinal fluid.
c   High-molecular-weight substances cross the microdialysis membrane and can be measured in the dialysate.
d   Lactate/pyruvate ratios are sensitive markers of brain tissue hypoxia and ischaemia.
e   Low levels of glutamate have been found in areas of contusion or secondary ischaemic brain injury.

Question 31: Intracranial pressure monitoring (ICP):

a   Normal resting ICP is 7-20mmHg.
b   ICP monitoring is recommended in all patients with a closed head injury, and a Glasgow Coma Scale (GCS) score less than or equal to 8.
c   With intraventricular ICP monitoring, the catheter transducer is placed at the level of the heart.
d   ICP monitoring is routinely useful in the management of acute stroke.
e   Transducer drift is high with intraparenchymal ICP monitors.

Question 32: In relation to intracranial perfusion, the following statements are true:

a   Cerebral perfusion pressure (CPP) = mean arterial pressure (MAP) - (intracranial pressure [ICP] + central venous pressure [CVP]).
b   The brain receives 50ml/100g/min blood.
c   Cerebral blood flow (CBF) increases by 10% for each mmHg rise in partial pressure of carbon dioxide.
d   Thiopentone reduces both CBF and intracranial pressure (ICP).
e   Autoregulation ensures a constant CBF between MAPs 60-160mmHg.

Question 33: Concerning the electroencephalogram (EEG):

a   An isoelectric EEG with burst suppression is the aim in barbiturate coma for raised intracranial pressure (ICP).

b   EEG is an important tool in the diagnosis of status epilepticus.

c   Most EEG activity is between 20 to 200mV.

d   Is unhelpful in distinguishing pseudoseizures.

e   Myoclonic status epilepticus following anoxic brain injury has an associated EEG pattern.

Question 34: Regarding illicit substances:

a   Naloxone 0.4-2mg should be used in severe heroin intoxication.

b   Cutting agents are often chemicals added to street drugs to dilute and maximise profit.

c   Delirium from gamma hydroxybutyrate (GHB) withdrawal should be treated with neuroleptics.

d   Endocarditis in intravenous drug abusers usually involves the left side of the heart.

e   A 'body packer' may present with a decreased conscious level after a flight.

Question 35: In relation to patients with weakness on critical care:

a   In myasthenia gravis, IgG autoantibodies block the presynaptic acetylcholine receptors at the nicotinic neuromuscular junction.

b   Rapid onset of symmetrical ascending flaccid paralysis with fever is seen in botulism.

c   Intensive care-acquired weakness often involves the cranial nerves.

d   Intravenous immunoglobulin (IVIG) is more effective than plasma exchange in the management of Guillain-Barré syndrome.

e   A negative inspiratory force <30cmH$_2$O and expiratory force <40cmH$_2$O may indicate the need for mechanical ventilation.

Question 36: Amitriptyline overdose:

a   May present with coma and miotic pupils.
b   Sodium bicarbonate is often used in severe cases, to achieve a pH 7.50-7.55.
c   Lipid emulsion 20% (1.5ml/kg) may be effective for cardiotoxicity unresponsive to other measures.
d   In mixed overdose with benzodiazepines, flumazenil should be given.
e   Cardiogenic shock may be treated with intravenous glucagon (5-10mg) followed by infusion.

Question 37: Concerning phosphodiesterase inhibitors:

a   Milrinone is a selective Type V inhibitor.
b   The mechanism of action of phosphodiesterase inhibitors is by preventing degradation of cyclic adenosine monophosphate (cAMP) and/or cyclic guanosine monophosphate (cGMP).
c   Type III inhibitors have a short half-life.
d   Sildenafil citrate may be effective in pulmonary hypertension.
e   Aminophylline is a non-selective phosphodiesterase inhibitor.

Question 38: Concerning transcranial Doppler sonography (TCD):

a   TCD allows calculation of red cell flow velocity in the circle of Willis.
b   The middle cerebral artery (MCA) carries 60% of carotid blood flow.
c   TCD technique is easy to undertake at the bedside.
d   Is useful in detection of vasospasm following subarachnoid haemorrhage.
e   A Lindegaard ratio of <3 suggests vasospasm.

Question 39: Sympathomimetics:

a   Metaraminol use often causes a fall in cardiac output.
b   Ephedrine is prone to tachyphylaxis.
c   Phenylephrine is a potent $\beta 1$-adrenoceptor agonist.
d   Dopexamine stimulates $\beta 2$-adrenoceptors and dopamine (D1) receptors.
e   Levosimendan increases intracellular calcium concentration causing a positive inotropic effect.

Question 40: In relation to opioids:

a   Following prolonged infusion, remifentanil is associated with a long-context sensitive half-life.
b   Codeine phosphate is safe to give intravenously.
c   The metabolite, morphine-6-glucoronide, is 20 times more potent than morphine, and accumulates in renal failure.
d   Alfentanil has a slower onset of action, when compared to fentanyl.
e   Tramadol may cause seizures.

Question 41: In the diagnosis of death, the following are true:

a   Death is the irreversible loss of consciousness.
b   Following cardiorespiratory arrest the patient should be observed for a minimum of 10 minutes before death confirmation.
c   Absence of a central pulse and heart sounds on auscultation can confirm death clinically.
d   Any return of cardiorespiratory function during the period of observation, warrants a further 5 minutes of observation from the next point of cardiorespiratory arrest.
e   Pupils need to be fixed and dilated for death confirmation.

Question 42: Concerning focused echocardiography in emergency life support:

a   At pulse check, the subcostal view may allow quick assessment for reversible causes of pulseless electrical activity (PEA) or asystolic arrest.
b   Ejection fraction (EF) is left ventricular end-systolic volume (LESV) minus left ventricular end-diastolic volume (LEDV) divided by left ventricular end-diastolic volume (LEDV) x 100.
c   The parasternal short axis view of the left ventricle (LV) is useful for looking at regional wall abnormalities supplied by all three coronary arteries.
d   In a spontaneously breathing patient, normal right atrial (RA) pressure corresponds to an inferior vena cava (IVC) diameter (1.2-1.7cm) and ≥50% collapse with respiration on the subcostal view.
e   Pericardial effusions can be classified into small or large.

111

Question 43: When considering aeromedical transfer:

a   Gas expansion rarely causes issues for pre-hospital aeromedical evacuation.

b   Staff without appropriate training may do occasional aeromedical transfers.

c   Air transfer is always faster than road transfer.

d   Oxygen requirement for a transfer is equal to transport time in minutes x ([minute ventilation x FiO_2] + ventilator driving gas).

e   Vibration may interfere with a patient's homeostatic autoregulation.

Question 44: In relation to status epilepticus in children, the following are true:

a   Febrile convulsions are a common cause of seizures between 6 months to 5 years of age, and may be prolonged in duration.

b   Midazolam (0.5mg/kg) may be given buccally in the immediate management, if no intravenous access is initially obtained.

c   Repeated boluses of intravenous lorazepam (0.1mg/kg) should be used if seizures are ongoing (10-20 minutes), following initial treatment.

d   Fosphenytoin (15-20mg/kg) may be given intraosseously (IO).

e   Rapid sequence induction with thiopentone or propofol, as induction agents, should be performed in refractory status epilepticus.

Question 45: Complications of HIV anti-retroviral therapy (ART) include:

a   Immune reconstitution syndrome (IRS).

b   Osteonecrosis.

c   Lipodystrophy syndrome.

d   Stevens-Johnson syndrome.

e   Hepatic impairment.

Question 46: Influenza A:

a   Influenza A is a DNA virus.

b   Neuraminidase facilitates the release of newly replicated viruses from infected cells.

c   Haemagglutinin allows attachment of the virus to host respiratory epithelium.

d   Influenza A is characterised by cough, fever, myalgia and sore throat.

e   It is best detected using PCR (polymerase chain reaction) techniques.

Question 47: Elevated serum levels of creatine kinase (CK) may be seen in:

a   Statin use.
b   Bacterial myositis.
c   Sarcoidosis.
d   Rhabdomyolysis.
e   Hypothyroidism.

Question 48: In relation to viral haemorrhagic fever (VHF):

a   Viral haemorrhagic fevers are produced from one of five virus families.
b   They are all spread via aerosolized particles.
c   Most viruses are identified through rapid enzyme immunoassays.
d   Supportive management in intensive care is the mainstay of treatment.
e   Ribavirin is indicated in Lassa fever only.

Question 49: Patients taking etanercept or infliximab are at increased risk of:

a   Typical bacterial infections.
b   Miliary tuberculosis.
c   Listeriosis-associated meningoencephalitis.
d   *Pneumocystis jiroveci* pneumonia.
e   Coccidioidomycosis infection.

Question 50: During the 2009 H1N1 influenza A pandemic:

a   Zanamivir (Relenza®) is administered via the oral route.

b   Oseltamivir is an M2 channel blocker and given in a dose 75mg twice a day.

c   The Sequential Organ Failure Assessment (SOFA) score was suggested by the UK Government as a critical care admission triage tool.

d   Pregnancy was an independent predictor of mortality.

e   Transfer to an extracorporeal membrane oxygenation (ECMO) centre, in patients with H1N1-related acute respiratory distress syndrome (ARDS) was associated with lower hospital mortality.

Question 51: Bioterrorism:

a   The clinical features of botulism are due to excessive release of acetylcholine at the neuromuscular junction.

b   Routes of exposure to *Clostridium* botulinum include inhalation, ingestion and person-to-person transmission.

c   Immunocompromised patients with botulism should not receive the trivalent antitoxin.

d   Sarin inhibits acetylcholinesterase.

e   Treatment of sarin toxicity includes the use of atropine and fomepizole.

Question 52: Concerning resuscitation of the pregnant patient:

a   A left lateral tilt of 15-30° should be used in all pregnant women undergoing cardiopulmonary resuscitation.

b   The incidence of a failed intubation in the pregnant population is approximately twice that of the non-pregnant population.

c   Peri-mortem Caesarean delivery should be performed within 5 minutes of cardiac arrest.

d   The American Heart Association recommend that chest compressions are performed in the same manner as the non-pregnant patient.

e   The Polio Macintosh laryngoscope blade is mounted at 135° to the handle.

Question 53: Pressures and temperature:

a   The critical pressure is the pressure required to liquefy a vapour above its critical temperature.

b   Absolute pressure equals the gauge pressure plus atmospheric pressure.

c   Charles' law states that at a constant pressure, the volume of a fixed mass of gas is directly proportional to the absolute temperature.

d   Henry's law states that at a constant pressure, the amount of gas dissolved in a solvent is proportional to its temperature above the solvent.

e   The boiling point of oxygen is -118°C.

Question 54: Amniotic fluid embolism (AFE):

a   Usually presents with seizures.

b   Is an embolic process.

c   Results in permanent neurological impairment in the majority of survivors.

d   Causes a reduction in systemic vascular resistance.

e   The diagnosis of AFE is one of exclusion.

Question 55: Regarding liver transplantation:

a   Survival at 12 months after liver transplantation for acute liver failure is approximately 65%.

b   The mortality rate whilst awaiting a liver transplant is approximately 30% at 1 year.

c   Most liver retrievals are performed in category I or II donation after circulatory death (DCD) donors.

d   The operative technique utilising vena cava preservation negates the need for veno-venous bypass.

e   Peri-operative thromboelastography may show an increased LY30 and LY60.

Question 56: Prediction of neurological outcome after cardiac arrest:

a   Can be based on the circumstances of the arrest.

b   A Prognosis After Resuscitation (PAR) score greater than 5 predicts a good neurological outcome.

c   The Lance Adams syndrome is associated with a good neurological outcome.

d   Raised levels of neurone-specific enolase after cardiac arrest is associated with a poor neurological outcome.

e   Can be reliably performed using clinical signs in patients who have undergone therapeutic hypothermia at 72 hours post-cardiac arrest.

Question 57: Postpartum haemorrhage (PPH):

a   Can be divided into primary and secondary PPH.

b   Genital tract trauma is the commonest cause.

c   When due to uterine atony, it should be treated with a rapid bolus of 10 units of intravenous oxytocin.

d   Hypotension is a late sign.

e   The use of intra-operative blood cell salvage in obstetrics is contraindicated.

Question 58: Regarding trauma management:

a   Acute coagulopathy of trauma is the result of hypothermia, acidaemia and coagulation factor dilution.

b   Hyperventilation of trauma patients increases mortality.

c   The Trauma Associated Severe Haemorrhage score uses five parameters to predict the need for massive transfusion.

d   Diagnostic peritoneal lavage (DPL) is now contraindicated as a diagnostic modality during the primary survey of trauma patients.

e   Serial lactate measurements can be used for prognostication in major trauma.

Question 59: Tranexamic acid (TXA) and Factor VIIa:

a TXA reduces the risk of death in bleeding trauma patients.

b The dose of TXA used in the CRASH 2 trial was 2g over 10 minutes followed by 1g over 8 hours.

c Factor VIIa requires the presence of tissue factor to activate Factors IX and X.

d Early use of recombinant Factor VIIa decreases transfusion requirements in trauma patients.

e There is level one evidence that recombinant Factor VIIa decreases mortality in trauma patients requiring massive transfusion.

Question 60: Chest trauma:

a Thoracic injury is responsible for 25% of all trauma-related deaths.

b In the supine position, pleural air may be demonstrated radiologically by a deep sulcus sign.

c Chest X-ray signs of a peri-aortic haematoma include: a widened mediastinum >6cm at the level of the aortic knuckle.

d The thoracic aorta is fixed at the following points: aortic valve, ligamentum arteriosum and origin of the renal arteries.

e Rupture of the left hemidiaphragm is more common than rupture of the right hemidiaphragm.

Question 61: Hyperchloraemic acidosis:

a Results in a raised anion gap.

b May occur secondary to severe diarrhoea.

c Occurs more commonly in patients receiving total parenteral nutrition (TPN).

d May occur due to impaired renal excretion of chloride ions in renal tubular acidosis (RTA).

e Is effectively treated with intravenous furosemide.

Question 62: During controlled ventilation:

a   Airway pressure generated depends on the compliance and resistance of the respiratory system and circuit.

b   The inspiratory pressure waveform is constant during volume ventilation.

c   In time triggering, breaths are delivered according to a pre-set frequency.

d   Triggering is when the ventilator incorrectly cycles to inspiration.

e   Cycling is used to dictate when the inspiratory phase is complete.

Question 63: Considering randomised controlled trials (RCTs):

a   They are prospective in design.

b   They utilise hypothetico-deductive reasoning.

c   They are useful in the validation of screening tests.

d   They are useful for studying disease prognosis.

e   May be open to bias in critical care studies due to difficulties with blinding interventions.

Question 64: Considering the hierarchy of evidence and clinical trials:

a   Primary research papers are considered the highest level of evidence.

b   Case control studies rank higher than cohort studies.

c   Evidence ranking may be affected by methodological rigour and the likelihood of bias.

d   Cohort studies rank lower than case control studies.

e   Randomised controlled trials (RCTs) with definitive results must display confidence intervals that do not overlap the threshold of clinically significant effect.

Question 65: Concerning donation after circulatory death (DCD) in critical care patients:

a   Following withdrawal of active treatment, critical care patients may be suitable for solid organ donation provided cardiorespiratory death occurs within 5 hours of treatment withdrawal.

b   Death following withdrawal of treatment should be confirmed by two members of the critical care team.

c   Members of the transplant team should be present during discussions with families regarding withdrawal of treatment.

d   Organs retrieved from DCD donors have worse long-term outcomes than those donated from brainstem death (DBD) donors.

e   Agreement from the coroner/non-UK equivalent should be obtained prior to discussion with the family to discuss the potential for organ donation.

Question 66: Critical care ventilation:

a   During volume-controlled ventilation, the difference in peak and plateau pressures reflects the pressure required to overcome resistive forces.

b   The plateau pressure during pressure-controlled ventilation reflects the pressure required to overcome elastic forces during inspiration.

c   Auto-triggering describes the ventilator incorrectly cycling to inspiration.

d   Desirable tidal volume should be based on the patient's actual body weight.

e   A lung protective strategy employs tidal volumes of 8-10ml/kg.

Question 67: When managing burns:

a   The extent of burn injury can be assessed using the 'Rule of Sevens'.

b   The Parkland formula states that 4ml colloid solution x kg body weight x % total body surface area (TBSA) burn should be given in the first 24 hours.

c   Nutritional supplementation with trace elements reduces morbidity and length of stay.

d   Parenteral nutrition should be started early if there is failure of enteral feeding.

e   Management may include the use of urinary acidification.

Question 68: Biochemical features of acute renal failure secondary to rhabdomyolysis include:

a   Metabolic alkalosis.
b   Hyperkalaemia.
c   Hyperuricaemia.
d   Hypoalbuminaemia.
e   Hypercalcaemia.

Question 69: The following statements in relation to myxoedema coma are true:

a   Bradycardia, hypoglycaemia and hypothermia are common clinical manifestations.
b   Thyroid function tests classically show low serum T3 and T4 (total and free), together with a reduced thyroid stimulating hormone (TSH) level.
c   Treatment involves rapid repletion of circulating thyroid hormones.
d   Thiamine replacement is indicated when treating myxoedema coma.
e   Vasoactive agents can be safely used in the management of myxoedema coma.

Question 70: Weaning from mechanical ventilation:

a   Weaning is the process of liberation from mechanical ventilation.
b   Delay in weaning prolongs critical care stay, increases costs and is associated with a higher mortality.
c   Synchronised intermittent mandatory ventilation (SIMV) alone is considered a poor weaning strategy.
d   The ongoing need for inotropes precludes weaning.
e   No universal consensus exists for weaning.

Question 71: High-frequency ventilation:

a   A high-pressure jet (10-50psi) is used in high-frequency oscillatory ventilation (HFOV).
b   Lung compliance is improved by maintaining the lung on its deflation limb on the dynamic pressure-volume curve.

c   Peak airway pressures are increased.
d   Oxygenation and carbon dioxide elimination are decoupled in HFOV.
e   The OSCILLATE trial found a higher mortality associated with HFOV use.

Question 72: Potassium:

a   Alkalosis promotes a shift of potassium from the intracellular fluid to the extracellular fluid.
b   β2-agonists promote intracellular movement of potassium through the action of cyclic adenosine monophosphate (cAMP).
c   Electrocardiogram (ECG) changes seen in hyperkalaemia include the development of prominent U-waves.
d   In severe hypokalaemia, potassium can be replaced at a rate of 40mmol per hour.
e   10ml of 10% calcium chloride contains twice as much calcium as 10ml of 10% calcium gluconate.

Question 73: Calcium:

a   40% of calcium in the extracellular fluid is bound to protein.
b   The Chvostek sign describes spasm of the muscles of the hand and forearm following occlusion of the brachial artery.
c   The total plasma calcium value is corrected for albumin by adding 0.02mmol/L calcium for each g/L albumin below 40g/L.
d   Calcitonin secretion is increased by hypercalcaemia and catecholamines.
e   Rasburicase and allopurinol decrease the formation of uric acid.

Question 74: Positive end-expiratory pressure (PEEP):

a   In severe acute respiratory distress syndrome (ARDS), a PEEP >15cmH$_2$O improves mortality.
b   PEEP increases functional residual capacity
c   Hepatic and renal blood flow is increased with higher levels of PEEP.
d   PEEP application increases intrathoracic pressure, diminishing venous return to the right heart.
e   An observed increase in lung compliance suggests alveolar recruitment.

Question 75: Regarding critical care nutrition:

a   Commencing enteral nutrition within 24 hours of intensive care admission is associated with a significant reduction in mortality.

b   Trophic feeding compared to full feeding during the first week of intensive care admission, is associated with worse functional outcomes in patients with acute lung injury.

c   During the early phase of critical care, a protein intake (0.5g/kg/day) is recommended.

d   Selenium supplementation is of no benefit in septic patients.

e   The timing of parenteral nutrition prescription remains uncertain.

Question 76: End-stage liver disease and liver transplantation:

a   The Model for End-Stage Liver Disease (MELD) was developed to predict survival in those awaiting liver transplantation.

b   Hepatopulmonary syndrome is a contraindication to liver transplantation.

c   A thorough pre-operative assessment will always identify cardiac dysfunction if present.

d   The Child Pugh score is calculated by attributing points to the following criterion: serum bilirubin, serum albumin, international normalised ratio (INR), presence and extent of ascites, and presence and degree of encephalopathy.

e   The post-reperfusion syndrome almost always resolves with appropriate fluid loading and electrolyte management.

Question 77: The following statements are true regarding thyroid storm:

a   Fever (>38.8°C) is a cardinal feature.

b   Biochemically a normal serum thyroid stimulating hormone (TSH), together with a significantly elevated serum T3 and T4 (total and free), is found.

c   Oral propranolol or intravenous β1-selective blockers are the preferred agents for heart rate control.

d   Treatment with steroids is contraindicated.

e   Medications which inhibit thyroid hormone release, rather than those which decrease thyroid hormone synthesis, should be used.

Question 78: Regarding prone position ventilation:

a The PROSEVA study group showed no mortality benefit at 28 days in severe acute respiratory distress syndrome (ARDS).

b Alveolar recruitment is improved with better drainage of secretions.

c A more homogenous ventilation distribution is achieved, due to favourable changes in thoraco-abdominal compliance.

d Proning increases extravascular lung water.

e The optimal duration of prone positioning is 24 hours.

Question 79: Hartmann's solution contains:

a 131mmol/L of sodium (Na^+).

b 4mmol/L of potassium (K^+).

c 154mmol/L of chloride (Cl^-).

d Bicarbonate.

e 9kcal of energy in 1L.

Question 80: Sedation and delirium in critical care:

a Specific treatment of delirium improves 1-year mortality.

b Routine monitoring of sedation may improve patients' outcomes.

c The Richmond Agitation-Sedation Scale (RASS) ranges from 1 to 7, with a score of 4 representing a calm and alert patient.

d The Intensive Care Delirium Screening Checklist (ICDSC) reports a dichotomous assessment at a single time point.

e When assessing 'inattention' using the Confusion Assessment Method ICU (CAM-ICU), 0-2 errors are allowed to score as negative.

Question 81: Nutritional requirements:

a The Parkland formula is used to predict caloric requirements.

b 25-30kcal/kg/day is the estimated daily energy requirement.

c The typical daily sodium requirement is 0.7-1mmol/kg/day.

d The typical daily carbohydrate requirement is 3-4g/kg/day, of which 60% should be glucose in parenteral nutrition.

e The typical daily calcium requirement is 0.4mmol/kg/day.

Question 82: The APACHE II scoring system:

a   Is an index of disease severity.

b   There are 10 variables that make up the Acute Physiology Score (APS).

c   In addition to the APS, there are age points and chronic health points.

d   Is assessed over the initial 48 hours of admission to critical care.

e   Has been validated for use in children.

Question 83: Vitamins and amino acids:

a   A non-essential amino acid is one that cannot be synthesised and must be supplied in diet.

b   In patients with severe organ failure, it is recommended that the non-essential amino acid, glutamine, is started within the first 24 hours of intensive care unit admission.

c   700-900mg is the recommended daily allowance for vitamin C.

d   Thiamine deficiency may cause wet beri-beri.

e   Rebound hypoglycaemia may occur on cessation of parenteral nutrition.

Question 84: Magnesium:

a   In addition to its role in the management of eclampsia and pre-eclampsia, magnesium may also be used as a tocolytic.

b   The usual dose of magnesium sulphate in the treatment of acute asthma is 2-4g as an intravenous infusion over 20 minutes.

c   Neuroprotective mechanisms of magnesium include stimulation of release of excitatory amino acids.

d   Neuroprotective mechanisms of magnesium include blockade of the N-methyl-D-aspartate glutamate receptor.

e   Magnesium is recognised as first-line treatment for torsades de pointes.

Question 85: Pulse oximetry:

a   Beer's law states that the intensity of transmitted light through a substance decreases exponentially as the concentration of the substance increases.

b   Lambert's law states that the intensity of transmitted light increases exponentially as the distance travelled through a substance increases.

c   The pulse oximeter probe has one light-emitting diode.

d   Red light has a wavelength of 590nm.

e   The isobestic point is the wavelength at which two substances absorb a particular wavelength of light to the same extent.

Question 86: Non-invasive ventilation (NIV):

a   Decreases work of breathing and may aid weaning from mechanical ventilation.

b   Can reduce the need for intubation and hospital morbidity.

c   Failure is associated with a higher mortality in respiratory failure.

d   Greatest benefit is seen in acute hypercapnic chronic obstructive pulmonary disease (COPD) exacerbation or cardiogenic pulmonary oedema.

e   Severe acidosis is a contraindication.

Question 87: Selection criteria for transplantation in patients with acute liver failure (ALF):

a   The Japanese and Clichy criteria include the cause of acute liver failure as a criterion.

b   Age, encephalopathy and coagulopathy are common to the main prognostic models in use.

c   Ongoing suicidal intent and psychiatric disorders are contraindications to transplantation.

d   The King's College criteria are the most well-characterised evaluation system.

e   The Clichy-Villejuif criteria include Factor V levels.

Question 88: Regarding lactate:

a   Pyruvate is converted to lactic acid by lactate oxidase under anaerobic conditions.

b   Normal serum lactate is between 1.5 and 4mmol/L.

c   In distributive shock, hyperlactaemia is always caused by hypoxia.

d   Type I lactic acidosis occurs in the presence of hypoxia.

e   In septic shock, targeting a reduction in lactate of at least 5% over a 2-hour period, was associated with a decrease in hospital mortality.

Question 89: Normal values on an electrocardiogram include:

a   A PR interval of 0.08 seconds.

b   A QRS duration of 0.16 seconds.

c   A QT interval of 0.44 seconds.

d   An axis of -45°.

e   The QT interval is corrected using the formula QTC = QT/heart rate.

Question 90: Capnography:

a   Phase I reflects mixed dead space and alveolar gas.

b   Inspired CO_2 can be inferred from the waveform.

c   Phase III is called the plateau phase and reflects alveolar emptying.

d   The normal plateau is a horizontal line.

e   Capnography may display three wave forms during accidental oesophageal intubation.

Answer overview: Paper 2

Question:	a	b	c	d	e		Question:	a	b	c	d	e
1	T	F	F	T	F		46	F	T	T	T	T
2	T	T	T	T	T		47	T	T	T	T	T
3	F	T	T	F	F		48	T	F	T	T	T
4	F	T	T	T	F		49	T	T	T	T	T
5	T	T	T	T	T		50	F	F	T	F	T
6	F	F	F	T	T		51	F	F	F	T	F
7	F	F	T	F	F		52	F	F	T	F	T
8	F	T	T	F	T		53	F	T	T	F	F
9	F	T	T	T	F		54	F	F	F	F	T
10	T	T	T	F	F		55	T	F	F	T	T
11	T	T	F	F	F		56	F	F	T	T	F
12	T	T	T	F	F		57	T	F	F	T	F
13	F	F	F	F	F		58	F	T	F	F	T
14	T	T	T	T	T		59	T	F	F	T	F
15	F	F	T	F	T		60	T	T	F	F	T
16	F	F	T	T	T		61	F	T	T	T	F
17	T	F	F	T	F		62	T	F	T	F	T
18	T	T	F	T	F		63	T	T	F	F	T
19	T	F	T	T	F		64	F	F	T	F	T
20	T	F	T	T	F		65	F	F	F	F	T
21	F	F	T	F	F		66	T	F	T	F	F
22	T	F	T	F	F		67	F	F	T	F	F
23	T	T	F	T	T		68	F	T	T	T	F
24	T	F	F	T	T		69	T	F	T	F	F
25	T	F	T	T	F		70	T	T	T	F	T
26	F	T	T	F	T		71	F	F	F	T	T
27	T	F	T	T	T		72	F	T	F	T	F
28	F	F	T	T	T		73	T	F	T	T	F
29	F	T	T	F	F		74	F	T	F	T	T
30	T	F	F	T	F		75	F	F	F	F	T
31	F	T	F	F	F		76	F	F	F	T	F
32	T	T	F	T	T		77	T	F	T	F	F
33	T	T	F	F	T		78	F	T	T	F	F
34	T	T	F	F	T		79	T	F	F	F	T
35	F	F	F	F	T		80	F	T	F	F	T
36	F	T	T	F	T		81	F	T	F	T	F
37	F	T	F	T	T		82	T	F	T	F	F
38	T	F	F	T	F		83	F	F	F	T	T
39	T	T	F	T	F		84	T	F	F	T	T
40	F	F	T	F	T		85	T	F	F	F	T
41	F	F	T	T	T		86	T	T	T	T	F
42	T	F	T	T	F		87	F	T	T	T	T
43	T	F	F	F	T		88	F	F	F	F	F
44	T	T	T	T	T		89	F	F	T	F	F
45	T	T	T	T	T		90	F	T	T	F	T

2 MCQ Paper 2: Answers

Answer 1: Cricothyroidotomy (surgical or cannula): True a & d

T   Transfixing the trachea during cricothyroidotomy may damage the oesophagus posteriorly.

F   Complications occur in >20% cricothyroidotomies, threatening life in <5% cases.

F   Narrow-bore cricothyroidotomy is contraindicated in complete upper airway occlusion as expiratory gas cannot escape rapidly enough to allow expiration. This may subsequently cause barotrauma, surgical emphysema and/or failed ventilation.

T   Surgical cricothyroidotomy is the gold standard technique with a high success rate. A four-step technique is recommended (identify cricothyroid membrane, stab incision and enlargement/blunt dissection, caudal traction on cricoid cartilage with tracheal hook, tube insertion and cuff inflation).

F   Haemorrhage is likely particularly with a wide-bore airway. Insertion should be continued and completed quickly, as it is likely to tamponade any bleeding.

1.   Popat M. The unanticipated difficult airway: the can't Intubate, can't ventilate scenario. Johnston I, Harrop-Griffiths W, Gemmell L, Eds. In: *AAGBI Core Topics in Anaesthesia* 2012; 4: 44-55.

2.   The Difficult Airway Society (DAS). http://www.das.uk.com/files/cvci-Jul04-A4.pdf.

Answer 2: The minimum standards for monitoring during general anaesthesia include: All True

Capnography, pulse oximetry, a monitor of oxygen supply, continuous electrocardigraphy (ECG) monitoring, tidal volume and airway pressure measurement/alarms are recommended minimum standards of monitoring during general anaesthesia by the Association of Anaesthetists of Great Britain and Ireland (AAGBI).

1.   The Association of Anaesthetists of Great Britain and Ireland (AAGBI). Recommendations for standards of monitoring during anaesthesia and recovery, 4th Edition, 2007. http://www.aagbi.org/sites/default/files/standardsofmonitoring07.pdf.

Answer 3: Management of tracheostomy and laryngectomy emergencies: True b & c

F   Initial manual or hand ventilation of a potentially displaced tracheostomy may cause massive surgical emphysema and impede resuscitative efforts and so is not advised. Attaching the Mapleson C or Water's circuit with capnography to the tracheostomy tube, whilst the patient is making spontaneous ventilatory effort, is extremely useful as it can quickly establish that the tracheostomy is indeed in the airway and is patent/semi-patent through lung ventilation and CO_2 exhalation.

T   This should be done even in laryngectomy patients as the distinction between a patient with a tracheostomy and a patent upper airway and a patient with a laryngectomy with no patent upper airway, may not be known at the time of resuscitative efforts and initial assessment.

T   Use of a soft suction catheter is an effective way of assessing tracheostomy patency.

F   During primary emergency oxygenation, a laryngeal mask or supraglottic airway device over the tracheostomy/laryngectomy stoma site may prove life-saving and should be considered early.

F   For secondary emergency oxygenation, intubation of the stoma can be undertaken in adults with a size 6.0 endotracheal tube or small tracheostomy tube. A size 7.0 endotracheal tube is not advised in the first instance as this may be too large. The priority here is to obtain a patent airway for oxygenation and ventilation, with success being more likely with a size 6.0 tube. An Aintree catheter may be very useful as one can oxygenate and even ventilate down it. A fibre-optic scope, bougie and/or airway exchange catheter may be considered in this drastic situation.

1. http://www.tracheostomy.org.uk.
2. McGrath BA, Bates L, Atkinson D, Moore JA. Multidisciplinary guidelines for the management of tracheostomy and laryngectomy airway emergencies. *Anaesthesia* 2012; 67: 1025-41.

Answer 4: Cerebrospinal fluid (CSF): True b-d

F   CSF is produced by the choroid plexus in the lateral and 3rd ventricles.

T   CSF is produced at a rate of 0.4ml/min by the choroid plexus, hence about 576ml per day.

T   CSF pressure is 6-10cmH$_2$O in the lateral position and 20-40cmH$_2$O in the sitting position.

T   CSF volume around the spinal cord is approximately 35ml.

F   Despite changes in CSF volume, intracranial pressure will remain stable under normal circumstances (5-15mmHg).

1. Moss E. The cerebral circulation. *Br J Anaesth CEPD Rev* 2001; 1(3): 63-71.
2. Tameem A, Krovvidi, H. Cerebral physiology. *Contin Educ Anaesth Crit Care Pain* 2013; 13(4): 113-8.
3. Smith T, Pinnock C, Lin T. *Fundamentals of Anaesthesia*, 3rd ed. Cambridge, UK: Cambridge University Press, 2009.

Answer 5: Central venous pressure (CVC) catheter position on chest X-ray: All True

T   The central line tip should be in the superior vena cava (SVC) or at the junction of the SVC and right atrium.

T   The tip should ideally be outside the pericardial reflection.

T   The tip should be at or above the carina.

T   If a subclavian vein catheter is allowed to lie with its tip abutting the wall of the SVC, it may cause the patient pain. Rarely, such placement may cause venous perforation and/or accelerated thrombus.

T   The true intravenous CVC position cannot be inferred from a plain chest X-ray, due to close proximity of the SVC to the pleura, ascending aorta and other structures.

1.   Waldmann C, Soni N, Rhodes A. *Oxford Desk Reference Critical Care*. Oxford, UK: Oxford University Press, 2008.

Answer 6: Pleural aspiration and chest drain management: True d & e

F   With bronchopleural fistulas (BPF), haemothoraces and viscous/highly purulent empyemas, large chest drains are preferred.

F   Thoracic ultrasound at the bedside immediately prior to needle/drain insertion is safer and recommended. Prior ultrasound marking in a different location or time may be hazardous, particularly if the patient position changes prior to doing the procedure.

F   The neurovascular bundle runs along the inferior border of the rib.

T   The 'safe triangle' is defined by the anterior border of latissimus dorsi, lateral border of pectoralis major, base superior to the horizontal level of the nipple and apex below the axilla.

T   To avoid the neurovascular bundle inferior to the rib border, a 2-3cm incision above the upper edge of the rib is recommended for a thoracostomy site.

1.   Waldmann C, Soni N, Rhodes A. *Oxford Desk Reference Critical Care*. Oxford, UK: Oxford University Press, 2008.

Answer 7: In neutropenic sepsis: True c

F   Intensive care management in England was required in less than 5% of neutropenic sepsis cases. Mortality from neutropenic sepsis ranges between 2-21%.

F   Neutropenic sepsis is diagnosed when the neutrophil count is <0.5 x 10^9 per litre, and a temperature >38°C or other signs/symptoms consistent with significant sepsis are present.

T   Neutropenic sepsis is a medical emergency and is an anticipated consequence of cancer treatment, in particular, chemotherapy. It can occur following radiotherapy.

F   Fluoroquinolone prophylaxis is recommended in adult patients with acute leukaemia, stem cell transplants or solid tumours in whom neutropenia is anticipated following chemotherapy for a certain period.

F   Piperacillin with tazobactam (Tazocin®) is recommended as the initial empiric antibiotic. Aminoglycosides, such as gentamicin, should not be used either as monotherapy or dual therapy for the initial treatment of suspected neutropenic sepsis, unless there are patient-specific or local microbiological indications.

1.   National Institute for Health and Care Excellence (NICE). Neutropenic sepsis: prevention and management of neutropenic sepsis in cancer patients. NICE Clinical Guideline 151, 2013. London, UK: NICE, 2013. http://www.nice.org.uk.

Answer 8: Left ventricular assist devices (LVAD): True b, c & e

F   A right ventricular assist device (RVAD) takes blood from the right atrium and injects into the pulmonary artery.

T   A LVAD improves heart function and reduces cardiac work.

T   In one trial, patients with refractory heart failure who received a VAD, 79% survived to transplant compared to 46% who did not. One-year survival was also significantly improved with 70% of VAD patients surviving compared to 30% in patients who did not receive a VAD.

F   Compared to medical therapy in patients ineligible for heart transplant, LVAD implantation was found in the REMATCH trial and post-analysis, to improve survival and overall functional status.

T   Non-pulsatile devices, i.e. continuous flow devices, have largely superseded pulsatile flow devices. Currently, both are still available for implantation.

1.   Harris P, Kuppurao L. Ventricular assist devices. *Contin Educ Anaesth Crit Care Pain* 2012; 12(3): 145-51.

2.   Copeland JG, Smith RG, Arabia FA, *et al*. Cardiac replacement with a total artifical heart as a bridge to transplantation. *N Engl J Med* 2004; 351: 859-67.

3.   Rose EA, Gelijns AC, Moskowitz AJ, *et al*. Long-term use of a left ventricular assist device for end-stage heart failure. REMATCH study group. *N Engl J Med* 2001; 345: 1435-43.

4. Lietz K, Long JW, Kfoury AG, *et al*. Outcomes of left ventricular assist device implantation as destination therapy in the Post-REMATCH era. *Circulation* 2007; 116: 497-505.

5. Krishnamani R, DeNofrio D, Konstam MA. Emerging ventricular assist devices for long-term cardiac support. *Nature Rev Cardiol* 2010; 7: 71-6.

Answer 9: Disseminated intravascular coagulation (DIC): True b-d

F   Thrombocytopenia, hypofibrinogenaemia, elevated fibrin degradation products and prolonged activated partial thromboplastin time (APTT), prothrombin time (PT) and thrombin clotting time (TCT) supports the diagnosis of DIC.

T   DIC can be chronic and overt. Chronic DIC is usually due to a compensated state (malignancy) with increased turnover of haemostatic components.

T   Management of DIC involves prompt removal or treatment of the cause. Fresh frozen plasma (FFP) can be given for treatment of prolonged APTT and PT. Cryoprecipitate will replace depleted fibrinogen levels (aim to correct >1.0). Factor IIa replacement may be considered. If no bleeding is present, heparin may be considered in the management of chronic DIC.

T   PT, APTT, bleeding time and platelet count are generally decreased in DIC. Fibrinogen levels are often low.

F   Stage I DIC usually presents with a hypercoagulable state with a decreased R- and K-time and increased maximum amplitude (MA) and alpha angle on the thromboelastogram (TEG) (see Figure 2.1). Secondary fibrinolysis on the trace is often seen. Type II DIC may present with a prolonged R-time.

1. http://lifeinthefastlane.com/education/ccc/disseminated-intravascular-coagulation.

2. Toh CH, Dennis M. Disseminate intravascular coagulation: old disease, new hope. *Br Med J* 2005; 327: 974-7.

3. Curry ANG, Pierce JMT. Conventional and near-patient tests of coagulation. *Contin Educ Anaesth Crit Care Pain* 2002; 7(2): 45-50.

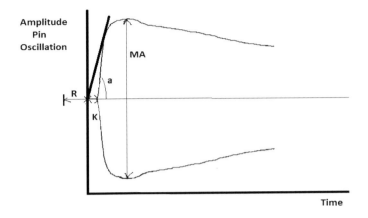

Figure 2.1. TEG analysis: DIC – secondary fibrinolysis.

Answer 10: Regarding temperature management following cardiac arrest: True a-c

T   The TTM trial showed that therapeutic hypothermia to 33°C conferred no additional benefit compared to a targeted temperature of 36°C post-cardiac arrest, with comparable mortality and neurological outcome in both groups.

T   This answer is controversial. Studies published in 2002 in the *New England Journal of Medicine* recommended therapeutic hypothermia (32-34°C) after ventricular fibrillation (VF) arrest. The TTM trial has reopened this debate and questioned the role of therapeutic hypothermia. Currently, the role of therapeutic hypothermia in critical care is unclear, with most clinicians on the strength of available literature still using a target temperature of 32-34°C in practice for at least 24 hours post-cardiac arrest, with rewarming to 36°C if cardiac instability occurs secondary to hypothermia. Further trials are warranted.

T   Fever is associated with worse neurological outcome post-cardiac arrest.

F   The TTM trial found no harm with a target temperature of 33°C compared with 36°C.

F   Cooling can suppress neurological signs, therefore it is recommended to wait >72 hours from rewarming before prognostication.

1. Nielson N, Wetterslev J, *et al*. Targeted Temperature Management at 33°C versus 36°C after cardiac arrest. *New Engl J Med* 2013; 369: 2197-206.
2. Bernard SA, Gray TW, Buist MD, *et al*. Treatment of comatose survivors of out-of-hospital cardiac arrest with induced hypothermia. *New Engl J Med* 2002; 346: 557-63.
3. The Hypothermia after Cardiac Arrest Study Group. Mild therapeutic hypothermia to improve the neurologic outcome after cardiac arrest. *New Engl J Med* 2002; 346: 549-56. Erratum 346: 1756.
4. Arrich J, Holzer M, Havel C, *et al*. Hypothermia for neuroprotection in adults after cardiopulmonary resuscitation. *Cochrane Database Syst Rev* 2012; 9: CD004128.
5. Taccone FS, Cronberg T, Friberg H, *et al*. How to assess prognosis after cardiac arrest and therapeutic hypothermia. *Crit Care* 2014; 18: 202.

Answer 11: Therapeutic hypothermia (<36°C): True a & b

T   Shivering increases O_2 consumption by 40-100% and is linked to an increased risk of cardiac events.

T   Hypothermia causes insulin resistance.

F   Cooling decreases metabolism by 7-10% per 1°C decrease below 37°C.

F   The risk of ventricular tachycardia (VT) and arrhythmias increases when the temperature is less than 28-30°C.

F   In the majority of patients myocardial contractility increases with hypothermia. Some patients, however, do get myocardial dysfunction.

1. Waldmann C, Soni N, Rhodes A. *Oxford Desk Reference Critical Care*. Oxford, UK: Oxford University Press, 2008.

Answer 12: Tumour lysis syndrome: True a-c

T   Tumour lysis syndrome is most associated with acute leukaemias and high-grade lymphomas, especially Burkitt's lymphoma.

T   It often occurs after chemotherapy but can also occur spontaneously. Occasionally, tumour lysis syndrome is seen with single-therapy dexamethasone treatment.

T   Hyperkalaemia, acidosis and renal failure are common life-threatening presentations of tumour lysis syndrome. Hyperphosphataemia, hypocalcaemia, increased serum and urine uric acid may also be present. Aggressive fluid hydration, management of hyperkalaemia, rasburicase and occasionally renal replacement therapy, form the mainstay of treatment.

F   Forced alkaline diuresis has variable efficacy and can be contraindicated where renal failure already exists, particularly if the patient is anuric and fluid overloaded.

F   Increased cell turnover associated with leukaemia and high-grade lymphomas, results in increased purine metabolism. Cancer therapy results in tumour cell lysis and release of purine metabolites and uric acid load. When the kidney becomes saturated with uric acid, crystals form in renal tubules and the distal collecting ducts causing renal failure. Rasburicase, a recombinant urate oxidase enzyme, catalyses the oxidation of poorly soluble uric acid, to the more water-soluble allantoin, reducing hyperuricaemia and renal failure risk.

1.   Beed M, Levitt M, Bokhari SW. Intensive care management of patients with haematological malignancy. *Contin Educ Anaesth Crit Care Pain* 2010; 10(6): 167-71.

Answer 13: Arterial pressure monitoring: All False

F   The radial artery more frequently delivers the blood supply to the digits (dominant vessel) compared with the ulnar artery.

F   Although not discriminatory in assessing arterial blood flow, Allen's test may indicate an issue with ulnar collateral blood supply if positive on radial artery compression and may warrant further investigation and caution.

F   The systolic blood pressure in the dorsalis pedis artery will be 10-20mmHg or so higher than central circulation. Systolic pressure increases from the aorta to the periphery. The pulse pressure is also likely to be higher in the dorslis pedis, but with no difference in mean pressures. Diastolic pressure decreases from the aorta to the periphery and the pulse pressure widens.

F   Cyclical variations in blood pressure are only seen during mechanical ventilation. Such variations are exacerbated in hypovolaemia. Systolic pressure variation (SPV) >10mmHg can be an indicator of hypovolaemia. The area under the arterial pressure trace is an indicator of cardiac output.

F   Mean arterial pressure (MAP) = diastolic blood pressure + 1/3 pulse pressure (SBP-DBP).

1.   Waldmann C, Soni N, Rhodes A. *Oxford Desk Reference Critical Care*. Oxford, UK: Oxford University Press, 2008.

2.   http://europepmc.org/abstract/MED/9424450/reload=0;jsessionid=2HIxd0uMq OGTfKtYCqrr.0.

3.   Spoerel WE, Deimling P, Aitken R. Direct arterial pressure monitoring from the dorsalis pedis artery. *Can Anaesth Soc J* 1975; 22(1): 91-9.

Answer 14: Adult congenital heart disease (CHD): All True

T   Over 90% of children with CHD amenable to treatment (device closure or surgery) survive to adulthood.

T   From the Concor programme, atrial septal defects (ASD) (17%) were the most common defect in adult patients in the Dutch registry. This was followed by ventricular septal defects (VSD) (14%), Tetralogy of Fallot (11%) and coarctation of the aorta (10%). Transposition of the great arteries (TGA) and Marfan's syndrome are rarer (5%).

T   Arrhythmias are a common complication of adult CHD. Loss of sinus rhythm may lead to decompensation, stasis, thromboembolism and sudden death. Anti-arrhythmic drugs are often poorly tolerated. Anticoagulation should be considered before DC cardioversion.

T   Left to right shunts with unrestricted blood flow to the lungs, result in pulmonary veno-occlusive disease. Eisenmenger's syndrome represents end-stage pulmonary hypertension and is defined as a reversal of the shunt (right to left) with cyanosis. 20% of Eisenmenger patients die during a medical procedure.

T   Transposition of the great arteries (TGA) is treated with a switch procedure, either atrially with formation of baffles (Mustard-Senning) or at the arterial level (arterial switch). Late complications of the Mustard-Senning procedure are right ventricular failure, atrial arrhythmias, tricuspid regurgitation and/or obstructed-leaky atrial baffles. The more recent arterial switch operation appears to have better outcomes so far, but still may be complicated by pulmonary stenosis, impaired coronary perfusion and aortic root dilatation with aortic regurgitation.

1. Kelleher AA. Adult congenital heart disease (grown up congenital heart disease). *Contin Educ Anaesth Crit Care Pain* 2012; 12(1): 28-32.

Answer 15: Upper gastrointestinal (GI) endoscopy: True c & e

F   Gastroduodenal erosions are responsible for 8-15% of acute upper GI bleeding only. Peptic ulcer disease is the most common cause in 35-75% of upper GI bleeding cases.

F   The Rockall score predicts intervention and mortality post-endoscopy.

T   The modified Glasgow score/Blatchford score predicts bleeding risk and the need for endoscopy.

F   The National Institute for Health and Care Excellence (NICE), UK, recommends that adrenaline alone should not to be used as monotherapy for non-variceal/ulcer injection. Adrenaline may be used with mechanical clips, thermal coagulation or fibrin injection of ulcers.

T   Proton pump inhibitors should be given to patients with non-variceal upper gastrointestinal bleeding and those with stigmata of recent haemorrhage shown at endoscopy. Acid suppression is not recommended before endoscopy, unless endoscopy is likely to be delayed.

1. Bersten AD, Soni N. *Oh's Intensive Care Manual*, 6th ed. Butterworth Heinemann Elsevier, 2009.

2. Waldmann C, Soni N, Rhodes A. *Oxford Desk Reference Critical Care*. Oxford, UK: Oxford University Press, 2008.

3. National Institute for Health and Clinical Excellence (NICE). Acute upper gastrointestinal bleeding: management. NICE Clinical Guideline 141, 2012. London, UK: NICE, 2012. http://www.nice.org.uk/cg141.

Answer 16: Electrical bioimpedance cardiac output monitoring: True c-e

F   Electrical bioimpedance cardiac output monitoring is useful in stable patients, but can become increasingly inaccurate for cardiac output estimation, in the presence of severe fluid shifts, arrhythmias and changes in ventilation, i.e. the critically ill.

F   Electrical bioimpedance cardiac output monitoring is non-invasive.

T   Vascular blood flow induces electrical impedance variation, which can be measured.

T   Thoracic changes in electric bioimpedance can be used to estimate cardiac output.

T   Electrodes placed on the limbs can be used to measure whole body electrical bioimpedance or on the thorax to measure thoracic bioimpedance. An algorithm with bioimpedance monitoring is used to estimate changes in cardiac output. The rate of change of impedance during the systolic phase of the cardiac cycle is measured; subsequently, an estimation of the stroke volume (SV) and the cardiac output (CO) is derived using a mathematical calculation.

1.   Waldmann C, Soni N, Rhodes A. *Oxford Desk Reference Critical Care*. Oxford, UK: Oxford University Press, 2008.

2.   Drummond KE, Murphy E. Minimally invasive cardiac output monitors. *Contin Educ Anaesth Crit Care Pain* 2012; 12(1): 5-10.

3.   Alhashemi JA, Cecconi M, Hofer CK. Cardiac output monitoring: an integrative perspective. *Crit Care* 2011; 15(2): 214.

Answer 17: Severe acute pancreatitis: True a & d

T   Aggressive fluid therapy within the first 12-24 hours following admission with severe acute pancreatitis is recommended by the American College of Gastroenterology, after which continuing such aggressive fluid therapy is unlikely to be beneficial and may cause harm.

F   Use of routine empirical antibiotics in severe acute pancreatitis is not recommended and should be given only in patients with infected pancreatic or extra-pancreatic necrosis or systemic infection who deteriorate or fail to improve after 7-10 days of hospitalisation.

F   Contrast-enhanced computed tomography (CT) and/or magnetic resonance imaging (MRI) should be reserved for patients in whom the diagnosis is unclear or who fail to improve clinically within the first 48-72 hours after hospital admission.

T   Early enteral nutrition is recommended in severe acute pancreatitis. Parenteral nutrition should be avoided unless enteral feeding is contraindicated. Enteral nasogastric versus nasojejunal feeding in pancreatitis appears to be comparable in safety and efficacy.

F   In stable patients with infected necrotic pancreatitis, surgical/radiological and/or endoscopic procedures should be delayed for more than 4 weeks, to allow liquefaction of the contents and the development of a fibrous wall around the necrosis. Early intervention is associated with greater mortality.

1.   Tenner S, Baillie J, DeWitt J, Vege SS. American College of Gastroenterology guideline: management of acute pancreatitis. *Am J Gastroenterol* 2013; 108(9): 1400-15.

Answer 18: Preload status: True a, b & d

T   Transmural pressure in the heart is proportional to cardiac chamber dilatation.

T   Cardiac transmural pressure is the result of the difference between intravascular and extravascular pressures. As the pericardial pressure normally equals zero, the filling pressure will usually equate to ventricular end-diastolic mean pressure.

F   Central venous pressure monitoring is a poor indicator of preload and overall filling; this is borne out in both clinical and experimental trial data.

T   Global end-diastolic volume index (GEDVI) represents the blood in heart chambers and is normally 650-800ml/m^2.

F   In old cardiac output monitoring systems, two indicators were used to calculate GEDVI and ITBVI — dye dilution intravascular and thermal dilution. Nowadays, the PiCCO system uses thermal dilution alone to calculate GEDVI. ITBVI is then calculated indirectly, ITBVI= GEDVI x 1.25.

1.   Waldmann C, Soni N, Rhodes A. *Oxford Desk Reference Critical Care*. Oxford, UK: Oxford University Press, 2008.
2.   Marik PE, Monnet X, Teboul JL. Hemodynamic parameters to guide fluid therapy. *Ann Intensive Care* 2011; 1: 1.

Answer 19: Uncommon liver disorders: True a, c & d

T   Reye's syndrome represents an abrupt failure of mitochondria with an unknown cause. There is an association with an acute viral prodrome, followed by acute encephalopathy which may progress to hepatic failure and metabolic decompensation. In the past, aspirin use in children was a frequent cause.

F   HELLP syndrome is frequently associated with severe pre-eclampsia/eclampsia but can present in the absence of these disorders. It often presents in the last trimester of pregnancy or immediately after delivery. Hepatic complications of HELLP caused by microangiopathy with sinusoidal obstruction can result in hepatic necrosis, infarction, haemorrhage and haematomas. Hepatic rupture is rare occurring in 1/40,000 to 1/250,000 cases.

T α1-antitrypsin (A1AT) deficiency is an autosomal recessive disorder. A1AT is a serine protease inhibitor that controls inflammatory cascades. It is synthesized in the liver and is the main cause of liver disease in children. A1AT deficiency predisposes to the development of emphysema and chronic liver failure including hepatocellular carcinoma. Liver transplantation may be considered in A1AT-deficient patients with decompensated cirrhosis.

T   Wilson's disease is a rare autosomal recessive disorder with toxic accumulation of copper in the liver and central nervous system. Serum copper and ceruloplasmin is usually decreased with increased 24-hour urinary copper excretion. A liver biopsy is often found to have a high copper content. Chelation of copper with penicillamine or trientine dihydrochloride forms the mainstay of management. Wilson's disease accounts for about 9% of emergency liver transplants for acute liver failure.

F   Budd-Chiari syndrome occurs when the <u>hepatic vein</u> is obstructed by thrombosis or tumour causing ischaemia, hepatocyte damage, liver failure and/or cirrhosis. Therapeutic strategies include anticoagulation, transjugular intrahepatic portocaval shunting (TIPS) or liver transplantation.

1.   McGovern MC, Glasgow JFT, Stewart MC. Reye's syndrome and aspirin: lest we forget. *Br Med J* 2001; 322: 1591-2.

2.   Mihu D, Costin N, Mihu CM, *et al.* HELLP syndrome - a multisystem disorder. *J Gastrointestin Liver Dis* 2007; 16(4): 419-24.

3.   Longmore M, Wilkinson I, Davidson EH, *et al. Oxford Handbook of Clinical Medicine*, 8th ed. Oxford, UK: Oxford University Press, 2010.

Answer 20: Selective oral decontamination (SOD) and selective digestive decontamination (SDD): True a, c & d

T   SDD has been found to convincingly reduce respiratory tract infections and ICU mortality. However, due to concerns over the emergence of micro-organism resistance, SDD use is not widely used in clinical practice. SDD and SOD remain hotly debated with no overall consensus. There is growing evidence of benefit with SOD/SDD in critical care.

F   For SDD, cefotaxime is usually given intravenously for 4 days in addition to medication given for oropharyngeal decontamination.

T   Oral decontamination may be done with oral chlorhexidine gluconate and is recommended by the Surviving Sepsis Campaign 2012. However, polymyxin E, tobramycin and amphotericin B are other agents that are more frequently given for SOD via a paste or NG suspension. Other agents such as gentamicin, nystatin and vancomycin have also been used in some centres.

T   The Surviving Sepsis Campaign recommends the introduction of SOD/SDD in an attempt to reduce the incidence of ventilator-associated pneumonia (VAP).

F   A number of meta-analyses have found no relation between the use of SOD or SDD and the development of antimicrobial resistance in pathogens. Future research is needed to assess long-term ICU outcomes and resistance rates following SOD/SDD use.

1.   D'Amico R, Pifferi S, Torri V, *et al.* Antibiotic prophylaxis to reduce respiratory tract infections and mortality in adults receiving intensive care. *Cochrane Database Syst Rev* 2009; 4: CD000022.

2.   Oostdijk EAN, de Wit GA, Bakker M, *et al.* Selective decontamination of the digestive tract and selective oropharyngeal decontamination in intensive care unit patients: a cost effectiveness analysis. *Br Med J* 2013; 3: e002529.

3.   Dellinger RP, Levy MM, Rhodes A, *et al.* Surviving Sepsis Campaign: international guidelines for management of severe sepsis and septic shock: 2012. *Intensive Care Med* 2013; 39(2): 165-228.

4.   Daneman N, Sarwar S, Fowler RA, Cuthbertson BH, the SuDDICU Canadian Study Group. Effect of selective decontamination on antimicrobial resistance in intensive care units: a systemic review and meta-analysis. *Lancet Infect Dis* 2013; 13(4): 328-41.

Answer 21: Hepatitis B (HBV): True c

F   Hepatitis B is a DNA virus. Hepatitis C and E are RNA viruses.

F   Most primary infection in adults, whether symptomatic or not, is self-limiting with clearance of virus from the blood and liver and development of immunity. Less than 5% of cases do not resolve resulting in persistent infection. Again this may be symptomatic or asymptomatic.

T   Hepatitis B surface antigen (HBsAg) is generally the first marker of HBV infection. Persistence of this antigen for more than 6 months suggests chronic HBV infection. Anti-HBs or HBsAg antibody is a neutralising antibody which suggests recovery and/or immunity to HBV and is the only marker detectable after HBV immunisation to convey immunity.

F   Interferon-alfa is immunomodulatory, which impairs HBV replication and upregulates MHC class I antigens on hepatocytes augmenting recognition by cytotoxic T-lymphocytes. Lamivudine directly blocks HBV replication by targeting viral reverse transcriptase and is not immunomodulatory. Lamivudine is better tolerated than interferon-alfa.

F   Hepatocellular carcinoma is 100x more common in chronic HBV infection, with HBsAg- and HBeAg-positive patients having the highest risk.

1.   Ganem D, Prince AM. Hepatitis B virus infection - natural history and clinical consequences. *New Engl J Med* 2004; 350: 1118-29.

2.   Jia-Horng K. Diagnosis of hepatitis B virus infection through serological and virological markers. *Expert Rev Gastroenterol Hepatol* 2008; 2(4): 553-62.

Answer 22: Transjugular intrahepatic portosystemic shunt (TIPS): True a & c

T   TIPS is the percutaneous formation of a tract between the hepatic vein and the intrahepatic segment of the portal vein. It is done to reduce portal venous pressure in portal hypertension and decompensated liver cirrhosis.

F   Severe encephalopathy is an absolute contraindication for TIPS. Accepted indications include varices that are refractory to endoscopic and medical management, refractory ascites and hepatic pleural effusions.

T   A portosystemic gradient of less than 12mmHg following TIPS and immediate control of variceal-related bleeding (if for varices) is deemed a success.

F   TIPS stenosis is a frequent occurrence, warranting close surveillance and Doppler ultrasonography. At 2 years, primary patency after TIPS placement has been reported to be about 40%.

F   Hepatic encephalopathy can complicate TIPS insertion. If this occurs, 15% of cases may be managed with medical therapy alone, but if severe, the TIPS may need to be narrowed or embolised.

1.   Puppala S, *et al*. Transjugular intrahepatic portosystemic shunt. Medscape reference, 2014. http://emedicine.medscape.com/article/1423244-overview.

Answer 23: Hepatitis C (HCV) therapy: True a, b, d & e

T   Hepatitis C RNA virus uncommonly leads to acute liver failure (<1% cases).

T   Inteferon-alfa is a potent inhibitor of HCV replication that acts by inducing host genes that have antiviral function.

F   Ribavirin is a nucleoside analogue which is used with peginterferon-alfa. It has synergistic effects which improves inhibition of HCV replication. Cyclophilin A is a crucial component of HCV replication and is a target of the inhibitor, cyclosporin A, which has been found to be effective in cell culture.

T   Boceprevir or telaprevir are protease inhibitors that inhibit the enzyme NS3/4A serine protease, which is responsible for cleaving HCV polyprotein during viral replication.

T   Boceprevir or telaprevir are most efficacious in combination with peginterferon and ribavirin for HCV genotype 1. Anaemia is a common side effect of both.

1.   Wang DW, Yin YM, Yao YM. Advances in the management of acute liver failure. *World J Gastroenterol* 2013; 19(41): 7069-77.

2.   Liang TJ, Ghanv MG. Current and future therapies for hepatitis C virus infection. *New Engl J Med* 2013; 368: 1907-17.

3.   http://www.nlm.nih.gov/medlineplus/druginfo/meds/a605018.html.

Answer 24: Regarding lithium dilution cardiac output (LiDCO) monitoring: True a, d & e

T   The LiDCO measures cardiac output via lithium transpulmonary dilution techniques. Lithium chloride (150mM) is injected into the venous circulation and a concentration time gradient is generated by an *ex vivo* ion-selective electrode attached to the peripheral arterial line. The cardiac output is calculated from the lithium dose and the area under the concentration curve prior to recirculation using the equation: cardiac output = lithium dose (mmol) x 60/area x (1-packed cell volume) (mmol/s).

F   0.3mmol of lithium is injected into a central or peripheral vein and used to calculate cardiac output.

F   The LiDCO sensor is connected to a normal arterial line only.

T   LiDCO allows continuous cardiac output monitoring and is proven reliable in ICU patients.

T   As well as cardiac output monitoring, LiDCO allows analysis of pulse pressure and stroke volume variation.

1.   Waldmann C, Soni N, Rhodes A. *Oxford Desk Reference Critical Care.* Oxford, UK: Oxford University Press, 2008.

2.   Drummond KE, Murphy E. Minimally invasive cardiac output monitors. *Contin Educ Anaesth Crit Care Pain* 2012; 12(1): 5-10.

3.   LiDCO. Cardiac output monitoring. www.lidco.com/clinical/lidco_science/lithium_dilution.php.

4.   Alhashemi JA, Cecconi M, Hofer CK. Cardiac output monitoring: an integrative perspective. *Crit Care* 2011; 15(2): 214.

Answer 25: Nasogastric (NG) and nasojejunal (NJ) feeding tubes: True a, c & d

T   Enteral nutrition is associated with a reduced risk of bacterial and toxin translocation as gut integrity is maintained.

F   Large-volume aspirates >500ml pose an increased risk of aspiration and may require feed reduction or cessation and/or pro-kinetic administration. Inappropriate cessation of enteral nutrition should be avoided, particularly if there are gastric residual volumes <500ml in the absence of other signs of intolerance. Often the gastric residual volume cut-off for enteral nutrition varies between critical care units. Cut-off is a balance of potential aspiration risk with higher residual volumes to potential complications if enteral feed is stopped.

T   NJ feeding is indicated post-gastro-oesophageal surgery. It is also relatively indicated in acute pancreatitis, post-Whipple surgery and in patients with gastric atony. Feeding route in acute pancreatitis is highly debated. The American College of Gastroenterology consensus is that enteral feeding is recommended in severe pancreatitis, with the NG versus NJ route being comparable in efficacy and safety.

T   NG tubes should not be passed more than 65cm, as further distance is associated with an increased risk of complications.

F   NJ tubes can be difficult to place and often require endoscopy, radiological assistance or placement at the time of surgery to ensure the tube is in the jejunum.

1.   Waldmann C, Soni N, Rhodes A. *Oxford Desk Reference Critical Care*. Oxford, UK: Oxford University Press, 2008.

2.   Martindale RG, McClave SA, Vanek VW, *et al.* Guidelines for the provision and assessment of nutrition support therapy in the adult critically ill patient: Society of Critical Care Medicine and American Society for Parenteral and Enteral Nutrition. *Crit Care Med* 2009; 37(5): 1757-61.

3.   Tenner S, Baillie J, DeWitt J, *et al.* American College of Gastroenterology guideline: management of acute pancreatitis. *Am J Gastroenterol* 2013; 108(9): 1400-15.

Answer 26: Intra-abdominal hypertension: True b, c & e

F   Normal intra-abdominal pressure (IAP) in the critically ill is 5-7mmHg. This varies with respiration and many other factors.

T   Intra-abdominal hypertension is graded by the World Society of Abdominal Compartment Syndrome (WSACS) 1-4: Grade I=IAP 12-15mmHg, Grade 2=IAP 16-20mmHg, Grade 3=IAP 21-25mmHg, Grade 4=IAP >25mmHg. Abdominal compartment syndrome is an IAP >20mmHg in association with new organ dysfunction.

T   IAP can be measured via the intravesical route using a simple Foley urinary catheter connected to a three-way tap and pressure transducer. With the patient in the supine position, a urinary catheter is placed and all residual urine drained. The catheter is then clamped distal to the point of pressure measurement. The pressure transducer is then connected to the urinary catheter and zeroed at the iliac crest in the mid-axillary line. No greater than 25ml of saline is then instilled into the bladder. Measurement should be taken 30-60s after fluid instillation and at the end of expiration, in the absence of active abdominal muscle contraction.

F   Abdominal perfusion pressure (APP) = mean arterial pressure (MAP) - intra-abdominal pressure (IAP). APP = (MAP-IAP). Previously, the WSACS recommended that the APP be maintained above 60mmHg as this had been correlated with improved outcomes, with an APP <50mmHg being associated with significant pathological disturbances affecting all body systems. However, in the updated 2013 guidance, the WSACS acknowledge that APP may be thought of as the abdominal analogue to cerebral perfusion pressure, but due to lack of evidence, could make no recommendation on how APP measurement and target APP should be used during resuscitation or management of the critically ill.

T   One study found that up to 25% of patients with an 'open abdomen' following laparotomy in trauma, developed secondary acute abdominal compartment syndrome despite the abdomen being open with temporary closure using a Bogota bag/plastic membrane. In the 'open abdomen', the abdominal cavity is simply larger with temporary closure, so increasing IAP can still cause acute compartment syndrome, warranting the continued need to measure IAPs.

1.   Berry N, Fletcher S. Abdominal compartment syndrome. *Contin Educ Anaesth Crit Care Pain* 2012; 12(3): 110-5.

2.   Waldmann C, Soni N, Rhodes A. *Oxford Desk Reference Critical Care*. Oxford, UK: Oxford University Press, 2008.

3.   Kirkpatrick AW, Roberts DJ, De Waele J, *et al*. Intra-abdominal hypertension and the abdominal compartment syndrome: updated consensus definitions and clinical practice guidelines from the World Society of the Abdominal Compartment Syndrome. *Intensive Care Med* 2013; 39: 1190-206.

Answer 27: Caffeine: True a, c-e

T   Caffeine: Cola contains 30-40mg/330ml, energy sports drinks, e.g. Red Bull™ 80mg/250ml, ground coffee 60-180mg/150ml, tea 20-60mg/150ml and plain chocolate 50mg/50g. Diet pills may contain large amounts of caffeine >250mg/tablet!

F   Tremors and hyperreflexia may occur with caffeine overdose. Other reported effects include: tachycardia, hypertension (+/- reflex bradycardia), cardiac arrhythmias, cardiac arrest, myocardial ischaemia and infarction, hyperpyrexia, hyperglycaemia, hypokalaemia, agitation, confusion, delirium and cerebral haemorrhage. Raised creatine phosphokinase (CK), rhabdomyolysis and renal failure can occur in extreme cases.

T   Peak plasma concentrations of caffeine occur 5-90 minutes after ingestion.

T   A fatal dose of caffeine is often quoted as 150-200mg/kg (5-10g) – though some people have been reported to have survived much higher doses.

T   Diazepam (0.1-0.3mg/kg) should be considered as first-line therapy, when treating the symptoms of caffeine toxicity. Glyceral trinitrate (GTN), calcium channel or β-blockers may be required for severe hypertension. Other severe complications should be managed and treated according to usual resuscitation guidelines. Specialist guidance (e.g. Toxbase® and/or clinical pharmacology opinion) should be sought, especially when managing severe cases.

1.   www.toxbase.org.

Answer 28: Detection of fluid responsiveness: True c-e

F   Clinical evaluation of a patient is a poor and unreliable indicator of fluid need and fluid responsiveness, though it remains integral to an overall assessment.

F   Central venous pressure (CVP) and pulmonary artery occlusion pressure (PAoP) predict fluid responsiveness poorly, though trend analysis may be useful.

T   In ventilated patients, pulse pressure variation or stroke volume variation from arterial waveform analysis can predict fluid responsiveness.

T   In patients who are spontaneously breathing, subsequent changes in intrathoracic pressure make pulse pressure variation analysis difficult.

T   Passive straight leg raising (PSLR) may be useful as an indicator of fluid responsiveness in spontaneously breathing and ventilated patients.

1.   Waldmann C, Soni N, Rhodes A. *Oxford Desk Reference Critical Care*. Oxford, UK: Oxford University Press, 2008.

2.   Marik PE, Monnet X, Teboul JL. Hemodynamic parameters to guide fluid therapy. *Ann Intensive Care* 2011; 1: 1.

Answer 29: Radiation poisoning and exposure: True b & c

F   A Gray (Gy) is defined as the absorption of 1J of ionising radiation by 1kg of matter. A Sievert (Sv) is a derived unit of dose equivalent radiation and quantifies the biological effect by taking into account the energy of a particular radiation type when compared with gamma rays.

T   Nausea and vomiting, fatigue and low appetite occur with exposure at doses of 0.5-1.5Gy. The threshold for death occurs at doses of approximately >1.5Gy. Without immediate medical support, an exposure to over 3-5Gy results in a 50% death rate within 60 days. An exposure to >10-20Gy results in death in about 100% in 2 weeks, primarily due to gastrointestinal and central nervous system failure.

T   Physician exposure per patient is estimated to be about 0.0134mSv following fluoroscopic exposure in theatre. Behind a lead apron exposure is reduced to 0mSv.

F   Skin burns often occur with exposure >3Gy.

F   A chest X-ray is associated with a 0.02mSv dose and has a lifetime cancer risk (in 16-69-year-olds) of 1 in 1,000 000. A CT of the chest and abdomen delivers a dose of 8-10mSv and is associated with a 1 in 2000 to 1 in 2500 lifetime cancer risk (age 16-69).

1.   Taylor J, Chandramohan M, Simpson K. Radiation safety for anaesthetists. *Contin Educ Anaesth Crit Care Pain* 2012; 13(2): 59-62

Answer 30: In relation to brain tissue oxygenation and microdialysis: True a & d

T   Brain tissue oxygen maintained >25mmHg is associated with better outcomes.

F   A microdialysis catheter has a fine double-lumen probe. At its tip it is lined with a semi-permeable dialysis membrane. The probe tip is placed into parenchymal tissue with the fine catheter placed into the lateral ventricle. It is perfused with fluid isotonic to the tissue interstitium to allow microdialysis and brain substance chemical analysis.

F   Low-molecular-weight <20kDa substances cross the microdialysis membrane and can be measured.

T   Lactate/pyruvate ratios are sensitive markers of brain tissue hypoxia and ischaemia.

F   High levels of glutamate have been found in areas of contusion or secondary ischaemia.

1.   Tisdall MM, Smith M. Cerebral microdialysis: research technique or clinical tool. *Br J Anaesth* 2006; 97(1): 18-25.

Answer 31: Intracranial pressure monitoring (ICP): True b

F   Normal ICP is about 7-15mmHg. An ICP >15mmHg is considered to be high.

T   The Brain Trauma Foundation recommends that ICP monitoring be undertaken in all patients with a closed head injury and Glasgow Coma Scale (GCS) score of <8.

F   For zeroing, an intraventricular catheter transducer is placed at the level of the foramen of Munro, which is roughly sited at the level of the external auditory meatus.

F   ICP monitoring has little benefit in acute stroke over clinical monitoring. It may be employed in malignant middle cerebral artery (MCA) infarction syndromes where hemicraniectomy is being considered.

F   Transducer drift of intraparenchymal monitors is low and they do not require routine replacement.

1.   Smith M. Monitoring intracranial pressure in traumatic brain injury. *Anesth Analg* 2008; 106: 240-8.

2.   Waldmann C, Soni N, Rhodes A. *Oxford Desk Reference Critical Care*. Oxford, UK: Oxford University Press, 2008.

3.   Vahedi K, Hofmeijer J, Jüttler E, *et al*. Early decompressive surgery in malignant infarction of the middle cerebral artery: a pooled analysis of three randomised controlled trials. *Lancet Neurol* 2007; 6: 215-22.

Answer 32: In relation to intracranial perfusion, the following statements are true: True a, b, d & e

T   Cerebral perfusion pressure (CPP) = MAP - (ICP+CVP), where mean arterial pressure = MAP, intracranial pressure = ICP and central venous pressure = CVP. Some CPP calculations exclude central venous pressure measurement as its effects are thought to be negligible.

T   The brain receives 15% of cardiac output and 20% of the total body oxygen supply. The brain receives 50ml/100g/min blood.

F   Cerebral blood flow increases by 3-4% for each mmHg increase in partial pressure of carbon dioxide ($PaCO_2$).

T   Thiopentone reduces both cerebral blood flow (CBF) and intracranial pressure (ICP) by suppressing the metabolic activity of the brain.

T   Autoregulation ensures a constant CBF between a MAP of 60-160mmHg. Following any brain insult (e.g. trauma, infection), autoregulation may be lost, with brain perfusion being highly dependent on adequate mean arterial pressure.

1.   Tameem A, Krovvidi H. Cerebral physiology. *Contin Educ Anaesth Crit Care Pain*
      2013; 13(4): 113-8.
2.   Waldmann C, Soni N, Rhodes A. *Oxford Desk Reference Critical Care*. Oxford, UK:
      Oxford University Press, 2008.

Answer 33: Concerning the electroencephalogram (EEG): True a, b & e

T   Burst suppression on EEG is the aim when inducing barbiturate (thiopentone) coma for refractory raised intracranial pressure (ICP).

T   EEG is an important diagnostic tool for confirming status epilepticus. This includes subclinical epilepsy and excluding pseudoseizures and functional disorders.

F   Most EEG activity is between 20-200µV. ('microV')

F   An EEG can be extremely useful in distinguishing seizures from pseudoseizures and functional disorders.

T   Generalised, repetitive spikes, sharp waves or triphasic waves at roughly 1-second intervals are seen with myoclonic status epilepticus and may represent a poor prognosis.

1.   Rosenthal ES. The utility of EEG, SSEP, and other neurophysiologic tools to guide
      neurocritical care. *Neurotherapies* 2012; 9: 24-36.

Answer 34: Illicit substances: True a, b & e

T   Intravenous naloxone 0.4-2mg may be given for heroin overdose, and then repeated within 2 minutes if no response is seen.

T   Cutting agents are chemicals added to street drugs to dilute and maximise profit. These substances may be toxic in their own right.

F   The use of neuroleptics (quetiapine and olanzapine) is not recommended in the management of GHB withdrawal psychosis, as it may lower the seizure threshold. Large doses of diazepam are often required and specialist input should be sought.

F   Intravenous drug abusers may present with venous thrombosis, abscess formation and endocarditis (which predominantly involves the right side of the heart due to venous return).

T   A 'body packer' will ingest carefully wrapped packages of illicit drugs, in order to evade security checks. These packages may rupture causing profound toxicity and death. A decreased conscious level in a patient following a flight (particularly from a region in the world where drug trafficking is common) needs consideration of 'body packing' within the differential diagnosis.

1. Nicholson Roberts T, Thompson JP. Illegal substances in anaesthetic and intensive care patients. *Contin Educ Anaesth Crit Care Pain* 2013; 13(1): 42-6.

Answer 35: In relation to patients with weakness on critical care: True e

F   In myasthenia gravis, IgG autoantibodies block the postsynaptic acetylcholine receptors at the nicotinic neuromuscular junction. The AchR antibodies reduce the number of functional receptors. A decreased amplitude in action potentials in the postsynaptic region is seen causing failure of muscle contraction. Myasthenia presents as weakness of voluntary muscle, which worsens on exercise (fatigability) and is relieved by rest. Management involves: anticholinesterase therapy (pyridostigmine), immunosuppressives (corticosteroids, cyclosporine, azathioprine), thymectomy, plasma exchange, intravenous immunoglobulin and avoidance of exacerbating drugs (e.g. polymyxin antibacterials, aminoglycosides, procainamide, quinine, β-blockers, magnesium and pencillamine).

F   Botulism is caused by *Clostridium* botulinum toxin causing the syndrome of an afebrile, descending, symmetrical, flaccid paralysis of motor or autonomic nerves. Management is supportive with critical care admission, if severe, and administration of antitoxin.

F   Intensive care-acquired weakness is diagnosed in the critically ill when no other plausible aetiology has been found. It is classified into three types: critical illness polyneuropathy (CIP), critical illness myopathy (CIM) or critical illness neuromyopathy (CINM). Those with CIM are further subdivided histologically. All have similar presentations at least 1 week following severe critical illness. A diagnosis is made if the weakness developed after critical illness onset and is not related to underlying critical illness condition, there is generalised symmetrical flaccid weakness that generally spares the cranial nerves and there is decreased muscle power (Medical

Research Council [MRC] score <48 noted on >2 occasions) or dependence on mechanical ventilation. Management strategies are limited with no interventions having been shown to improve outcome. Supportive care and rehabilitation is the central tenet of treatment. It is estimated that 65% of patients who develop ICU-acquired weakness will be dead within 1 year (45% die during their hospital admission).

F IVIG and plasma exchange have been proven to be equally effective for the treatment of Guillain-Barré syndrome (GBS) and may hasten recovery.

T A vital capacity <15ml/kg or <1 litre or reduction by 50% from baseline, a negative inspiratory force <30cmH$_2$O and expiratory force <40cmH$_2$O and nocturnal desaturations may indicate the need for mechanical ventilation.

1. Thavasothy M, Hirsch N. Myasthenia gravis. *Contin Educ Anaesth Crit Care Pain* 2002; 2(2): 88-90.
2. Shah AK, Goldenberg WD, Lorenzo N, *et al*. Myasthenia gravis. Medscape reference, 2013. http://emedicine.medscape.com/article/1171206-overview#showall.
3. Wenham T, Cohen A. Botulism. *Contin Educ Anaesth Crit Care Pain* 2008; 8(1): 21-5.
4. Appleton R, Kinsella J. Intensive care unit-acquired weakness. *Contin Educ Anaesth Crit Care Pain* 2012; 12(2): 62-6.
5. Andary MT, Oleszek JL, Maurelus K, *et al*. Guillain-Barré syndrome. Medscape reference, 2014. http://emedicine.medscape.com/article/315632-overview#showall.
6. Patwa HS, Chaudhry V, Katzberg H, *et al*. Evidence-based guideline: intravenous immunoglobulin in the treatment of neuromuscular disorders: Report of the Therapeutics and Technology Assessment Subcommittee of the American Academy of Neurology. *Neurology* 2012; 78: 1009-15.
7. Guest T. Neurological causes of muscle weakness in critical care. Anaesthesia Tutorial of the Week 79, 2007. www.aagbi.org/education/educational-resources/tutorial-week.

Answer 36: Amitriptyline overdose: True b, c & e

F Amitriptyline toxicity is due to anticholinergic effects (dilated mydriatic pupils), cardiac sodium channel blockade and α-1 adrenoceptor blockade. It also blocks presynaptic uptake of amines and blocks cardiac potassium channels. Serotonin syndrome is characterised by the triad of altered mental status, neuromuscular hyperactivity and autonomic instability. Mental status changes may include: agitation, confusion, delirium, and hallucinations, drowsiness and coma. Neuromuscular features occur: profound shivering, tremor, teeth grinding, myoclonus and hyperreflexia. Autonomic instability includes: tachycardia, fever and hypertension or hypotension, flushing, diarrhoea and vomiting. In severe toxicity cases, seizures, hyperthermia, rhabdomyolysis, renal failure and coagulopathies may occur. All patients following overdose should be observed for a minimum of 6 hours.

T   50mmol of sodium bicarbonate is equivalent to: 333ml 1.26%, 300ml 1.4%, 100ml of 4.2% or 50ml 8.4% $NaHCO_3$. Alkalinisation with sodium bicarbonate is used to treat QRS prolongation, with doses of magnesium being used to treat cases with a prolonged QT interval.

T   Prolonged resuscitation in the event of cardiac arrest (at least 1 hour) caused by amitriptyline overdose is recommended, as good outcomes can still be achieved. Lipid emulsion (Intralipid® 20%) 1.5ml/kg over 1 minute, may be effective for cardiotoxicity unresponsive to bicarbonate and resuscitation. The initial bolus is then followed by an infusion 15-30ml/kg/hr for 30-60 minutes to an initial maximum of 12ml/kg. The initial bolus may be repeated 2-3 times as per guidelines.

F   Administration of the reversal agent flumazenil for benzodiazepines in mixed overdose with amitriptylline, is likely to precipitate seizures and further deterioration.

T   Refractory hypotension, heart failure, cardiogenic shock due to amitriptyline overdose, can be treated with intravenous glucagon 5-10mg with an infusion of 50-150µg/hr.

1.   www.toxbase.org.
2.   Ward C, Sair M. Oral poisoning: an update. *Contin Educ Anaesth Crit Care Pain* 2010; 10(1): 6-11.
3.   http://www.aagbi.org/sites/default/files/la_toxicity_2010_0.pdf.

Answer 37: Concerning phosphodiesterase inhibitors: True b, d & e

F   Milrinone is a selective phosphodiesterase III inhibitor. It prevents degradation of cAMP and possibly cGMP in cardiac and vascular smooth muscle. Increasing cAMP within the myocardium increases slow calcium ion release and concentration, resulting in a positive inotropic effect. In vascular smooth muscle, calcium ion flux is altered causing vasodilation. Milrinone can be considered as an inodilator.

T   Phosphodiesterase inhibitors can prolong or enhance the effects of physiological processes mediated by cAMP or cGMP, by preventing their breakdown by phosphodiesterases.

F   Type III phosphodiesterase inhibitors, such as milrinone and enoximone, have long half-lives (4 to 6 hours), preventing minute by minute adjustment.

T   Sildenafil is a Type V inhibitor and may be effective in severe pulmonary hypertension (prevents breakdown of cGMP, increasing vasorelaxation in the pulmonary vascular bed). It is also used in the treatment of erectile dysfunction.

T   Aminophylline is a non-selective phosphodiesterase inhibitor of all five phosphodiesterase isoenzymes, which hydrolyse cAMP and possibly cGMP, increasing their intracellular levels. It causes bronchodilatation, improved diaphragmatic contractility and positive inotropic and chronotropic effects.

1.   Peck TE, Hill SA, Williams M. *Pharmacology for Anaesthesia and Intensive Care*, 3rd ed. Cambridge, UK: Cambridge University Press, 2008.

2.   Vincent JL, De Backer D. Circulatory shock. *New Engl J Med* 2013; 369: 1726-34.

Answer 38: Concerning transcranial Doppler sonography (TCD): True a & d

T   TCD allows calculation of the red cell flow velocity in the circle of Willis.

F   The MCA carries 75-80% of carotid blood flow. An ischaemic stroke in this region is classed as a total anterior circulation infarct (TACI).

F   Although TCD can be performed at the bedside, it requires expertise to ensure consistency and reliability in the interpretation of results.

T   TCD can identify MCA and basilar artery vasospasm with high sensitivity and specificity. It is routinely used for this purpose, within neurocritical care units.

F   A Lindegaard ratio (ratio between flow velocity in the MCA and that of the ipsilateral carotid artery), which exceeds >3 or a flow velocity over 120cm/s is suggestive of vasospasm.

1.   Waldmann C, Soni N, Rhodes A. *Oxford Desk Reference Critical Care*. Oxford, UK: Oxford University Press, 2008.

2.   Naqvi J, Yap KH, Ahmad G, Ghosh J. Transcranial Doppler ultrasound: a review of the physical principles and major applications in critical care. *Int J Vasc Med* 2013; 2013: 629378.

Answer 39: Sympathomimetics: True a, b & d

T   Metaraminol use often causes a fall in cardiac output despite an increase in overall recorded blood pressure, due to increased systemic vascular resistance and afterload caused by α1-receptor agonism. Metaraminol exhibits some weak β-adrenoceptor activity also.

T   Ephedrine acts on both α- and β-adrenoceptors. It has both direct and indirect sympathomimetic actions and inhibits monoamine oxidase, increasing endogenous noradrenaline levels. It can be prone to tachyphylaxis as noradrenaline stores become depleted.

F   Phenylephrine is a potent α1-adrenoceptor agonist. It causes a rapid rise in systemic vascular resistance and blood pressure. It has no β-adrenoceptor effects.

T   Dopexamine stimulates β2-adrenoceptors and dopamine D1-receptors predominantly. It has minimal effect on D2 and β1-adrenoceptors. It has positive inotropic effects and, reduces afterload due to β2-peripheral stimulation and subsequent vasodilatation.

F   Levosimendan is indicated in acutely decompensated heart failure. It is a positive inotrope and potent vasodilator. Its main actions are through calcium sensitization and stabilisation of cardiac troponin and actin-myosin, rather than through direct increase of intracellular calcium concentration.

1. Peck TE, Hill SA, Williams M. *Pharmacology for Anaesthesia and Intensive Care,* 3rd ed. Cambridge, UK: Cambridge University Press, 2008.
2. Bangash MN, Kong ML, Pearse RM. Use of inotropes and vasopressor agents in critically ill patients. *Br J Pharmacol* 2012; 165: 2015-33.

Answer 40: In relation to opioids: True c & e

F   Remifentanil, a μ-opioid receptor agonist, has a short half-life of 3-4 minutes. It is metabolised by plasma esterases and has a very short context-sensitive half-life (i.e. regardless of infusion duration, remifentanil does not accumulate).

F   Codeine phosphate may be given orally, subcutaneously, rectally, and intramuscularly. The intravenous route is associated with massive histamine release causing significant hypotension and hypoxia. Intravenous administration is thus not recommended.

T   Morphine is an agonist at μ-opioid, κ-opioid and δ-opioid receptors. Morphine is metabolised by hepatic glucoronidation to morphine-6-glucoronide (10%, which is 20 times more potent than morphine) and morphine-3-glucoronide (90%, inactive analgesic). Both are excreted renally and may accumulate in renal failure. Morphine has a half-life of 3 to 7 hours. Side effects include nausea, constipation, respiratory depression, histamine release, itch and hypotension.

F   Alfentanil has a pKa of 6.5 with 89% present in the unionised form. Fentanyl has a pKa of 8.4 so only 9% is unionised at body pH 7.4. Alfentanil has a lower lipid solubility but faster onset of action than fentanyl, when given in equipotent doses, due to its pKa properties.

T   Tramadol has agonist properties at all opioid receptors. Tramadol may interact with drugs that inhibit central serotonin or noradrenaline reuptake (e.g. tricyclic antidepressants, selective serotonin reuptake inhibitors) causing seizures.

1. Cox RG. Hypoxaemia and hypotension after intravenous codeine phosphate. *Can J Anaesth* 1994; 41(12): 1211-3.
2. Reade MC, Finfer S. Sedation and delirium in the intensive care unit. *New Engl J Med* 2014; 370: 444-54.

3.   Peck TE, Hill SA, Williams M. *Pharmacology for Anaesthesia and Intensive Care*, 3rd ed. Cambridge, UK: Cambridge University Press, 2008.

Answer 41: In the diagnosis of death, the following are true: True c & d

F   Irreversible loss of consciousness in itself does not entail individual death, e.g. persistent vegetative state. A patient must have lost the irreversible capacity to breathe in addition, for death to be diagnosed.

F   The individual should be observed for a minimum of 5 minutes following cardiorespiratory arrest before confirming death.

T   The absence of a central pulse and heart sounds on auscultation is used clinically to confirm the absence of mechanical cardiac function and cardiorespiratory death. In hospital, in addition to these clinical findings, death may be confirmed with asystole on the electrocardiogram, an absent arterial line pulsation or absence of heart contractility on echocardiography.

T   Any return of cardiorespiratory function during 5 minutes of observation warrants a further 5 minutes of observation, from the next point where cardiorespiratory arrest occurs.

F   Following 5 minutes of observation, pupillary reflexes to light need to be absent (regardless of size), with absent corneal reflexes and no motor response to supra-orbital pressure.

1.   Academy of Medical Royal Colleges. A code of practice for the diagnosis and confirmation of death, 2008. http://www.aomrc.org.uk/publications/statements/doc details/42-a-code-of-practice-for-the-diagnosis-and-confirmation-of-death.html.

Answer 42: Concerning focused echocardiography in emergency life support: True a, c & d

T   Within the 10-second pulse check during cardiopulmonary resuscitation (CPR), for a patient in a non-shockable rhythm (PEA/asystole), a FEEL echo using the subcostal view may allow cardiac images to be obtained. These images can then be reviewed whilst CPR continues to assess for potential reversible causes of the arrest. These include severe hypovolaemia, a dilated right heart (thromboembolic event), gross pericardial effusion (tamponade), severe ventricular dysfunction (need for inotropes) and new regional wall abnormalities (ischaemic myocardium).

F   Normal ejection fraction is 55-75%. EF= LEDV-LESV/LEDV x 100, where LEDV-LESV = stroke volume (SV).

T   The parasternal short axis view of the left ventricle (LV) shows areas of myocardium supplied by all three coronary vessels and is ideally suited for assessing for ischaemic regional wall abnormalities. New regional wall abnormalities associated with haemodynamic instability are suggestive of an acute myocardial ischaemic event. An assessment of LV contractility can also be made: normal or dyskinetic, hypokinetic, akinetic and hyperkinetic regional wall abnormalities may be found.

T   On subcostal view, in a <u>spontaneously</u> breathing patient, cyclic variations in pleural pressure are transmitted to the right atrium, which in turn produces cyclic variation in venous return that is increased by inspiration, leading to an inspiratory reduction of about 50% in inferior vena cava (IVC) diameter normally. IVC diameter (1.2-1.7cm) and ≥50% collapse with respiration, corresponds with a normal right atrial (RA) pressure in spontaneously breathing patients. In patients who are <u>mechanically</u> ventilated, the inspiratory phase increases pleural pressure which is transmitted to the right atrium reducing venous return. This causes an inversion of the cyclic changes in IVC diameter, leading to increases in the inspiratory phase and decreases in the expiratory phase. Dilatation of the IVC, indicating high right atrial pressure (e.g. secondary to fluid overload or pulmonary hypertension), abolishes these variations. Respiratory variation in IVC diameter is only seen in mechanically ventilated patients normally or when right atrial pressure is low and may be used as a surrogate to assess a patient's volumetric status. In a ventilated patient, with signs of circulatory insufficiency, this cyclic variation in IVC diameter may be a rough indication of hypovolaemia and need for fluid volume.

F   Pericardial effusions can be classified into small <0.5cm, moderate <0.5-2cm and large >2cm. Unclotted blood in the pericardium appears as a circumferential echolucent space. Tamponade occurs when pressure in the pericardium exceeds pressures in the heart impairing cardiac filling.

1.   www.FEEL-Uk.com.

2.   Jardin F, Beauchet A. Ultrasound examination of the venae cavae. http://www.fmp-usmba.ac.ma/umvf/UMVFmiroir/sahel/application-cardiologie/l-echocardiographie-en-reanimation/index3fbd.html?option=com_content&task=view&id=36&Itemid=93.

Answer 43: When considering aeromedical transfer: True a & e

T   Gas expansion of cavities due to altitude (e.g. worsening of a pneumothorax) is rarely an issue for most pre-hospital evacuation by air, as altitudes are often below 2000m. Above altitudes of 2000m, gas expansion and cabin pressure become more of an issue.

F   Staff involved in aeromedical transport must have both high-level expertise and knowledge in managing the patient's condition and have appropriate aeromedical training including safety training, aeromedical evacuation procedures and basic on-board communication skills (particularly for helicopters).

F   Air transfer over long distances or when access is difficult, may be faster than road. However, the perceived speed of air transfer can be slowed down by logistical aspects. These include loading and unloading of a patient and subsequent inter-vehicle transfer times.

F   Oxygen requirement for transfer = 2x transport time in minutes (double for safety) x ([MV x FiO_2] + ventilator driving gas). Minute volume (MV) is in litres per minute and FiO_2 from 0.21 (room air) to 1.0 (100% FiO_2) and ventilator driving gas in litres per minute.

T   Vibration (helicopter) and noise can cause blurred vision, shortness of breath, motion sickness and fatigue. It can also cause disruption of the body's ability to autoregulate, particularly in burns patients. Vibration can lead to wound-fracture disruption increasing the need for analgesia, sedation and resuscitation. Routine observations can become extremely difficult. Feeling a pulse or listening to a chest can sometimes be impossible, and the need for trained and experienced personnel is paramount.

1.   Griffiths A, Lowes T, Henning J. Pre-hospital Anaesthesia Handbook. London, UK: Springer-Verlag, 2010.

2.   http://www.aagbi.org/sites/default/files/interhospital09.pdf.

3.   Ellis D, Hooper M. *Cases in Pre-hospital and Retrieval Medicine.* Churchill
      Livingstone Elsevier, 2010.

Answer 44: In relation to status epilepticus in children, the following are true: All True

T   Febrile convulsions are the most common cause of seizures between 6 months to 5 years of age, and may be prolonged in duration. Other causes include central nervous system infection (status epilepticus is a rare feature of acute infection), metabolic abnormalities (hypoglycaemia, hyponatraemia, hypocalcaemia and hepatic encephalopathy), anticonvulsant withdrawal, trauma, poisoning, systemic hypertension and pseudo epilepsy.

T   Lorazepam (0.1mg/kg IV) or diazepam (0.5mg/kg PR) or midazolam (0.5mg/kg buccal) should be used for immediate management (within 0-10 minutes).

T   Repeated lorazepam (0.1mg/kg IV) or paraldehyde (0.4mg/kg PR) should be used if seizures are ongoing (10-20 minutes) following initial treatment.

T   Fosphenytoin (15-20mg/kg) may be given via the intravenous (IV) or intraosseous (IO) routes. Phenytoin 18mg/kg may also be given IV or IO. These drugs form the 3rd stage of treatment for refractory status epilepticus (>15 minutes since seizure commencement). Phenobarbitone 20mg/kg IV or further doses of paraldehyde (0.4mg/kg PR) may also be given.

T   Rapid sequence induction with thiopentone or propofol, as induction agents, should be performed in refractory status epilepticus.

1.   Cavanagh S, Liversedge T. Status epilepticus in children. Anaesthesia Tutorial of the
      Week 248, 2012. www.aagbi.org/education/educational-resources/tutorial-week.

Answer 45: Complications of HIV anti-retroviral therapy (ART) include: All True

T   Immune reconstitution syndromes (IRS) can occur on initiation of ART due to an improvement in immune function, resulting in a marked inflammatory response to opportunistic pathogens (including *Mycobacterium avium* complex [MAC], *Pneumocystis pneumonia* [PCP], tuberculosis, *Cytomegalovirus* [CMV], cryptococcus and other infections e.g. *Herpes zoster*). There is currently no strong evidence for the prevention and management of IRS. Some strategies include antibiotic prophylaxis and delaying ART in cases of severe opportunistic infection.

T Osteonecrosis has been reported in advanced HIV disease or following prolonged combination ART.

T Metabolic effects of ART include fat redistribution, insulin resistance and dyslipidaemia. The use of nucleoside reverse transcriptase inhibitors (NRTIs), stavudine in particular, has been implicated in a lipodystrophy syndrome.

T Nevirapine, a non-nucleoside reverse transcriptase inhibitor, is associated with a high incidence of rash, including Stevens-Johnson syndrome. Stevens-Johnson syndrome is also seen with protease inhibitors.

T Many ART drugs cause hepatic impairment.

1. Jacobson MA. Clinical implications of immune reconstitution in AIDS. HIV Insite, 2006. UCSF. http://hivinsite.ucsf.edu.

2. Chow DC, Day LJ, Souza SA, Shikuma CM. Metabolic complications of HIV therapy, 2006. HIV Insite. UCSF. http:hivinsite.ucsf.edu.

3. The British National Formulary (BNF) 66. Joint Formulary Committee 66 (September 2013). BMJ Publishing Group Ltd and Royal Pharmaceutical Society. http://www.bnf.org/bnf/index.htm.

Answer 46: Influenza A: True b-e

F Influenza A is an RNA virus.

T Influenza A is described by surface glycoproteins, haemagglutinin (H) and neuraminidase (N). 16 types of haemagglutinin and 9 types of neuraminidase exist. Influenza B is the second type of influenza virus (i.e. A or B).

T Haemagglutinin allows attachment of the virus to host respiratory epithelium.

T Influenza A is characterised by cough, fever, myalgia and sore throat.

T   Reverse transcriptase polymerase chain reaction RT-PCR testing, from nasopharyngeal swabs or aspirates, is the best method of diagnosis.

1.   Gwavava C, Lynch G. Intensive care management of pandemic (H1N1) influenza. Anaesthesia Tutorial of the Week 2009, 2011. www.aagbi.org/education/educational -resources/tutorial-week.

2.   Parsons PE, Wiener-Kronish JP. *Critical Care Secrets*, 5th ed. Missouri, USA: Elsevier Mosby, 2013.

Answer 47: Elevated serum levels of creatine kinase (CK) may be seen in: All True

T   Elevated CK may be seen with drug- or toxin-induced muscle injury or inflammation. Common drugs which may cause an elevated CK include: statins, colchicine, alcohol, cocaine, zidovudine and steroids.

T   Any infective cause of myositis will cause an elevated CK.

T   Autoimmune or rheumatologic disorders may cause an elevated CK (e.g. vasculitis, sarcoidosis, dermatomyositis and polymyalgia).

T   A finding of elevated CK is characteristic of patients with massive rhabdomyolysis.

T   Hypothyroidism and hyperthyroidism may be both associated with an elevated CK level.

1.   Parsons PE, Wiener-Kronish JP. *Critical Care Secrets*, 5th ed. Missouri, USA: Elsevier Mosby, 2013.

Answer 48: Viral haemorrhagic fever (VHF): True a, c-e

T   Viral haemorrhagic fevers are produced from one of five virus families: arenaviruses, bunyaviruses, filoviruses, flaviviruses and rhabdoviruses.

F   Evidence from viral haemorrhagic fever outbreaks strongly suggest that the routes of transmission are through direct contact with blood or body fluids (through mucous membranes or broken skin) and/or indirect contact with environments contaminated with splashes, droplets of blood or body fluids. Experts agree that there is no circumstantial or epidemiological evidence of an aerosol transmission risk from VHF patients.

T   Most VHF viruses are identified through rapid enzyme immunoassays.

T   Supportive management of VHF is the mainstay of treatment. Resuscitation, fluids and blood products are often required.

T   Ribavirin is indicated in the management of Lassa fever only.

1.   Hamele M, Poss WB, Sweney J. Disaster preparedness, pediatric considerations in primary blast injury, chemical and biological terrorism. *World J Crit Care Med* 2014; 3(1): 15-23.

2.   Department of Health. Management of Hazard Group 4 viral haemorrhagic fevers and similar human infectious diseases of high consequence, 2012. Advisory Committee on Dangerous Pathogens. http://www.ficm.ac.uk/news-events/ebola-and-critical-illness.

3.   Fowler RA, Fletcher T, Fischer WA, *et al*. Caring for critically ill patients with Ebola virus disease. Perspectives from West Africa. *Am J Resp Crit Care Med* 2014; 190(7): 733-7.

Answer 49: Patients taking etanercept or infliximab are at increased risk of: All True

T   Use of biologic agents such as TNF-α antagonists (e.g. etanercept, infliximab) is associated with important side effects which should be considered in the critically ill. Typical and atypical bacterial infections are increased with such biologic agents.

T   Miliary tuberculosis and reactivation of latent tuberculosis is associated with biologic agents.

T   Meningoencephalitis and severe sepsis can be caused by listeriosis and is associated in patients taking biologic agents.

T   There is an increased risk of *Pneumocystis jiroveci* pneumonia (PCP) in the immunocompromised patient.

T   Disseminated fungal infections are more common in patients who are immunocompromised or on biologic agents. There is an increased risk of histoplasmosis and coccidioidomycosis infection in these patient groups.

1.   Parsons PE, Wiener-Kronish JP. *Critical Care Secrets*, 5th ed. Missouri, USA: Elsevier Mosby, 2013.

Answer 50: During the 2009 H1N1 influenza A pandemic: True c & e

F   Zanamivir is given intravenously and is used when the enteral absorption of oral oseltamivir is poor or in cases of resistant virus.

F   Oseltamivir is an oral neuraminidase inhibitor, which is active against both influenza A and B. It is dosed at 75mg bd for 5 days, doubled in severe infection (150mg bd for 10 days). Ribavirin may also be used in conjunction. M2 channel blockers (rimantadine) are not routinely used to treat influenza, due to neurotoxicity.

T   The SOFA score was suggested by the UK Department of Health as a critical care triage tool. Triage suggested included patients with a SOFA score >11 and certain inclusion/exclusion criteria would not be admitted to critical care, and also withdrawal of care would be considered at 48 hours and on subsequent days for patients with SOFA scores >11. Retrospective survey data post-pandemic suggested if this approach had been undertaken, withdrawal of care would have potentially occurred in several patients who subsequently survived after a short period of ventilation.

F   Influenza infection whilst pregnant (particularly during the 3rd trimester) carries a high rate of complications and increased need for hospitalisation (4-7 x risk).

T   Referral and transfer of H1N1-related ARDS to an ECMO centre was associated with a lower hospital mortality compared with non-ECMO referred patients, even if the referred patients did not ultimately receive ECMO.

1.   Gwavava C, Lynch G. Intensive care management of pandemic (H1N1) influenza. Anaesthesia Tutorial of the Week 2009, 2011. www.aagbi.org/education/educational -resources/tutorial-week.

2.   Noah MA, Peek GJ, Finney SJ, et al. Referral to an extracorporeal membrane oxygenation center and mortality among patients with severe 2009 influenza A (H1N1). JAMA 2011; 306(15): 1659-68.

3.   Zangrillo A, Zoccai GB, Landoni G, et al. Extracorporeal membrane oxygenation (ECMO) in patients with H1N1 influenza infection: a systemic review and meta-analysis including 8 studies and 266 patients receiving ECMO. Crit Care 2013; 17: R30.

Answer 51: Bioterrorism: True d

F   *Clostridium* botulinum produces a neurotoxin, which acts at the presynaptic terminal of the neuromuscular junction to prevent acetylcholine release, causing a flaccid paralysis.

F   Person-to-person transmission does <u>not</u> occur.

F   Children, pregnant women and immunocompromised patients with botulism should still receive antitoxin. There is a small risk of a hypersensitivity reaction and anaphylaxis.

T   Sarin inhibits acetylcholinesterase. Clinical features of sarin toxicity include miosis, rhinorrhitis, bronchospasm, weakness, convulsions, respiratory arrest and death.

F   Atropine is used to antagonise the muscarinic effects of sarin. Pralidoxime mesilate reactivates anticholinesterase at nicotinic sites and may be used in treatment. Fomepizole is used as an antidote in suspected methanol or ethylene glycol poisoning.

1.   Bersten AD, Soni N. *Oh's Intensive Care Manual*, 6th ed. Butterworth Heinemann Elsevier, 2009.

2.   Wenham T, Cohen A. Botulism. *Contin Educ Anaesth Crit Care Pain* 2008; 8(1): 21-5.

Answer 52: Concerning resuscitation of the pregnant patient: True c & e

F   A left lateral tilt of 15-30° should be used in those who are known to be of 20 weeks' gestation and above, those in whom gestation is unknown but the uterus is clearly visible and in those who are less than 20 weeks' gestation but have a visible uterus or uterus palpable at the level of the umbilicus due to polyhydramnios or multiple pregnancy. Manual displacement of the uterus with one or two hands can be used instead of a left lateral tilt.

F   The incidence of a failed intubation in obstetrics is estimated to be around eight times that of the non-pregnant population, when looking at data from general anaesthetics.

T   The Society of Obstetric Anesthesia and Perinatology recommend that in maternal cardiac arrest, rapid peri-mortem Caesarean section be undertaken, with timing of incision within 4 minutes and neonatal delivery within 5 minutes of cardiac arrest. A recent review by Einav *et al* found a positive association between peri-mortem Caesarean delivery within 10 minutes and an improved maternal outcome.

F In maternal arrest, the American Heart Association recommends that chest compressions should be performed slightly higher on the sternum due to the elevation of the diaphragm and abdominal contents. In comparison, the Resuscitation Council UK does not recommend doing chest compressions differently, with the location of chest compressions during maternal arrest being debated.

T The Polio Macintosh laryngoscope blade is mounted at 135° to the handle. This feature makes it useful for intubation in pregnant patients with breast hypertrophy. A short handled laryngoscope can also be used.

1. American Heart Association. Part 10.8: Cardiac arrest associated with pregnancy, 2010. http://m.circ.ahajournals.org/content/112/24_suppl/IV-150.full.
2. Resuscitation Council (UK). Advanced life support, 6th ed. London, UK: Resuscitation Council (UK), 2011. www.resus.org.uk.
3. Smith T, Pinnock C, Lin T. *Fundamentals of Anaesthesia*, 3rd ed. Cambridge, UK: Cambridge University Press, 2009.
4. The Society of Obstetric Anesthesia and Perinatology. Consensus statement on the management of cardiac arrest in pregnancy, 2012. http://soap.org/CPR-statement-draft-5-28-13.pdf.
5. Einav S, Kaufman N, Sela HY. Maternal cardiac arrest and peri-mortem Caesarean delivery: evidence or expert-based? *Resuscitation* 2012; 83(10): 1191-200.

Answer 53: Pressures and temperature: True b & c

F The critical pressure is the pressure required to liquefy a vapour at its critical temperature.

T This is true total pressure.

T Charles' law states that at a constant pressure, the volume of a fixed mass of gas is directly proportional to the absolute temperature.

F Henry's law states that at a constant temperature, the amount of gas dissolved in a solvent is proportional to its partial pressure above the solvent.

F This is the critical temperature of oxygen (-118°C). The boiling point is -183°C.

1.   Davis PD, Kenny GNC. *Basic Physics and Measurement in Anaesthesia*, 5th ed. Edinburgh, UK: Butterworth Heinemann, 2003.

Answer 54: Amniotic fluid embolism (AFE): True c & e

F   AFE often presents with sudden hypoxia, cardiovascular collapse and coagulopathy. Chest pain, confusion, foetal distress, cough, headache and seizures are less common presentations.

F   The pathophysiology is unclear, but an immune process is thought to be responsible for the syndrome.

T   The majority of patients who suffer AFE die within the first hour. It is thought approximately 85% of survivors suffer permanent neurological damage.

F   Amniotic fluid and cells entering the circulation cause an increase in both pulmonary and systemic vascular resistance.

T   It used to be thought that the findings of amniotic fluid and foetal tissue within the maternal circulation at post mortem was pathognomonic of AFE, but it is now known that foetal squames can be detected in the maternal circulation during normal labour without AFE developing.

1.   Dedhia JD, Mushambi MC. Amniotic fluid embolism. *Contin Educ Anaesth Crit Care Pain* 2007; 7(5): 152 6.

Answer 55: Regarding liver transplantation: True a, d & e

T   One-year survival following liver transplantation for acute liver failure is approximately 65%. This is less than following transplantation for chronic liver failure.

F   Data from the United Kingdom between April 2010 to March 2011 shows that at 1 year post-registration on the transplant list, 12% of patients had died or had been removed from the list due to clinical deterioration.

F   In the United Kingdom during 2012-2013, there were 825 organ donors who donated their livers for transplant: 640 donated after brainstem death (DBD) and 185 after circulatory death (DCD). DCD donors can be grouped by the Maastricht classification (see Table

2.1). Liver and lungs for transplant can currently only be taken from controlled donors (category III-IV).

Table 2.1. Maastricht classification.

Maastricht classification	Donor status	Controlled/uncontrolled donation
I	Dead on arrival to hospital	Uncontrolled
II	Unsuccessful resuscitation	Uncontrolled
III	Awaiting cardiac arrest	Controlled
IV	Cardiac arrest after brainstem death	Controlled
V	Cardiac arrest in a hospital inpatient	Uncontrolled

T   This is known as the 'piggyback technique'. Advantages of this technique include haemodynamic stability and negation of the need for veno-venous bypass.

T   Activation of the fibrinolytic system during the anhepatic and post-reperfusion stages of liver transplantation may occur in some recipients. LY30 and LY60 on a thromboelastogram measure the percentage decrease in amplitude at 30 and 60 minutes post-maximum amplitude of the clot and give a measure of the degree of fibrinolysis.

1.   Waldmann C, Soni N, Rhodes A. *Oxford Desk Reference Critical Care*. Oxford, UK: Oxford University Press, 2008.

2.   NI IS Blood and Transplant. Organ donation and transplantation activity report 2012/2013. Available at http://www.organdonation.nhs.uk/statistics/transplant_activity_report/current_activity_reports/ukt/activity_report_2012_13.pdf.

3.   Ridley S, Bonner S, Bray K, *et al.* UK guidance for non-heart-beating donation. *Br J Anaesth* 2005; 95(5): 592-5.

4.   Bersten AD, Soni N. *Oh's Intensive Care Manual*, 6th ed. Butterworth Heinemann Elsevier, 2009.

Answer 56: Prediction of neurological outcome after cardiac arrest: True c & d

F   There may be an association between circumstances and neurological outcome, but this is not definite.

F   The PAR score is used to predict non-survival, not neurological outcome.

T   The Lance Adams syndrome is associated with intentional myoclonus and preservation of consciousness, as opposed to myoclonic status which is associated with poor neurological outcome.

T   Neurone-specific enolase is a biochemical marker that is released following cerebral damage and is detected in blood and cerebrospinal fluid.

F   In a small study of patients who had undergone therapeutic hypothermia post-cardiac arrest, a small number of patients with poor clinical signs (absent corneal or pupillary reflexes or myoclonic status epilepsy) on day 3 regained awareness. Currently, expert view is that extreme caution should be used, when using clinical signs alone at 72 hours post-cardiac arrest to predict neurological function in patients who have undergone therapeutic hypothermia. Further studies are required to fully elucidate the effect of therapeutic hypothermia on markers of poor neurological function post-cardiac arrest.

1.   Temple A, Porter R. Predicting neurological outcome and survival after cardiac arrest. *Contin Educ Anaesth Crit Care Pain* 2012; 12(6): 283-7.

2.   Porter R, Goodhart I, Temple A. Predicting survival in cardiac arrest patients admitted to intensive care using the Prognosis After Resuscitation score. *Crit Care* 2011; 15(Suppl 1): 299.

3.   Cronberg T, Horn J, Kuiper MA, *et al*. A structured approach to neurologic prognostication in clinical cardiac arrest trials. *Scand J Trauma Resusc Emerg Med* 2013; 21: 45.

4.   Al Thenayan E, Savard M, Sharpe M, *et al*. Predictors of poor neurologic outcome after induced mild hypothermia following cardiac arrest. *Neurology* 2008; 71: 1535-7.

Answer 57: Postpartum haemorrhage (PPH): True a & d

T Primary PPH occurs within 24 hours of childbirth, with secondary PPH occurring between 24 hours and 6 weeks' postpartum.

F Postpartum haemorrhage (PPH) is usually due to uterine atony.

F A rapid bolus of 10 units of intravenous oxytocin has been associated with cardiovascular collapse. A slow intravenous bolus of 5 units should be given instead.

T Due to the physiological changes of pregnancy, several litres of blood may be lost before signs of hypovolaemia present.

F The National Institute for Health and Care Excellence has advised that this technique can be used, but noted the theoretical safety concerns regarding infusion of foetal cells and amniotic fluid.

1. Bersten AD, Soni N. *Oh's Intensive Care Manual*, 6th ed. Butterworth Heinemann Elsevier, 2009.

2. Thomas C, Madej T. Obstetric emergencies and the anaesthetist. *Contin Educ Anaesth Crit Care Pain* 2002; 2(6): 174-7.

3. National Institute for Health and Care Excellence. Intraoperative blood cell salvage in obstetrics. NICE Clinical Guideline IPG144, 2015. London, UK: NICE, 2015. http://guidance.nice.org.uk/IPG144/Guidance/pdf.

Answer 58: Regarding trauma management: True b & e

F These factors contribute to the acute coagulopathy of trauma, but other factors are now known to be involved, including activation of fibrinolytic pathways and tissue injury-related generation of thrombin-thrombomodulin complexes.

T Without signs of imminent cerebral herniation, normoventilation to a $PaCO_2$ of 5.0 to 5.5kPa is recommended.

F The Trauma Associated Severe Haemorrhage score uses seven parameters: systolic blood pressure, haemoglobin, intra-abdominal fluid, complex long bone and/or pelvic fractures, heart rate, base excess and gender.

F Diagnostic peritoneal lavage (DPL) is recommended as one of the diagnostic modalities to be considered during the primary survey of a patient in haemorrhagic shock with an unidentified source of bleeding. Clinical examination, radiography and ultrasonography are utilised more often, but DPL may occasionally be required.

T   The use of serial lactate measurement in trauma patients is well established.

1.   Spahn DR, Bouillon B, Cerny V, *et al.* Management of bleeding and coagulopathy following major trauma: an updated European guideline. *Crit Care* 2013; 17(2): R76.

Answer 59: Tranexamic acid (TXA) and Factor VIIa: True a & d

T   In the CRASH 2 trial, all-cause mortality was 14.5% in the TXA group and 16% in the placebo group. The risk of death due to bleeding was 4.9% versus 5.7% in favour of TXA. These findings were significant.

F   The loading dose of TXA was 1g followed by a further dose of 1g over 8 hours.

F   Factor VIIa can activate Factors IX and X on the platelet membrane in the absence of tissue factor.

T   Early use of recombinant Factor VIIa has been found to decrease transfusion requirements in trauma patients.

F   There is no evidence that recombinant Factor VIIa decreases mortality in trauma patients requiring massive transfusion.

1.   CRASH 2 trial collaborators. Effect of tranexamic acid on death, vascular occlusive events, and blood transfusion in trauma patients with significant haemorrhage (CRASH 2): a randomised, placebo-controlled trial. *Lancet* 2010; 376: 23-32.

2.   Duchesne JC, Mathew KA, Marr AB, *et al.* Current evidence-based guidelines for factor VIIa use in trauma: the good, the bad and the ugly. *Am Surg* 2008; 74(12): 1159-65.

3.   Perkins JG, Schreiber MA, Wade CE, Holcomb JB. Early versus late recombinant factor VIIa in combat trauma patients requiring massive transfusion. *J Trauma* 2007; 62(5): 1095-9.

Answer 60: Chest trauma: True a, b & e

T   25% of all trauma-related deaths are caused by thoracic injury.

T   This occurs where air collects antero-inferiorly. A pneumothorax may also be demonstrated by increased radiolucency on one side of the chest compared to the other.

F   A widened mediastinum is defined as being greater than 8cm in width.

F   The thoracic aorta is fixed at the aortic valve, ligamentum arteriosum and at the diaphragmatic hiatus.

T   The right hemidiaphragm is congenitally stronger and protected by the liver.

1.   Waldmann C, Soni N, Rhodes A. *Oxford Desk Reference Critical Care*. Oxford, UK: Oxford University Press, 2008.

2.   Bersten AD, Soni N. *Oh's Intensive Care Manual*, 6th ed. Butterworth Heinemann Elsevier, 2009.

Answer 61: Hyperchloraemic acidosis: True b, c & d

F   Hyperchloraemic acidosis occurs due to either a loss of strong cations such as sodium or a relative increase in anions such as chloride. It produces a normal anion gap acidosis.

T   Profuse diarrhoea may result in large sodium losses into the gut lumen and produce a hyperchloraemic acidosis.

T   Iatrogenic administration of excess chloride via TPN or infusions of normal saline, are the most common causes of a hyperchloraemic acidosis.

T   In renal tubular acidosis (RTA), chloride excretion is impaired and a hyperchloraemic acidosis may result.

F   Furosemide may occasionally be used in renal tubular acidosis (RTA) with a plasma pH of >7.35 but has no routine role in the management of hyperchloraemic acidosis.

1.   Waldmann C, Soni N, Rhodes A. *Oxford Desk Reference Critical Care*. Oxford, UK: Oxford University Press, 2008.

Answer 62: During controlled ventilation: True a, c & e

T   Airway pressure generated during controlled ventilation depends on the compliance and resistance of the respiratory system and circuit.

F   Inspiratory flow is constant (square wave) during volume-controlled ventilation.

T   In time triggering, breaths are delivered according to a pre-set frequency.

F   Triggering is when the ventilator detects a drop in airway pressure or flow that occurs when a patient makes a spontaneous breath, instigating the ventilator to deliver a positive pressure inspiratory breath.

T   Volume, time and flow can be used to cycle the ventilator.

1.   Waldmann C, Soni N, Rhodes A. *Oxford Desk Reference Critical Care*. Oxford, UK: Oxford University Press, 2008.

Answer 63: Considering randomised controlled trials (RCTs): True a, b & e

T   RCTs are always prospective in their design.

T   RCTs seek to disprove rather than prove a hypothesis. This is known as hypothetico-deductive reasoning.

F   Cross-sectional surveys provide a better means of assessing screening tests than RCTs.

F   Longitudinal surveys of inception cohort studies provide a better means of studying disease prognosis.

T   All RCTs are open to bias due to blinding, but this can be a particular problem in critical care studies.

1.   Greenhalgh T. *How to Read a Paper - the Basics of Evidence-based Medicine*. Oxford, UK: Wiley-Blackwell, 2014.

2.   Sackett DL, Wennberg JE. Choosing the best research design for each question. *Br Med J* 1997; 315(7123): 1636.

3.   Stewart LA, Parmar MK. Bias in the analysis and reporting of randomized controlled trials. *Int J Technol Assess Health Care* 1996; 12(2): 264-75.

Answer 64: Considering the hierarchy of evidence and clinical trials: True c & e

F   Secondary research papers such as systematic reviews and meta-analyses of randomised controlled trials are considered to be the highest form of evidence.

F   The hierarchy of evidence is as follows: 1) systematic reviews and meta-analyses; 2) RCTs with definitive results; 3) RCTs with non-definitive results; 4) cohort studies; 5) case-controlled studies; 6) cross-sectional surveys; 7) case reports; 8) expert or personal opinion.

T   Serious methodological flaws or risk of bias may lead to downgrading of evidence according to the hierarchy.

F   See above.

T   For results of an RCT to be considered definitive, its confidence intervals must not overlap the threshold of clinically significant effect.

1.   Guyatt GH, Sackett DL, Sinclair JC, et al. Users' guides to the medical literature. IX. A method for grading health care recommendations. Evidence-Based Medicine Working Group. JAMA 1995; 274(22): 1800-4.

2.   Greenhalgh T. How to Read a Paper - the Basics of Evidence-based Medicine. Oxford, UK: Wiley-Blackwell, 2014.

Answer 65: Concerning donation after circulatory death (DCD) in critical care patients: True e

F   Critical care patients are only deemed suitable for solid organ donation after cardiac death, if they die within a set period of time after treatment withdrawal. The maximum functional warm ischaemic time for solid organs varies depending on organ. For example: kidney (120 minutes, extended up to 4 hours if kidney deemed to be viable), liver (30 minutes), lung (60 minutes, time to lung re-inflation critical) and pancreas (30 minutes).

F   Death should be confirmed within 5 minutes of loss of cardiorespiratory activity and requires confirmation by one doctor only.

F   Members of the transplant team should not be involved in any family discussions regarding withdrawal of treatment and should only meet the family once the decision to withdraw treatment has been made.

F   Long-term outcomes from kidneys retrieved from DCD donors are the same as those from brainstem dead (DBD) donors.

T   In England and Wales according to the UK Donation Ethics Committee (UKDEC): "For donation after circulatory death, the coroner must be consulted before the patient has died".

1.   American College of Critical Care Medicine & Society of Critical Care Medicine. Recommendations for nonheartbeating organ donation. A position paper by the Ethics Committee, American College of Critical Care Medicine, Society of Critical Care Medicine. *Crit Care Med* 2001; 29(9): 1826-31.

2.   Ridley S, Bonner S, Bray K, *et al.* UK guidance for non-heart-beating donation. *Br J Anaesth* 2005; 95(5): 592-5 .

3.   Weber M, Dindo D, Demartines N, *et al.* Kidney transplantation from donors without a heartbeat. *N Engl J Med* 2002; 25; 347(4): 248-5.

4.   UK Donation Ethics Committee (UKDEC) & Academy of Medical Royal Colleges. An ethical framework for controlled donation after circulatory death, 2011. http://www.aomrc.org.uk/doc_view/9425-an-ethical-framework-for-controlled-donation-after-circulatory-death.

5.   NHS Blood and Transplant. The role of HM coroner in relation to organ donation: England, Northern Ireland and Wales, 2014. http://www.odt.nhs.uk/donation/deceased-donation/organ-donation-services/role-of-hmc.

Answer 66: Critical care ventilation: True a & c

T   During volume-controlled ventilation, the difference in peak and plateau pressures reflects the pressure required to overcome resistive forces.

F   Volume-controlled ventilation only (VCV). During pressure-controlled ventilation (PCV), inspiratory pressures are constant, therefore, it is not possible to differentiate the elastic and resistive properties of the patient's lungs from observation of the airway trace.

T   Auto-triggering describes the ventilator incorrectly cycling to inspiration.

F   Tidal volumes generated should be based on ideal body weight.

F   The ARDS network termed 'lung protective ventilation' to be 6-7ml/kg tidal volumes. Lung protective ventilation has been shown to reduce mortality in acute lung injury, with possible benefits also seen in patients with normal lungs.

1.   Waldmann C, Soni N, Rhodes A. *Oxford Desk Reference Critical Care*. Oxford, UK: Oxford University Press, 2008.

2.   The Acute Respiratory Distress Syndrome Network. Ventilation with lower tidal volumes as compared with traditional tidal volumes for acute lung injury and the acute respiratory distress syndrome. *New Engl J Med* 2000; 342(18): 1301-8

Answer 67: When managing burns: True c

F   The burns injury can be assessed using the Wallace Rule of Nines.

F   The original Parkland formula specified Ringer's lactate as the solution of choice not colloid. For the initial 24-hour fluid resuscitation, the Parkland formula recommends: 4ml x body weight (kg) x % total body surface area (TBSA) burn should be given in the initial 24 hours from burns injury, with half given within the first 8 hours and the remaining half over 16 hours.

T   There is evidence that supplementation with zinc, copper and selenium is associated with a decrease in rates of nosocomial pneumonia, improved wound healing and decreased length of stay in severely burned patients. The use of glutamine in burns has also been associated with reduced infectious complications and length of stay. However, following the REDOXS study, glutamine use in critically ill patients <u>with</u> shock and multi-organ failure is not recommended, as it is associated with an increased mortality.

F   There is no benefit to commencing early parenteral nutrition in this situation.

F   Urinary alkalisation and <u>not</u> acidification may be beneficial where there is haemoglobinurea and/or myoglobinurea to increase excretion and prevent the development of acute renal failure from rhabdomyolysis.

1.   Casaer MP, Mesotten D, Hermans G, *et al.* Early versus late parenteral nutrition in critically ill adults. *New Engl J Med* 2009; 365: 506-17.

2.   Bersten AD, Soni N. *Oh's Intensive Care Manual*, 6th ed. Butterworth Heinemann Elsevier, 2009.

3.   Berger MM, Eggimann P, Heyland DK, *et al.* Reduction of nosocomial pneumonia after major burns by trace element supplementation: aggregation of two randomised trials. *Crit Care* 2006; 10(6): R153.

4.   Heyland D, Muscedere J, Wischmeyer PE, *et al.* A randomised trial of glutamine and antioxidants in critically ill patients. *New Engl J Med* 2013; 368(19): 1489-97.

Answer 68: Biochemical features of acute renal failure secondary to rhabdomyolysis include: True b-d

F   Classically in severe rhabdomyolysis, a metabolic acidosis occurs due to the release of organic acids and lactic acid production from ischaemic muscle.

T   As myocytes are damaged there is an efflux of intracellular contents into the circulation with hyperkalaemia, hyperuricaemia and hyperphosphataemia observed.

T   Hyperuricaemia caused by muscle and cell nuclei damage, may contribute directly to renal tubular damage.

T   Hypoalbuminaemia occurs due to proteinuria and protein leakage.

F   Hypercalcaemia is not a characteristic feature of rhabdomyolysis, but can be seen as a late complication.

1.   Barnard M. Rhabdomyolysis. Anaesthesia Tutorial of the Week 198, 2010. www.aagbi.org/education/educational-resources/tutorial-week.

2.   Hunter JD, Gregg K, Damani Z. Rhabdomyolysis. *Contin Educ Anaesth Crit Care Pain* 2006; 6(4): 141-3.

Answer 69: The following statements in relation to myxoedema coma are true: True a & c

T   Bradycardia, hypoglycaemia and hypothermia are common clinical manifestations of myxoedema coma. In addition to these, hypotension and hyponatraemia are often seen.

F   Thyroid function tests classically show low serum T4 and T3 (total and free), together with a significantly elevated thyroid stimulating hormone (TSH) level.

T   Mortality may be up to 80% with myxoedema coma, warranting the initiation of prompt and aggressive treatment, even before definitive diagnostic tests are complete. Specialist input relating to regimens for the treatment of myxoedema coma should be sought. Protocols vary with the administration of T4 alone or combined T4 and T3 regimens used. Concerns remain relating to T3 cardiac toxicity in the elderly.

F   Glucocorticoids (e.g. hydrocortisone 100mg qds) should be given along with thyroxine in patients with suspected myxoedema coma, as adrenal reserve may be decreased in severe hypothyroidism.

F   Caution should be exercised when using vasoactive agents in myxoedema coma, as they may be ineffective and precipitate dangerous cardiac arrhythmias. Drug metabolism may also be affected. For example, digoxin metabolism may be inadequate, leading to raised serum levels and a subsequent risk of toxicity.

1.   Fliers E, Wiersinga WM. Myxedema coma. *Rev Endocr Metab Disord* 2003; 4(2): 137-41.

2.   European Society of Intensive Care Medicine (ESICM); Patient-centered Acute Care Training (PACT). Electrolytes and homeostasis module. http://pact.esicm.org. European Society of Intensive Care Medicine.

Answer 70: Weaning from mechanical ventilation: True a, b, c & e

T   Weaning is the process of liberation from mechanical ventilation.

T   Delay in weaning prolongs critical care stay, increases costs and is associated with a higher mortality.

T   The use of synchronised intermittent mandatory ventilation (SIMV) alone from recent weaning trials is deemed the least efficient method for weaning. Combining SIMV with spontaneous breathing/pressure support may improve efficiency.

F   The ongoing need for inotropes does not preclude weaning.

T   There is no universal strategy or consensus currently for weaning critical care patients from mechanical ventilation. Further research and international collaboration is needed.

1.   Waldmann C, Soni N, Rhodes A. *Oxford Desk Reference Critical Care*. Oxford, UK: Oxford University Press, 2008.

2.   Lermitte J, Garfield MJ. Weaning from mechanical ventilation. *Contin Educ Anaesth Crit Care Pain* 2005; 5(4): 113-7.

Answer 71: High-frequency ventilation: True d & e

F   In high-frequency jet ventilation (HFJV), a high-frequency, high-pressure jet (10-50 pound/square inch, psi or 68.9-344.5kPa) is delivered via a small-bore cannula into the airway. Air is entrained into the airway by the high-pressure jet. Exhalation occurs passively.

F   During high-frequency ventilation the lung is maintained on its deflation limb on the static pressure-volume curve, improving lung compliance and alveoli recruitment.

F   Peak airway pressures are reduced with high-frequency ventilation, minimising barotrauma.

T   Oxygenation and carbon dioxide elimination are decoupled in high-frequency oscillatory ventilation (HFOV).

T   In the OSCILLATE trial, 548 patients from 39 centres were recruited. Mortality was 47% in HFOV vs. 35% receiving conventional ventilation. Increased sedative and muscle relaxant use was required in the HFOV group. In another trial conducted around the same time, the OSCAR trial found an identical 41% 30-day mortality. Increased sedative and muscle relaxant use was also found in the HFOV group.

1.   Waldmann C, Soni N, Rhodes A. *Oxford Desk Reference Critical Care*. Oxford, UK: Oxford University Press, 2008.

2.   Ferguson N, Cook DJ, Guyatt GH, *et al*; the OSCILLATE Trial Investigators. High-frequency oscillation in early acute respiratory distress syndrome. *New Engl J Med* 2013; 368(9): 795-805.

3.   Young D, Lamb SE, Shah S, *et al*; the OSCAR Study Group. High-frequency oscillation for acute respiratory distress syndrome. *New Engl J Med* 2013; 368: 806-13.

Answer 72: Potassium: True b & d

F   Acidosis and α-adrenergic agonists promote a shift of potassium from the intracellular fluid to the extracellular fluid. Alkalosis and insulin release (seen with hyperkalaemia) promotes the reverse, a shift of potassium from extracellular to intracellular fluid.

T $\beta2$-agonists promote intracellular movement of potassium through cyclic AMP-dependent activation of Na^+/K^+ pumps.

F   Prominent U-waves, small or inverted T-waves, a prolonged PR interval and depressed ST segments are electrocardiographic features of hypokalaemia. In comparison, tall tented T-waves, small P-waves, a wide QRS complex which may progress to a sinusoidal waveform and ventricular fibrillation are seen with severe hyperkalaemia.

T   Potassium 40mmol may be replaced over 1 hour via the central venous route, to avoid damage to peripheral veins. Continuous ECG and 1-4-hourly monitoring of plasma potassium levels is advised.

F   10ml of 10% calcium chloride contains nearly three times as much calcium than 10ml of 10% calcium gluconate (6.8mmol versus 2.325mmol, respectively).

1.   Bersten AD, Soni N. *Oh's Intensive Care Manual*, 6th ed. Butterworth Heinemann Elsevier, 2009.

2.   Sydney South West Area Health Service. Potassium chloride: safe use of intravenous potassium chloride (adult patients), 2007. Document no. SSW_GL2007_006. Available at https://www.sswahs.nsw.gov.au/pdf/policy/gl2007006.pdf.

Answer 73: Calcium: True a, c & d

T   40% of calcium in the body is bound to protein (mainly albumin), 47% is ionised and 13% is in a complex with citrate, sulphate and phosphate.

F   This is the Trousseau sign of latent tetany. The Chvostek sign refers to an abnormal reaction to the stimulation of the facial nerve. These signs may be elicited in patients with hypocalcaemia.

T   The total plasma calcium value is corrected for albumin by adding 0.02mmol/L calcium for each g/L albumin below 40g/L.

T   Calcitonin is secreted from the parafollicular cells of the thyroid gland, inhibits mobilisation of bone calcium and increases renal calcium and phosphate excretion.

F   Allopurinol decreases the formation of uric acid, whereas rasburicase promotes its degradation.

1.   Bersten AD, Soni N. *Oh's Intensive Care Manual*, 6th ed. Butterworth Heinemann Elsevier, 2009.

2.   Yentis SM, Hirsch NP, Smith GB. *Anaesthesia and Intensive Care A-Z. An Encyclopaedia of Principles and Practice*, 3rd ed. Edinburgh, UK: Elsevier Butterworth Heinemann, 2004.

3.   Parsons PE, Wiener-Kronish JP. *Critical Care Secrets*, 5th ed. Missouri, USA: Elsevier Mosby, 2013.

Answer 74: Positive end-expiratory pressure (PEEP): True b, d & e

F   In severe ARDS, high PEEP (>15cmH$_2$O) does not improve mortality. Some PEEP (around 5-10cmH$_2$O) is associated with improved oxygenation.

T   Application of PEEP increases functional residual capacity.

F   Decreased renal blood flow and reduced splanchnic and hepatic perfusion can occur with higher levels of PEEP.

T   PEEP application increases intrathoracic pressure, diminishing venous return to the right heart.

T   Following PEEP application, an observed increase in lung compliance is suggestive of alveolar recruitment.

1.   The National Heart, Lung and Blood Institute ARDS Clinical Trials Network. Higher versus lower positive end-expiratory pressures in patients with the acute respiratory distress syndrome. *New Engl J Med* 2004; 351: 327-36

2.   Waldmann C, Soni N, Rhodes A. *Oxford Desk Reference Critical Care*. Oxford, UK: Oxford University Press, 2008.

Answer 75: Regarding critical care nutrition: True e

F   For critically ill patients who are expected to remain in intensive care for over 48 hours, the need for nutrition is an accepted standard of care. However, the type of feeding route (enteral vs. parenteral), timing and energy deficit replacement is controversial and remains hotly debated. Many guidelines promote enteral nutrition over any form of standard care, including waiting for return of oral intake and intravenous dextrose. Further large randomised controlled trials are warranted to investigate enteral feeding versus delayed nutrition. Many studies have found that early enteral nutrition is associated with lower infectious complications and a reduction in overall cost.

However, recently, the CALORIES trial reported that among adult patients without contraindications to either enteral or parenteral route, when enteral nutrition and parenteral nutrition are initiated early and with similar caloric and protein doses, no significant difference in clinical outcomes including mortality and infectious complications was found.

F   Many studies have found that excess energy supply, in excess of energy needs, is associated with worse outcomes and complications in critical care patients. However, the question of how much enteral nutrition should be administered early during critical illness is unknown. The EDEN trial (ARDS network 2012) assessed 1000 patients with acute lung injury, who were given either a small amount of enteral feeding (trophic feeding) for 1 week in the intensive care unit or full enteral feeding from the time of admission. Despite the patients in the trophic feeding group accumulating a greater nutritional deficit than the full-feed group, there was no difference in acute or long-term functional outcomes in ALI. This result is comparable to other small randomised controlled trials which compared underfeeding to the full enteral feeding approach.

F   During the early phase of intensive care admission, a high protein intake (1.5g/kg/day) has been recommended, regardless of calorie intake, to overcome large muscle and protein losses during the first week of critical illness.

F   Intravenous selenium supplementation may be beneficial in septic patients, with a recent meta-analysis (Alhazzani *et al*, 2013) suggesting a mortality benefit.

T   The timing to prescribe parenteral nutrition is currently unclear. Most recommendations are that parenteral nutrition be used in patients where enteral nutrition is not tolerated or fails to match nutritional needs. Parenteral nutrition is not advised in patients who are expected to have a short critical care stay (<4 days) and likely to resume oral intake within 5 days. Further research is needed to investigate.

1.   Singer P, Doig GS, Pichard C. The truth about nutrition in the ICU. *Intensive Care Med* 2014; 40: 252-5.

2.   Doig GS, Heighes PT, Simpson F, *et al.* Early enteral nutrition, provided within 24h of injury or intensive care unit admission, significantly reduces mortality in critically ill

patients: a meta-analysis of randomised controlled trials. *Intensive Care Med* 2009; 35(12): 2018-27.

3. Macdonald K, Page K, Brown L, Bryden D. Parenteral nutrition in critical care. *Contin Educ Anaesth Crit Care Pain* 2013; 13(1): 1-5.

4. Caeser MP, Van den Berghe G. Nutrition in the acute phase of critical illness. *New Engl J Med* 2014; 370: 1227-36.

5. The National Heart, Lung and Blood Institute Acute Respiratory Distress Syndrome (ARDS) Clinical Trials Network. Initial trophic vs full enteral feeding in patients with acute lung injury: the EDEN randomised controlled trial. *JAMA* 2012; 307: 795-803.

6. Alhazzani W, Jacobi J, Sindi A, *et al*. The effect of selenium therapy on mortality in patients with sepsis syndrome: a systematic review and meta-analysis of randomised controlled trials. *Crit Care Med* 2013; 41(6): 1555-64.

7. Harvey SE, Parrott F, Harrison DA, *et al*; the CALORIES Trial Investigators. Trial of the route of early nutritional support in critically ill adults. *New Engl J Med* 2014; 371: 1673-84.

Answer 76: End-stage liver disease and liver transplantation: True d

F   MELD was initially developed to predict survival after a transjugular intrahepatic portosystemic shunt, but it has also been shown to be useful in predicting survival in those awaiting liver transplantation.

F   Hepatopulmonary and portopulmonary syndromes are active indications for liver transplantation.

F   Increased afterload in the early post-transplant period due to increased systemic vascular resistance may reveal cardiac dysfunction, which was not previously evident at pre-operative assessment.

T   The Child Pugh score is used to assess the prognosis of chronic liver disease.

F   Post-reperfusion syndrome occurs after reperfusion of the portal vein through the donor graft and can result in hypotension, bradycardia, vasodilatation, pulmonary hypertension, hyperkalaemia and cardiac arrest. It is usually transient, but in approximately 30% of patients it necessitates the use of vasopressors and/or inotropes.

1. Bersten AD, Soni N. *Oh's Intensive Care Manual*, 6th ed. Butterworth Heinemann Elsevier, 2009.

2.   Jackson P, Gleeson D. Alcoholic liver disease. *Contin Educ Anaesth Crit Care Pain* 2010; 10(3): 66-71.

Answer 77: The following statements are true regarding thyroid storm: True a & c

T   High fever is a characteristic finding. Tachycardia and tachypnoea are commonly seen in thyroid storm. Heart failure, cardiac ischaemia and arrhythmias may also develop. A goitre may be found clinically, but its presence is not necessary for diagnosis.

F   A significantly elevated serum T3 and T4 (total and free) and an undetectable TSH is the usual biochemical finding. Raised liver enzymes, hypercalcaemia, hyperglycaemia and leucocytosis may also be seen.

T   Oral or nasogastric propranolol (60-80mg every 4 hours) or intravenous β1-selective blockers (e.g. esmolol) are the preferred agents for heart rate control in thyroid storm. Esmolol infusions have been used with good effect, as the number of β1-receptors is markedly increased in thyroid storm (esmolol: loading 250-500µg/kg, followed by maintenance infusion 50-100µg/kg per min).

F   Administration of stress doses of glucocorticoids (e.g. hydrocortisone 100mg tds), are advised to support the circulation during thyroid storm.

F   Medications which inhibit thyroid hormone release (e.g. sodium iodide), in addition to those which decrease thyroid hormone synthesis (e.g. propylthiouracil), should be used in the management of thyroid storm.

1.   European Society of Intensive Care Medicine (ESICM). Patient-centered Acute Care Training (PACT). Electrolytes and homeostasis module. http://pact.esicm.org.
2.   Hinds CJ, Watson JD. *Intensive Care: A Concise Textbook*, 3rd ed. Saunders Ltd, 2008: 481-3.

Answer 78: Regarding prone position ventilation: True b & c

F   The PROSEVA study group found improved 28-day mortality (16% prone vs. 32.8% supine [p=0.001]) and 90-day mortality (23.6%

prone and 41% supine [p<0.001]) in severe ARDS (PaO_2/FiO_2 ratio <150mmHg).

T   The prone position improves alveolar recruitment and allows better drainage of chest secretions.

T   With proning a more homogenous ventilation distribution is achieved, due to favourable changes in thoraco-abdominal compliance.

F   Extravascular lung water is reduced following proning.

F   The optimal duration of proning is currently unknown. The PROSEVA study proned patients for at least 16 hours. The average number of proning sessions was 4+/-4 per patient.

1.   Guerin C, Reignier J, Richard JC, et al. Prone positioning in severe acute respiratory distress syndrome. New Engl J Med 2013; 368(2):159-68.

2.   Waldmann C, Soni N, Rhodes A. Oxford Desk Reference Critical Care. Oxford, UK: Oxford University Press, 2008.

3.   Edgcombe H, Carter K, Yarrow S. Anaesthesia in the prone position. Br J Anaesth 2008; 100(2): 165-83.

Answer 79: Hartmann's solution contains: True a & e

T   Hartmann's solution contains: 131mmol/L sodium (Na^+), 5mmol/L potassium (K^+), 2mmol/L calcium, 29mmol/L lactate and 111mmol/L chloride (Cl^-).

F   5mmol/L potassium.

F   Hartmann's contains 111mmol/L chloride (Cl^-), which is less than normal saline (0.9% saline). 0.9% saline contains 154mmol/L of chloride and sodium.

F   Hartmann's contains lactate which is metabolised via pyruvate to glucose in the liver or to carbon dioxide and water in tissues. It does not contain bicarbonate.

T   9kcal of energy is contained in 1L of Hartmann's.

1.   Myburgh JA, Mythen MG. Resuscitation fluids. New Engl J Med 2013; 369: 1243-51.

2.   Waldmann C, Soni N, Rhodes A. Oxford Desk Reference Critical Care. Oxford, UK: Oxford University Press, 2008.

Answer 80: Sedation and delirium in critical care: True b & e

F   Although there is an association with delirium and worse outcomes in the critically ill, no causal relationship has been established. Treatment is broadly empirical as the mechanisms for delirium have yet to be determined. At the present time, evidence that any specific treatment of delirium improves outcome is tenuous.

T   Routine monitoring of sedation level may improve patients' outcomes. Targeted and minimal sedation has been associated with reduced ventilator days and length of stay on the intensive care unit.

F   The Richmond Agitation-Sedation Score (RASS) ranges from -5 to +4, with more negative scores indicating deeper sedation and more positive scores indicating increasing agitation. A score of 0 represents a calm and alert patient. An alternative score is the Riker Sedation-Agitation Scale (SAS) which ranges from 1 to 7, with a score <4 indicating deeper sedation, a score of 4 indicating a calm and co-operative patient and scores of 5 and above indicating increasing agitation. In the critically ill, RASS and SAS are deemed equivocal sedation assessment scales.

F   It is estimated that critical care staff members fail to identify delirium in up to 75% of patients. Two tools in common use in critical care for identifying delirium are the Intensive Care Delirium Screening Checklist (ICDSC) and the Confusion Assessment Method ICU (CAM-ICU). The ICDSC includes signs that can be observed over a period of time. The CAM-ICU tool reports a dichotomous assessment at a single time point.

T   CAM-ICU assess four domains: mental status, inattention, altered level of consciousness using the RASS score and disorganised thinking. 0-2 errors when assessing inattention is deemed CAM-ICU negative. If >2 errors are made then further delirium assessment is undertaken. See the review by Connor *et al* for full details.

1.   Reade MC, Finfer S. Sedation and delirium in the intensive care unit. *New Engl J Med* 2014; 370: 444-54.

2.   Connor D, English W. Delirium in critical care. Anaesthesia Tutorial of the Week 232, 2011. www.aagbi.org/education/educational-resources/tutorial-week.

Answer 81: Nutritional requirements: True b & d

F   The Harris-Benedict equation is used to predict caloric requirements.

T   The estimated daily energy requirement is 25-30kcal/kg/day. This energy requirement may alter depending on clinical state. Indirect calorimetry is the gold standard for assessing individual energy needs, but is frequently unavailable.

F   The typical potassium daily requirement is 0.7-1mmol/kg/day, whereas sodium is 1-2mmol/kg/day.

T   The typical daily carbohydrate requirement is 3-4g/kg/day of which 60% should be glucose in parenteral nutrition. 40% of energy should be provided by lipids. The typical protein requirement is 1-2g/kg/day depending on illness.

F   The typical daily calcium and magnesium requirement is 0.1mmol/kg/day.

1.   Bersten AD, Soni N. *Oh's Intensive Care Manual*, 6th ed. Butterworth Heinemann Elsevier, 2009.

Answer 82: The APACHE II scoring system: True a & c

T   The Acute Physiology And Chronic Health Evaluation II (APACHE II) score is an index of disease severity (0-71 points).

F   There are 12 variables within the Acute Physiology Score: core temperature, mean arterial pressure (MAP), heart rate, respiratory rate, A-a gradient (if $FiO_2 \geq 0.5$) or PaO_2 (if Fio2 <0.5), arterial pH, serum Na^+, serum K^+, serum creatinine, haematocrit, leucocytes and neurological Glasgow Coma Score.

T   In addition to the Acute Physiology Score (APS), there are age points (scored 0-6) and chronic health points (scored 2 or 5).

F   The APACHE II score is derived from the degree of abnormality in the first 24 hours of ICU admission.

F   The APACHE II score has not been validated for use in children.

1.   Bouch DC, Thompson JP. Severity scoring systems in the critically ill. *Contin Educ Anaesth Crit Care Pain* 2008; 8(5): 181-5

2.   Knaus WA, Draper EA, Wagner DP, *et al*. APACHE II: a severity of disease classification system. *Crit Care Med* 1985; 13(10): 818-29.

Answer 83: Vitamins and amino acids: True d & e

F   An essential amino acid is one that cannot be synthesised and must be supplied in the diet. Such amino acids include: histidine, isoleucine, leucine, lysine, methionine, phenylalanine, threonine, tryptophan and valine.

F   Glutamine supplementation in patients requiring parenteral nutrition for longer than 10 days was in the past recommended. However, the recent REDOXS study (Heyland *et al*, 2013) found that patients who were in severe organ failure (shocked state, renal failure), who received high-dose glutamine (0.78g/kg/day) had an increased overall mortality. The SIGNET trial (Andrews *et al*, 2011) showed no benefit of low-dose glutamine (0.1 to 0.2g/kg/day) when given as part of parenteral feeding. Current evidence does not support glutamine supplementation early in critical illness as part of parenteral nutrition and, in particular, in patients with renal failure or two or more organ failure glutamine use may increase mortality.

F   700-900μg is the recommended daily allowance for vitamin C

T   Thiamine deficiency may cause wet or dry beri-beri or lactic acidosis.

T   Staff need to be aware of potential rebound hypoglycaemia on cessation of parenteral nutrition and assess/treat accordingly.

1.   Bersten AD, Soni N. *Oh's Intensive Care Manual*, 6th ed. Butterworth Heinemann Elsevier, 2009.

2.   Heyland D, Muscedere J, Wischmeyer PE, *et al*. A randomised trial of glutamine and antioxidants in critically ill patients. *New Engl J Med* 2013; 368: 1489-7.

3.   Andrews PJ, Avenell A, Noble DW, *et al*. Randomised trial of glutamine, selenium, or both, to supplement parenteral nutrition for critically ill patients. *Br Med J* 2011; 342: d1542.

4.   Caeser MP, Van den Berghe G. Nutrition in the acute phase of critical illness. *New Engl J Med* 2014; 370: 1227-36.

5.   Waldmann C, Soni N, Rhodes A. *Oxford Desk Reference Critical Care*. Oxford, UK: Oxford University Press, 2008.

Answer 84: Magnesium: True a, d and e

T   Magnesium has been used as a tocolytic (suppress premature labour), though the mechanism of action is not clear. Its use in eclampsia and pre-eclampsia is well recognised.

191

F   The British Thoracic Society (BTS) and Scottish Intercollegiate Guidelines Network (SIGN) recommend a dose of 1.2-2g as an intravenous infusion over 20 minutes.

F   Magnesium use has been studied in the treatment of delayed cerebral ischaemia seen in subarachnoid haemorrhage. Inhibition of the release of excitatory amino acids and blockade of the N-methyl-D-aspartate glutamate receptor are possible neuroprotective mechanisms.

T   See explanation above.

T   Torsades de pointes is a distinctive form of polymorphic ventricular tachycardia (VT) characterized by a gradual change in the amplitude and twisting of the QRS complexes around the isoelectric line. It is associated with a prolonged QT interval which can be acquired or congenital. Magnesium is recognised as initial therapy in the acute setting, as it reduces the amplitude of early after-depolarisations (EADs) by blocking calcium inflow and promoting resting repolarisation

1.   Parikh M, Webb ST. Cations: potassium, calcium, and magnesium. *Contin Educ Anaesth Crit Care Pain* 2012; 12(4): 195-8.

2.   Hunter JD, Sharma P, Rathi S. Long QT syndrome. *Contin Educ Anaesth Crit Care Pain* 2008; 8(2): 67-70.

Answer 85: Pulse oximetry: True a & e

T   Beer's law states that the intensity of transmitted light through a substance decreases exponentially as the concentration of the substance increases.

F   The intensity of transmitted light decreases as the distance travelled through a substance increases.

F   There are two light-emitting diodes: red and infrared.

F   Red light has a wavelength of 660nm and infrared 940nm.

T   The isobestic point is used as a reference point where light absorption is independent of saturation. The isobestic points for oxy and deoxyhaemoglobin are 590nm and 805nm.

1.   Waldmann C, Soni N, Rhodes A. *Oxford Desk Reference Critical Care*. Oxford, UK: Oxford University Press, 2008.

Answer 86: Non-invasive ventilation (NIV): True a-d

T   NIV decreases the work of breathing and may aid weaning from mechanical ventilation.

T   Can reduce the need for intubation and hospital morbidity.

T   Failure of NIV is associated with a higher mortality in respiratory failure.

T   The greatest benefit of NIV use is seen in patients with respiratory failure caused by acute COPD exacerbation or cardiogenic pulmonary oedema.

F   Severe respiratory acidosis (<pH 7.25) is not a contraindication for a short trial of NIV (1-2 hours) in a monitored environment, where prompt intubation and ventilation may be undertaken as rescue, if NIV fails. Coexistent severe metabolic with respiratory acidosis, may suggest a mixed aetiology and other organ dysfunction, resulting in a greater incidence of NIV failure.

1.   Waldmann C, Soni N, Rhodes A. *Oxford Desk Reference Critical Care*. Oxford, UK: Oxford University Press, 2008.

2.   McNeil GBS, Glossop AJ. Clinical applications of non-invasive ventilation in critical care. *Contin Educ Anaesth Crit Care Pain* 2012; 12(1): 33-7.

Answer 87: Selection criteria for transplantation in patients with acute liver failure (ALF): True b-e

F   The Clichy criteria and Japanese criteria do not include the cause of acute liver failure in their criteria for liver transplant selection.

T   Age, encephalopathy and coagulopathy are criteria common to all prognostic models e.g. King's College, Clichy and Japanese prognostic models.

T   Contraindications to transplantation include: substance abuse, psychiatric disorders, ongoing suicidal intent, severe sepsis and multi-organ failure.

T   The King's College criteria are the most well-characterised evaluation system. It assesses age, cause, encephalopathy grade, bilirubin level and coagulopathy.

T   The Clichy-Villejuif criteria, or Clichy criteria, are more commonly used in Northern Europe for the assessment of ALF patients for transplantation. It includes severe encephalopathy, age and coagulopathy.

1.   Wang DW, Yin YM, Yao YM. Advances in the management of acute liver failure. *World J Gastroenterol* 2013; 19(41): 7069-77.

2.   Bernal W, Wendon J. Acute liver failure. *New Engl J Med* 2014; 369: 2525-34.

Answer 88: Regarding lactate: All False

F   Glycolysis produces the metabolite pyruvate. In aerobic conditions, pyruvate is converted to acetyl CoA to enter the Krebs cycle. However, under anaerobic conditions pyruvate is converted to lactic acid via the enzyme lactate dehydrogenase (LDH).

F   Normal serum lactate is 0.5-2.2mmol/L.

F   In distributive shock, the pathophysiology is complex and associated hyperlactaemia may be the result of a combination of increased glycolysis, inhibition of lactate dehydrogenase, hypoxia and impaired liver function.

F   Lactic acidosis in the presence of hypoxia is termed Type A hyperlactaemia.

F   Jansen *et al* demonstrated that in patients with septic shock and a blood lactate level >3mmol/L, targeting a decrease of at least 20% over a 2-hour period was associated with a reduction in hospital mortality.

1.   Phypers B, Pierce JMT. Lactate physiology in health and disease. *Contin Educ Anaesth Crit Care Pain* 2006; 6(3): 128-32.

2.   Vincent JL, De Backer D. Circulatory shock. *New Engl J Med* 2013; 369: 1726-34.

3.   Jansen TC, van Bommel J, Schoonderbeek FJ, *et al*. Early lactate-guided therapy in intensive care unit patients: a multicenter, open-label, randomised controlled trial. *Am J Respir Crit Care Med* 2010; 182: 752-61.

4.   Waldmann C, Soni N, Rhodes A. *Oxford Desk Reference Critical Care*. Oxford, UK: Oxford University Press, 2008.

Answer 89: Normal values on an electrocardiogram include: True c

F   A normal PR interval is 0.12 to 0.2 seconds; a shortened PR interval suggests pre-excitation or junctional rhythm.

F   A normal QRS duration is 0.08 to 0.12 seconds; a prolonged QRS duration may be due to electrolyte abnormalities, hypothermia or bundle branch block.

T   The QT interval is measured from the start of the QRS complex to the end of the T-wave

F   This is left axis deviation.

F   The QT interval can be corrected for heart rate using the formula $QTC = QT/\sqrt{RR}$.

1.   Resuscitation Council (UK). Advanced life support, 6th ed. London, UK: Resuscitation Council (UK), 2011. www.resus.org.uk.

Answer 90: Capnography: True b, c & e

F   Phase I reflects anatomical dead space. Phase II is an S-shaped upswing which denotes mixed dead space and alveolar gases.

T   If rebreathing occurs, the baseline of the CO_2 trace will not reach zero. At this point inspired CO_2 can be calculated.

T   Phase III is called the plateau phase and reflects alveolar emptying.

F   There is often a slight upward slope, with the highest point reflecting end-tidal CO_2.

T   This situation is rare. If there is gas in the stomach, for example, if the patient has recently ingested fizzy drinks, this CO_2 may mask accidental oesophageal intubation due to the presence of a short-lived capnography waveform (often up to three waveforms), delaying recognition.

1.   Waldmann C, Soni N, Rhodes A. *Oxford Desk Reference Critical Care*. Oxford, UK: Oxford University Press, 2008.

3 MCQ Paper 3: Questions

Question 1: Differential diagnoses for delayed waking post-general anaesthesia include:

a   Hypoglycaemia.
b   Residual neuromuscular blockade.
c   Electrolyte disturbance.
d   Central cholinergic syndrome.
e   Hypothermia.

Question 2: Hazards of blood transfusion:

a   Patients who receive a blood transfusion have a dose-related increased risk of death.
b   Blood transfusion is associated with a worse outcome in transplant patients.
c   Leucodepletion may increase the risk of transfusion-associated lung injury (TRALI).
d   Transfusion of red cells older than 14 days is not associated with worse peri-operative outcomes.
e   Attention to transfusion rate, fluid balance and diuretic cover may reduce TRALI.

Question 3: In severe necrotising pancreatitis:

a   In the first 7-10 days pancreatic necrosis develops a surrounding fibrous wall.
b   Infected necrosis requires urgent debridement in stable patients.
c   Sterile necrosis is associated with less severe systemic involvement than infected necrosis.
d   Endoscopic debridement of necrotic tissue is preferred to open surgical management.
e   Many patients do not require surgical intervention.

Question 4: Regarding management of arrhythmias:

a   The initial management of supraventricular tachycardia (SVT) should be with intravenous adenosine 12mg.
b   Isoprenaline may be used for complete heart block with broad QRS, whilst awaiting transvenous pacing.
c   Intravenous amiodarone 900mg over 20-60 minutes is recommended in stable regular broad complex tachycardia.
d   Intravenous verapamil 2.5 to 5mg is safe in patients with stable ventricular tachycardia.
e   A potassium plasma concentration of 4 to 5mmol/L should be targeted in patients with cardiac arrhythmias.

Question 5: Hypertonic saline:

a   7.5% sodium chloride contains 1283mmol/L of Na^+.
b   Draws interstitial and intracellular water into the intravascular space.
c   Decreases cerebral swelling and intracranial pressure (ICP).
d   250ml of 7.5% sodium chloride is an inadequate initial resuscitation dose.
e   May cause severe hyponatraemia.

Question 6: Humidification:

a   Absolute humidity is defined as the weight of water vapour contained in a given volume of gas.

b   Relative humidity (RH) is the content of water in air at a specific temperature compared to the capacity of water that air can hold at the same temperature.

c   Gas arriving to the airway from the ventilator has a relative humidity of 10%.

d   The nose can humidify air up to a relative humidity of 60%.

e   Hygroscopic heat and moisture exchangers (HME) filter bacteria.

Question 7: The following are common pathological changes following brainstem death:

a   Severe hypotension.

b   Hyponatraemia.

c   Pulmonary oedema.

d   Thromboembolic events.

e   Metabolic alkalosis.

Question 8: When inserting a chest drain, the following statements are true:

a   The anatomical triangle considered 'safe' is bordered by the latissimus dorsi, pectoralis major and a line superior to the horizontal level of the nipple.

b   A small-bore chest tube, inserted with a Seldinger technique, is inappropriate for the management of a pneumothorax.

c   The administration of prophylactic antibiotics should be considered in trauma patients undergoing chest drain insertion.

d   Chest drain insertion is classically associated with minimal patient discomfort.

e   If suction is required, following chest drain insertion, this may be performed via an underwater seal at a level of 10-20cmH_2O.

Question 9: Heat:

a   The specific heat capacity is the amount of heat needed to raise the temperature of 1kg of a substance by 1°C.

b   The wet and dry bulb hygrometer directly measures relative humidity.

c   As the molar concentration of a solute increases, there is a proportional increase in the boiling point.

d   In the measurement of temperature, thermistors utilise the Seebeck effect.

e   An ultrasonic nebuliser can achieve an absolute humidity of over 100%.

Question 10: Drugs in pregnancy:

a   Ketamine should be avoided in early pregnancy.

b   Suxamethonium readily crosses the placenta.

c   Non-steroidal anti-inflammatory drug (NSAID) use in the third trimester may cause closure of the foramen ovale.

d   Suxamethonium may have a prolonged action in pregnancy.

e   The risk of antiepileptic drugs affecting the foetus are greatest in the first trimester.

Question 11: Biological terrorist attacks:

a   Category A biological weapons are those which can be easily disseminated.

b   A particle size of 0.6-5μm will result in deposition in the alveoli.

c   Anthrax is a Gram-positive, spore-forming coccus.

d   Appropriate treatment of anthrax includes the use of ciprofloxacin and doxycycline.

e   Following pulmonary exposure to anthrax, the incubation period is up to 14 days.

Question 12: Ventilator-associated pneumonia (VAP):

a   The most common pathogens are anaerobic Gram-negative bacilli.

b   The Clinical Pulmonary Infection Score utilises a points system with five categories.

c   Bronchoalveolar lavage (BAL) is more accurate than protected specimen brushings and tracheobronchial aspirates at diagnosing VAP.
d   There is evidence that the presence of C-reactive protein in serum and BAL fluid is a useful biomarker for the presence of VAP.
e   Invasive strategies to diagnose VAP do not alter mortality.

Question 13: Epidural catheters:

a   May be safely inserted 4 hours after a prophylactic dose of subcutaneous low-molecular-weight heparin (LMWH).
b   May be safely removed 4 hours after systemic unfractionated heparin (UFH) is stopped.
c   May be safely inserted 4 hours after a 75mg dose of aspirin.
d   May be safely removed 24 hours after fondaparinux dose.
e   May be performed safely in patients whose international normalised ratio (INR) is less than 1.4.

Question 14: With reference to thromboelastography (TEG):

a   The R value is the time from initiation to fibrin formation.
b   The K value is measured from the beginning of clot formation until the amplitude is equal to 20mm.
c   A maximum amplitude (MA) of <50mm suggests good clot strength.
d   A LY30 time of greater than 7.5% is characteristic of fibrinolysis.
e   The α-angle measures fibrin breakdown.

Question 15: Non-invasive ventilation (continuous positive airway pressure [CPAP]/bilevel positive airway pressure [BiPAP]) is contraindicated in:

a   Coma.
b   Mechanical bowel obstruction.
c   Recent upper GI surgery.
d   Cardiogenic pulmonary oedema.
e   Chest wall trauma.

Question 16: Phaeochromocytoma:

a 20% of cases are malignant.

b Is classically associated with multiple endocrine neoplasia (MEN) Type 1.

c 24-hour urinary collection for catecholamines and metanephrines has a high sensitivity but a low specificity for diagnosis.

d Hyperglycaemia, hypercalcaemia and erythrocytosis are laboratory features.

e In relation to pre-operative preparation for surgical resection of phaeochromocytoma, β-blockade should be instigated prior to α-blockade.

Question 17: Acute adrenocortical insufficiency (Addisonian crisis):

a Usually causes distributive shock.

b Septicaemia-induced Waterhouse-Friderichsen syndrome is not associated.

c Acute steroid withdrawal almost exclusively causes a glucocorticoid deficiency.

d In emergency treatment, the therapeutic use of dexamethasone allows adrenocorticotropic hormone (ACTH) stimulation testing later, without affecting or interfering with the measurement of serum cortisol levels.

e Hypoglycaemia, hypokalaemia and hypernatraemia are characteristic findings.

Question 18: Antimicrobial resistance (AMR):

a AMR is resistance to an antimicrobial where the organism in question was initially sensitive.

b Resistant organisms can include fungi, viruses and parasites in addition to bacteria.

c Misprescribing of antimicrobials can accelerate this natural phenomenon.

d Extended-spectrum β-lactamases (ESBLs) are responsible for a minority of resistant Gram-negative bacteria.

e *Candida krusei* is usually sensitive to fluconazole.

Question 19: Regarding emergency surgery for ruptured abdominal aortic aneurysm (AAA):

a   The law of Laplace is not applicable to aneurysm enlargement.
b   The v-POSSUM score is a useful predictor of patient outcomes.
c   If the clinical situation permits, induction of anaesthesia should occur after the patient is fully prepped and draped.
d   Aggressive fluid resuscitation is paramount.
e   Massive gastrointestinal haemorrhage may occur following rupture of an AAA.

Question 20: Regarding the neonatal circulation:

a   Blood leaves the placenta in a single umbilical vein.
b   The ductus arteriosus shunts umbilical venous blood through the liver.
c   Only one third of blood entering the inferior vena cava (IVC) passes into the right ventricle.
d   Blood returns to the placenta via two umbilical veins.
e   On clamping of the umbilical cord, reversal of the right to left flow through the ductus arteriosus occurs.

Question 21: Pulmonary artery catheters (PAC):

a   The PAC-man trial established a mortality benefit in using PAC.
b   PAC may be used to establish the aetiology of shock states.
c   Mitral valve regurgitation may cause error when using thermodilution to calculate cardiac output via a PAC.
d   The Fick principle is used to calculate cardiac output.
e   The area under the curve on a temperature versus time graph is inversely proportional to the cardiac output.

Question 22: Management of acute ST-elevation myocardial infarction (STEMI):

a   Ticagrelor and aspirin should be given once the diagnosis is made.

b   Primary percutaneous coronary intervention (PCI) is recommended within 90 minutes of first medical contact, if the patient initially arrives at a non-PCI-capable hospital.

c   An injectable anticoagulant should be used (e.g. bivalirudin).

d   Fibrinolytic therapy is recommended within 12 hours of symptom onset if primary PCI cannot be performed.

e   Resolution of ST-segment elevation of less than 50% at 30 minutes is deemed fibrinolysis failure.

Question 23: Complications following obesity surgery include:

a   Dumping syndrome.

b   Cholelithiasis.

c   Pulmonary embolism (PE) and deep vein thrombosis (DVT).

d   Diabetes mellitus.

e   Sepsis.

Question 24: Regarding oxygen delivery in adults:

a   0.0225ml of oxygen for each 1mmHg of partial pressure oxygen is carried in every 100ml of blood.

b   Approximately 250ml/min of oxygen is consumed at rest.

c   Oxygen content of blood is calculated by: [1.34 x Hb x SaO_2] + [0.02 x PaO_2 in kPa].

d   In normal circumstances, oxygen uptake by tissues is approximately 4.5ml of oxygen for every 100ml of blood delivered.

e   1.39ml oxygen per gram of haemoglobin is the directly measured maximum O_2-carrying capacity of blood and is called Hufner's constant.

Question 25: Scoring systems in acute liver disease:

a   The Model for End-stage Liver Disease (MELD) score encompasses age, bilirubin, albumin, international normalised ratio (INR) and creatinine within its model.

b   The Lille score is most accurate for predicting 6-month mortality in patients with alcoholic hepatitis.

c   The Maddrey discriminant function is used in viral hepatitis.

d   A Glasgow Alcoholic Hepatitis score of 9 or above carries a 28-day mortality in excess of 50%.

e   The Child-Pugh score is used for prognosis in acute liver failure.

Question 26: Dexmedetomidine:

a   Is an α2-adrenoceptor antagonist.

b   Is 200 times more specific for α2-receptors compared to α1-receptors.

c   Has no analgesic properties.

d   Is excreted mainly unchanged by the kidney.

e   Can cause hypertension.

Question 27: Management of acute aneurysmal subarachnoid haemorrhage (SAH):

a   Blood pressure should be maintained at less than 160mmHg systolic or 110mmHg mean arterial pressure in the acute setting.

b   Triple H therapy (hypertension, hypervolaemia and haemodilution) has been demonstrated to be beneficial post-aneurysmal SAH.

c   Enteral nimodipine should be started on diagnosis and continued for 21 days.

d   The International Subarachnoid Aneurysm Trial (ISAT) showed that endovascular coiling is associated with better outcomes than surgical clipping.

e   Mortality from acute SAH is approximately 50%.

Question 28: Regarding severe acute adult meningitis:

a   Bacterial seeding of the meninges commonly occurs via haematogenous spread.

b   Fever, headache and neck stiffness form the classic triad of presenting symptoms.

c   Adjuvant dexamethasone therapy reduces mortality and hearing loss, and improves neurological sequelae in acute bacterial meningitis.

d   The use of corticosteroids may predispose to delayed cerebral thrombosis.

e   Moderate hypothermia (32-34°C) is beneficial during initial treatment.

Question 29: Regarding pain:

a   Pain receptors responding to pressure and tissue damage are associated with myelinated C fibre endings.

b   C fibres synapse with cells in the substantia gelatinosa.

c   Transcutaneous electrical nerve stimulation activates Aβ fibres.

d   Ketamine exerts an analgesic effect through agonism at N-methyl-D-aspartate (NMDA) receptors.

e   Opioid receptors are G-protein coupled receptors.

Question 30: During adult cardiopulmonary resuscitation:

a   Drugs should be administered by the tracheal route if intravenous access is not immediately available.

b   Blood products can be delivered via the intraosseous (IO) route.

c   In a shockable rhythm, intravenous amiodarone 300mg should be delivered after the third shock.

d   The correct dose of atropine for the treatment of asystole or pulseless electrical activity is 3mg.

e   During defibrillation, current flow is directly proportional to transthoracic impedance.

Question 31: Pathophysiology of sepsis:

a   The pathophysiology of bacterial sepsis initiated by Gram-positive organisms involves lipopolysaccharides.

b   Interleukin 1, 2 and 6 have pro-inflammatory properties.

c   Cytokines increase the expression of enzyme-inducible nitric oxide synthase in endothelial cells.

d   Tumour necrosis factor causes cardiovascular insufficiency through a direct myocardial depressant effect.

e   A thromboelastogram from a patient with severe sepsis may show a reduced maximum amplitude.

Question 32: Haematological malignancies and critical care:

a   Granulocyte colony-stimulating factor (GCSF) may be used to promote lymphocyte recovery following bone marrow transplant (BMT).

b   The incidence of graft versus host disease (GVHD) increases with increasing age of donor and recipient.

c   Acute GVHD is graded from I to IV.

d   Cytokines do not play a role in the manifestations of graft versus host disease.

e   Respiratory failure is the commonest cause of death in patients undergoing bone marrow transplant.

Question 33: Following burn injury:

a   Cardiac output is immediately reduced.

b   Oedema formation is largely complete after 24 hours.

c   There is an immediate increase in metabolic rate.

d   Drugs which are renally excreted will accumulate.

e   The free fraction of benzodiazepines in plasma will increase.

Question 34: *Clostridium difficile*:

a   Risk factors include age >60 years and previous use of broad-spectrum antibiotics.

b   The use of intravenous vancomycin is warranted if oral or intravenous metronidazole is ineffective.

c   Diagnosis is confirmed by stool culture.

d   There is evidence for the use of probiotics to prevent *Clostridium difficile*-associated diarrhoea.

e   Is a Gram-positive, spore-forming, anaerobic, toxin-producing bacteria.

Question 35: Peripartum cardiomyopathy (PPCM):

a   PPCM resembles that of a dilated cardiomyopathy.

b   The ejection fraction is often less than 45%.

c   PPCM can present at any point during pregnancy.

d   Appropriate initial management of acute heart failure due to PPCM could include oxygen, non-invasive ventilation (NIV), intravenous furosemide and intravenous nitroglycerine.

e   PPCM resulting in dependence on inotropic agents and/or an intra-aortic balloon pump, would be appropriate indications for a left ventricular assist device (LVAD) consideration.

Question 36: In relation to medical statistics, and Type II errors:

a   A Type II error is the erroneous conclusion from a study that an intervention has no effect.

b   A Type II error may also be referred to as a false positive.

c   Type II errors may also be referred to as β-errors.

d   Type II errors often arise due to the underpowering of studies.

e   A Type II error occurs when a study concludes that an intervention has a significant effect when in fact it occurs due to chance.

Question 37: In relation to extracorporeal membrane oxygenation (ECMO):

a   Veno-arterial ECMO (VA ECMO) drains blood from the right atrium and returns it to a large vein.

b   Veno-venous ECMO (VV ECMO) is preferred to VA ECMO in the treatment of respiratory failure as normal pulmonary blood flow is maintained.

c   An ECMO circuit consists of a drainage cannula, pump, oxygenator, and an arterial-return cannula.

d   Haematology support is vital for the running of an ECMO service.

e   The well-publicised CESAR trial showed no benefit of ECMO in adults.

Question 38: Following liver transplantation:

a   'Small for size syndrome' is a consequence of portal hyperaemia.

b   Early anticoagulation is contraindicated.

c   Patients should be ventilated for at least 6 hours postoperatively.

d   Treatment strategies including inhaled nitric oxide and intravenous prostacyclin may be required.

e   An intra-abdominal pressure (IAP) of 12mmHg is abnormal.

Question 39: Appropriate treatments in the management of poisoning are:

a   Selective serotonin reuptake inhibitor (SSRI) overdose — benzodiazepines.

b   Iron overdose — multiple-dose activated charcoal.

c   Verapamil overdose — insulin.

d   Lithium overdose — haemodialysis.

e   Organophosphate overdose — atropine.

Question 40: In the management of traumatic brain injury (TBI):

a   There is level I evidence to support a cerebral perfusion pressure of ≥70mmHg.

b   Intracranial pressure should be monitored in all salvageable patients with a severe TBI and abnormal CT scan.

c   An appropriate initial dose of mannitol for the control of raised intracranial pressure in a 70kg male is 175ml of 20% mannitol.

d   Abnormalities in serum potassium are associated with induction and cessation of thiopentone barbiturate coma.

e   Therapeutic hypothermia has been shown to confer benefit in patients with traumatic brain injury.

Question 41: The following may cause a raised mean corpuscular volume (MCV) without anaemia on full blood count analysis (FBC):

a   Chronic alcohol excess.

b   Chronic obstructive pulmonary disease (COPD).

c   Methotrexate therapy.

d   Phenytoin therapy.

e   Hypothyroidism.

Question 42: Human albumin solution (HAS):

a   Is derived from plasma from one donor.

b   4.5% HAS is hyperoncotic.

c   20% HAS is mildly hypotonic.

d   Improved outcomes in critical care have been found with the use of HAS compared to saline.

e   May have an outcome benefit when used post-ascitic drainage.

Question 43: In relation to an empyema, the following statements are true:

a   Empyemas are predominantly caused by anaerobic bacteria.

b   An empyema tends to form 7 to 14 days after the onset of pneumonia.
c   An empyema with a pH of less than 7.4 requires urgent drainage.
d   Organised and loculated collections are best treated with intercostal drainage and antibiotics.
e   An empyema will often have a reduced lactate dehydrogenase (LDH) level (<1000IU/L) on fluid analysis.

Question 44: Acute tubulo-interstitial nephritis:
a   Most acute tubulo-interstitial nephritides are caused by hypersensitivity reactions to drugs rather than by direct toxicity.
b   Rifampicin is amongst the frequently implicated agents.
c   ACE-inhibitors are amongst the frequently implicated agents.
d   The absence of a rash is useful in excluding acute allergic interstitial nephritis.
e   Acute tubulo-interstitial nephritis caused by non-steroidal anti-inflammatory drugs (NSAIDs) may present with nephrotic syndrome.

Question 45: Sodium:
a   Sodium is the principal anion of the extracellular fluid (ECF).
b   The amount of total sodium (mmol) in the extracellular compartment exceeds that in the intracellular compartment.
c   A complication of hypertonic saline (3%) therapy is osmotic demyelination syndrome.
d   Hypernatraemia is always associated with hyperosmolality.
e   Factitious hyponatraemia may be associated with hyperlipidaemia.

Question 46: Regarding suxamethonium apnoea:
a   Plasma cholinesterase (pseudocholinesterase) reduces suxamethonium to succinyl monocholine and choline.
b   It may be worsened by ketamine use.
c   Inherited cholinesterase deficiency is associated with abnormal sex-linked recessive genes.
d   Treatment includes administration of dantrolene.
e   Halothane and caffeine are used to diagnose susceptibility.

Question 47: Regarding the diaphragmatic foramina:

a   The inferior vena cava (IVC) passes through the diaphragm at the level of T10.

b   The right phrenic nerve pierces the dome of the diaphragm.

c   The thoracic duct passes through at the level of T12.

d   The azygos vein and vagi pass through at T8.

e   The oesophagus passes through the diaphragm to the left of the midline at the level of T8.

Question 48: Macrophage activation syndrome (MAS):

a   Pancytopenia, liver failure, coagulopathy and multi-organ failure may be seen.

b   Is due to uncontrolled proliferation of CD8 lymphocytes and well-differentiated macrophages.

c   High serum ferritin levels are often seen.

d   MAS often causes a cytokine storm.

e   High-dose steroid therapy is contraindicated.

Question 49: Acute pancreatitis:

a   The Atlanta definition of 2013 describes two categories of severity (mild and severe).

b   Serum triglyceride should be obtained in the absence of gallstones and alcohol history.

c   Serum amylase is always raised in alcohol-induced acute pancreatitis.

d   Predictive scoring systems such as the Glasgow score and Bedside Index for Severity in Acute Pancreatitis (BISAP) are of limited prognostic value.

e   Corticosteroids should be given as part of acute management.

Question 50: The following are normal right heart pressures on pulmonary artery catheter (PAC) insertion:

a   Mean right atrial pressure of 0-7mmHg.

b   Right ventricular pressure of 15-25mmHg systolic and 0-8mmHg diastolic.

c   Mean pulmonary artery pressure of 25-35mmHg.

d   Mean pulmonary capillary wedge pressure (PCWP) of 6-12mmHg.

e   Pulmonary artery systolic pressure of 35-45mmHg.

Question 51: Considering jaundice:

a   It is clinically detectable when serum bilirubin exceeds 20µmol/L.

b   Sepsis can be a cause of prehepatic jaundice.

c   Unconjugated bilirubin appears in the urine.

d   May occur following an episode of hypotension on critical care.

e   Stools are often pale and urine dark in biliary obstruction.

Question 52: Oesophageal Doppler:

a   Peak velocity is a good estimate of myocardial contractility.

b   By age 70 peak velocity falls to less than 50cm/second.

c   Stroke distance (SD) is the area under the velocity-time curve and provides an estimate of stroke volume.

d   An increase in stroke volume of less than 5-10% with a fluid bolus suggests hypovolaemia.

e   A corrected flow time (FTc) greater than 400ms is due to hypovolaemia.

Question 53: Calcium channel blocker overdose:

a   Overdose of sustained release preparations may benefit from gastric decontamination even if given later than 1 hour post-ingestion.

b   May cause hypercalcaemia.

c   Symptomatic bradycardia does not respond to atropine.

d   Insulin and dextrose may be used in severe refractory hypotension.

e   Intralipid® 20% (1.5ml/kg) should be considered in the presence of unresponsive cardiotoxicity.

Question 54: The following are recognised effects of medication toxicity:

a   Nystagmus, ataxia and tremor with lithium.
b   Cyanosis with metoclopromide.
c   Serotonin syndrome development and nefopam.
d   Hyperadrenergic crisis with white wine in patients taking moclobemide.
e   Hypoglycaemia and metformin overdose.

Question 55: Management of a donation after brainstem death (DBD) organ donor:

a   DBD donors are more likely to donate multiple transplantable organs.
b   The most common physiological derangement in DBD donors is diabetes insipidus.
c   The incidence of donor loss before retrieval due to cardiovascular instability may be as high as 2%.
d   Thromboprophylaxis should be maintained.
e   Methylprednisolone (15mg/kg) use is associated with increased organ retrieval.

Question 56: Neonatal and paediatric intensive care:

a   In cold septic shock, noradrenaline use is recommended.
b   In persistent catecholamine-resistant shock, it is important to rule out and correct intra-abdominal pressures >12mmHg.
c   Tight glycaemic control in critically ill children improves clinical outcomes.
d   A restrictive blood transfusion policy (transfusion threshold haemoglobin level of 80g/L) is safe in patients with non-cyanotic congenital heart defects, undergoing elective cardiac surgery.
e   Targeting O_2 saturation levels below 90% in extremely preterm infants is associated with an increased risk of death.

Question 57: Signs of spinal cord injury (SCI) in the unconscious patient include:

a   Flaccid areflexia in the arms and/or legs.

b   Elbow flexion with inability to extend.
c   Unexplained tachycardia and hypertension.
d   Priapism.
e   Pain response below the suspected level of injury.

Question 58: Regarding pulmonary artery catheter (PAC) insertion via the internal jugular vein:

a   The distance to a right atrial trace from insertion is approximately 15-20cm.
b   The PAC balloon should be inflated once in the pulmonary artery.
c   The distance from insertion to a right ventricular (RV) pressure trace is approximately 40cm.
d   The distance from insertion to a pulmonary artery waveform is approximately 35-50cm.
e   The balloon should always be deflated before withdrawing the catheter.

Question 59: Regarding the mechanism of action of anticoagulant drugs:

a   Vitamin A is antagonised by warfarin.
b   Heparin inhibits anti-thrombin III, a protease inhibitor.
c   Low-molecular-weight heparins (LMWHs) act predominantly through inhibition of Factor Xa.
d   Danaparoid inhibits Factors Xa and IIa.
e   Rivaroxaban is a direct thrombin inhibitor.

Question 60: Regarding gastrointestinal (GI) perforation:

a   Boerhaave syndrome is a cause of upper gastrointestinal perforation.
b   Free gas under the diaphragm on chest X-ray is only present in 50% of cases of intraperitoneal perforation.
c   Peritonism may be absent in patients taking corticosteroids.
d   Colonic distension in pseudomembranous colitis may be decompressed with colonoscopy to prevent perforation.
e   The degree of sepsis seen post-GI perforation is dependent on anatomical location.

Question 61: Regarding the storage of blood products:

a   The addition of saline, adenine, glucose and phosphate enables packed red cells to be stored for 35 days.

b   Platelets are stored at 5°C and agitated.

c   ABO-incompatible platelets may be used in adults.

d   Fresh frozen plasma (FFP) is stored at -30°C.

e   Cryoprecipitate is prepared from a single donation and may be stored for up to 12 months.

Question 62: Spinal cord anatomy:

a   The posterior columns transmit pain and temperature sensation.

b   The spinothalamic tract conveys proprioception.

c   The spinal cord is attached to the coccyx by the filum terminale.

d   The solid spinal cord ends at L1/L2 in adults.

e   The arteria radicularis magna supplies the lower two thirds of the spinal cord.

Question 63: Causes of right ventricle (RV) failure include:

a   Acute pulmonary embolus.

b   Protamine.

c   Extensive lung resection.

d   Acute respiratory distress syndrome (ARDS).

e   Obstructive sleep apnoea.

Question 64: Liver function test abnormalities:

a   Albumin is a useful marker of synthetic liver function in the critically ill.

b   Aspartate aminotransferase (AST) is more specific for liver injury than alanine aminotransferase (ALT).

c   AST is the primary enzyme raised in cholestatic liver disease.

d   The normal range for serum ammonia is 15-45µg/dl.

e   Prothrombin time (PT) is indirectly a sensitive test of liver synthetic function.

Question 65: Regarding noradrenaline (norepinephrine):

a   Dose range is 0.1 to 2.0mg/kg/min.
b   Predominantly acts at α1-adrenergic receptors.
c   Is recommended as a first-line vasopressor in septic shock.
d   Up to 25% of noradrenaline is metabolised by the lungs.
e   Low-dose vasopressin compared to noradrenaline reduces mortality in septic shock.

Question 66: Acute intracerebral haemorrhage (ICH):

a   ICH accounts for 10-30% of all strokes.
b   Haematoma expansion of greater than 33% of original volume may occur shortly after onset of ICH.
c   Intensive lowering of blood pressure (SBP less than 140mmHg within 1 hour) improves mortality and severe disability.
d   Human prothrombin complex is indicated in those taking warfarin.
e   Early surgery should be undertaken in all patients with spontaneous superficial ICH without intraventricular haemorrhage.

Question 67: Considering salicylate poisoning:

a   Gastric lavage should be considered within 2 hours of ingestion.
b   Acidosis increases renal excretion.
c   In severe overdose, a normal anion gap may be attributed to a falsely high sodium concentration.
d   Tablet bezoars may significantly delay absorption and systemic effects.
e   Loss of hyperventilatory drive at intubation may precipitate deterioration and death.

Question 68: Physiology of pregnancy:

a   The plasma volume increases by 45%.
b   At term, the vena cava is completely occluded in 90% of supine pregnant patients.
c   Uterine blood flow at term is 20% of cardiac output.
d   Cardiac output is increased by 30% by the third trimester.
e   Functional residual capacity (FRC) decreases by up to 10%.

Question 69: In relation to the transplanted heart:

a   The Valsalva manoeuvre will not affect heart rate.
b   Volume loading will result in increased contractility.
c   There is a normal response to hypovolaemia and hypotension.
d   Adenosine is an appropriate first-line therapeutic treatment for supraventricular tachycardia.
e   Amiodarone and lidocaine are effective for the treatment of ventricular arrhythmias.

Question 70: The focused assessment with sonography in trauma (FAST) scan:

a   Is a five-view scan.
b   Will detect more than 100-250ml of free fluid.
c   Will reliably detect retroperitoneal haematoma.
d   Is capable of detecting gross injury to solid organs.
e   When selecting a transducer, increasing the frequency of the scan head reduces the depth accuracy of the image.

Question 71: High-frequency ventilation (HFV):

a   When compared to HFV, tidal volume must exceed dead space for effective ventilation during conventional ventilation.
b   During HFV, tidal volumes are near to or less than anatomical dead space.
c   Pendelluft is the principal mechanism of gas transport in HFV.
d   Taylor dispersion is the exchange of gas between adjacent lung units due to differing time constants.
e   Molecular diffusion is not important in HFV.

Question 72: Indications for extracorporeal membrane oxygenation (ECMO) include:

a   Cardiac failure/acute cardiogenic shock.
b   Severe pulmonary fibrosis.
c   Resuscitation/cardiorespiratory arrest.
d   Primary graft failure following heart or lung transplant.
e   To aid organ donation after circulatory death (DCD).

Question 73: 0.9% saline:

a   Contains the same sodium (Na^+) concentration as plasma.

b   Is isotonic.

c   Compared to chloride-restrictive fluid (e.g. Plasma-Lyte® or Hartmann's), the use of 0.9% saline is associated with a reduced renal replacement therapy need and reduced incidence of postoperative infection.

d   Can produce a hypochloraemic metabolic acidosis.

e   May cause abdominal discomfort.

Question 74: Potassium:

a   The vast majority of potassium stored within the human body is in the intracellular fluid, with skeletal muscle being the principal reservoir.

b   Hyperkalaemia is exacerbated in the alkalotic state.

c   Less than 50% of the potassium absorbed by the body is excreted by the kidneys.

d   β2-adrenergic agents augment activity at the Na^+/K^+-ATPase pump.

e   The enzyme sodium-potassium adenosine triphosphatase (Na^+/K^+-ATPase) pumps two potassium ions into the cell in exchange for three sodium ions pumped out.

Question 75: Contrast-induced nephropathy (CIN):

a   Prevalence studies have shown that CIN is the third commonest cause of hospital-acquired acute renal failure.

b   The volume of contrast used is not a risk factor for the development of CIN.

c   Regarding hydration strategies in preventing CIN, bicarbonate solutions may be more effective than saline.

d   In fluid restricted patients at risk of CIN, oral theophylline has been proposed as a management strategy.

e   Periprocedural prophylactic continuous veno-venous haemofiltration (CVVH) may be associated with a significant decrease in the number of patients with chronic renal failure developing CIN when exposed to contrast.

Question 76: Heart-lung interactions:

a   Lung underinflation and hyperinflation increase pulmonary vascular resistance.

b   Spontaneous inspiration increases intrathoracic pressure.

c   Artificial ventilatory inspiration increases intrathoracic pressure.

d   Lung inflation alters autonomic tone.

e   Spontaneous ventilatory effort against resistive or elastic load, decreases left ventricular stroke volume and manifests as pulsus paradoxus.

Question 77: Regarding the cranial nerves (CN):

a   The trochlear nerve provides motor supply to the superior rectus muscle.

b   Sensory nerve supply to the face, nose and mouth is supplied by the facial nerve.

c   Pathology associated with the internal carotid artery may present with a third cranial nerve (III) palsy.

d   Sensation to the anterior one third of the tongue is supplied by the glossopharyngeal nerve.

e   The optic nerve innervates the sphincter pupillae and ciliary muscles.

Question 78: Considering atrial fibrillation (AF):

a   AF affects approximately 1.5 to 2% of the general population.

b   The presence of AF is associated with a three-fold increase in the risk of stroke.

c   Vernakalant has been demonstrated to be superior to amiodarone in restoring sinus rhythm in stable patients.

d   Left atrial ablation is a reasonable first-line therapy in selected patients with paroxysmal AF and no structural heart disease.

e   Dronedarone should not be given to AF patients with moderate or severe heart failure.

Question 79: Acute acalculous cholecystitis (AAC):

a   Is inflammation of the gallbladder in the presence of gallstones.

b   Is most common in women after trauma or surgery.

c   Serial ultrasound surveillance for AAC should be considered in trauma patients with a high Injury Severity Score.

d   Cholecystectomy should be undertaken in AAC caused by anti-phospholipid syndrome and systemic lupus erythematosus (SLE).

e   Mortality of untreated AAC is low.

Question 80: Renal replacement therapy (RRT) may be used in the overdose management of:

a   Amitriptyline.

b   Aspirin.

c   Lithium.

d   Diltiazem.

e   Metformin.

Question 81: Concerning corrected flow time (FTc) measured by oesophageal Doppler:

a   An FTc less than 330ms may be due to excessive metaraminol use.

b   An FTc of up to 400ms may be normal in anaesthetised patients.

c   A normal FTc is 230 to 260ms.

d   A low peak velocity and FTc less than 330ms may be due to increased preload.

e   Goal-directed therapy using oesophageal Doppler protocols may improve outcomes for surgical patients.

Question 82: Acute ischaemic stroke (AIS):

a   Aspirin and clopidogrel in combination following minor AIS or transient ischaemic attack is not superior to aspirin treatment alone.

b   Statin therapy should be started immediately following AIS.

c   Patients presenting within 4.5 hours of onset of AIS should be considered for thrombolysis with intravenous tissue-type plasminogen activator (tPA).

d   Decompressive craniectomy may improve the outcome in patients with malignant middle cerebral artery (MCA) infarction.

e   Tight glycaemic control (glucose of 4-8mmol/L) is recommended post-AIS.

Question 83: Regarding spinal cord syndromes:

a   Damage or obstruction to the artery of Adamkiewicz may result in a central cord syndrome.

b   Conus medullaris syndrome produces extensive upper and lower motor neuron paralysis in the lower limbs.

c   Brown-Sequard syndrome typically affects the upper limbs more than the lower limbs.

d   Anterior cord syndrome typically presents with complete loss of sensation and motor function below the level of the lesion.

e   Cauda equina syndrome may present with saddle anaesthesia and bladder/bowel dysfunction.

Question 84: Starch-based intravenous fluids:

a   Are derived from bovine collagen.

b   Have the lowest risk of anaphylactoid reactions compared to other colloid fluids.

c   Are safe in critical care patients.

d   Are associated with an increased need for dialysis in the critically ill.

e   Itch occurs in up to 13% of patients receiving starch-based intravenous fluids.

Question 85: Regarding postoperative management following liver resection:

a   Up to 30% of liver resection patients will have a significant complication.

b   Ascites may cause hypovolaemia in the first 48 hours.

c   Persistent elevation in hepatic transaminases is common.

d   Paracetamol may be given in the first 48 hours postoperatively.

e   Hyperphosphataemia may indicate liver regeneration.

Question 86: Ventilator-induced lung injury (VILI):

a   Gross barotrauma manifesting as pneumothorax is a frequent complication of mechanical ventilation.

b   Atelectrauma occurs due to direct injury to the alveoli from over-distension.

c   Biotrauma occurs due to shearing injury to the alveoli, caused by repetitive collapse and opening.
d   Development of extra-alveolar air due to perivascular alveoli disruption is thought to be an initial mechanism of barotrauma.
e   Biotrauma in the lung increases leucocytes, tumour necrosis factor (TNF), Il-6 and Il-8 release.

Question 87: Regarding hepatic encephalopathy:
a   The West Haven system divides hepatic encephalopathy into five grades.
b   Only complicates acute liver failure.
c   Hyperammonaemia plays a critical role in pathogenesis.
d   Lactulose 30-60ml orally or via a nasogastric tube is recommended.
e   Rifaximin is licenced for prophylaxis.

Question 88: A pneumothorax:
a   Is more common in females than in males.
b   Always requires treatment with an intercostal drain.
c   When under tension will cause tracheal deviation towards the affected side.
d   May occur as a complication of tracheostomy insertion.
e   Is more common in smokers than non-smokers.

Question 89: Electrocution and radiation injuries:
a   Tetanic contractions of skeletal muscle occur with currents in excess of 15-20amps.
b   A current flow across the chest of 100mA can cause ventricular fibrillation.
c   Micro-shock can occur in the presence of a saline-filled central venous catheter, due to low current density at the heart.
d   One gray is the absorption of one joule of energy in the form of ionising radiation per kilogram of matter.
e   With regards to the effects of high-dose radiation, an exposure dose of one gray will result in a change in blood count.

Question 90: In relation to tracheostomy:

a   Haemorrhage from the innominate vessels is an early complication of insertion.

b   It is recommended that the first routine tracheostomy change be performed at day 3 after percutaneous tracheostomy.

c   Ultrasound scanning of the neck prior to percutaneous tracheostomy is mandatory.

d   Early tracheostomy improves long-term outcomes and reduces length of ICU stay.

e   Surgical tracheostomies are more cost-effective and result in fewer complications, when compared to the percutaneous route in ICU patients.

Answer overview: Paper 3

Question:	a	b	c	d	e		Question:	a	b	c	d	e
1	T	T	T	T	T		46	F	T	F	F	F
2	T	F	F	F	F		47	F	F	T	F	F
3	F	F	F	T	T		48	T	T	T	T	F
4	F	T	F	F	T		49	F	T	F	T	F
5	T	T	T	F	F		50	T	T	F	T	F
6	T	T	F	F	F		51	F	T	F	T	T
7	T	F	T	F	F		52	T	F	T	F	F
8	T	F	T	F	T		53	T	F	F	T	T
9	T	F	T	F	F		54	T	T	F	F	F
10	T	F	F	T	T		55	T	F	T	T	T
11	T	T	F	T	F		56	F	T	F	T	T
12	F	T	F	F	T		57	T	T	F	T	F
13	F	T	T	F	T		58	T	F	F	T	T
14	T	T	F	T	F		59	F	F	T	T	F
15	T	T	F	F	F		60	T	F	T	F	T
16	F	F	F	T	F		61	F	F	T	F	T
17	T	F	T	T	F		62	F	F	T	T	T
18	T	T	T	F	F		63	T	T	T	T	T
19	F	F	T	F	T		64	F	F	F	T	T
20	T	F	T	F	T		65	F	T	T	T	F
21	F	T	F	F	T		66	T	T	F	T	F
22	T	F	T	T	F		67	F	F	F	T	T
23	T	T	T	F	T		68	T	T	T	F	F
24	F	T	T	T	F		69	T	T	F	F	T
25	F	T	F	T	F		70	F	T	F	T	T
26	F	F	F	F	T		71	T	T	F	F	F
27	T	F	T	T	T		72	T	F	T	T	T
28	T	T	F	T	F		73	F	T	F	F	T
29	F	T	T	F	T		74	T	F	F	T	T
30	F	T	T	F	F		75	T	F	T	T	T
31	F	T	T	T	T		76	T	F	T	T	T
32	F	T	T	F	T		77	F	F	F	F	F
33	T	T	F	F	T		78	T	F	T	T	T
34	T	F	F	T	T		79	F	F	T	F	F
35	T	T	F	T	T		80	F	T	T	F	T
36	T	F	T	T	F		81	T	T	F	F	T
37	F	T	T	T	F		82	F	F	T	T	F
38	T	F	F	T	T		83	F	T	F	F	T
39	T	F	T	T	T		84	F	F	F	T	T
40	F	T	T	T	T		85	T	T	F	F	F
41	T	T	T	T	T		86	T	F	F	T	T
42	F	F	T	F	T		87	T	F	T	T	F
43	T	T	F	F	F		88	F	F	F	T	T
44	T	T	F	F	T		89	F	T	T	T	T
45	F	T	T	T	T		90	F	F	F	F	F

225

3 MCQ Paper 3: Answers

Answer 1: Differential diagnoses for delayed waking post-general anaesthesia include: All True

T   Delayed awakening — defined as failure to respond within 60 minutes after the cessation of anaesthesia or altered mental state post-anaesthesia — has a large differential list. Hypoglycaemia is a common but potentially serious cause that should be considered early.

T   Postoperative residual neuromuscular blockade occurs frequently and is often undiagnosed. A degree of neuromuscular blockade may persist despite return of the train of four. Hypothermia, administration of magnesium, delayed effects of neostigmine, and gentamicin use may all result in prolonged neuromuscular blockade and delayed recovery.

T   Hyponatraemia and hypercalcaemia may cause altered mental state and delayed recovery post-anaesthesia.

T   Central cholinergic syndrome is rare but may occur and delay recovery post-anaesthesia. Physostigmine 0.5mg intravenously should be considered if this syndrome is suspected.

T   Hypothermia, acidaemia, cerebrovascular events, seizures and infection are other common causes of delayed waking post-general anaesthesia.

1.   Ruskin KJ, Rosenbaum SH. *Anaesthesia Emergencies*. Oxford, UK: Oxford University Press, 2011: Chapter 10.

2.   Lobaz S, Sammut M, Damodaran A. Sugammadex rescue following prolonged rocuronium neuromuscular blockade with 'recurarisation' in a patient with severe renal failure. *Br Med J Case Reports* 2013; doi:10.1136/bcr-2012-007603.

Answer 2: Hazards of blood transfusion: True a

T   Blood transfusion is associated with an increased risk of death, infection, length of critical care stay, organ dysfunction and hospital stay. The cause of this association is unclear, but anaemia in part is a marker of disease severity.

F   The immunomodulatory effects of blood transfusion are well described and may be associated with better outcomes in renal, cardiac and liver transplantation. Worse outcomes may be seen in patients with cancer, with an associated increased incidence of cancer recurrence, peri-operative infection and metastatic spread of primary tumours following blood transfusion.

F   TRALI is a new acute lung injury characterised by acute dsypnoea with hypoxia and bilateral pulmonary infiltrates, with non-cardiogenic pulmonary oedema occurring within 6 hours of transfusion. The use of leucodepleted fresh frozen plasma (FFP), FFP from male donors only, pooled plasma donations (to dilute any antibodies present) and screening and subsequent exclusion of donors who are at high risk of having anti-leucocyte antigen antibodies, are all strategies that have been employed to reduce TRALI incidence.

F   Transfusion of older red cells (>14 days) is associated with an increased risk of postoperative complications and reduction in survival compared to fresher red cells (<14 days). This may be related to storage lesions that reduce structural and functional characteristics of red cells.

F   Transfusion-associated circulatory overload (TACO) often presents with acute respiratory distress, pulmonary oedema, tachycardia, increased blood pressure and evidence of positive fluid balance after transfusion. Tight fluid balance and diuresis may prevent its development. The pathogenesis of TACO is different to that of TRALI, which cannot be prevented by such measures.

1.   Clevenger B, Kelleher A. Hazards of blood transfusion in adults and children. *Contin Educ Anaesth Crit Care Pain* 2013; 14(3): 112-8.

Answer 3: In severe necrotising pancreatitis: True d & e

F   Within the first 7-10 days pancreatic necrosis is seen as a diffuse semi-solid inflammatory mass with no obvious demarcation. A fibrous organising wall around necrotic areas tends to develop 4 weeks after the initial onset of disease and as such necrotic pancreatic tissue is more amenable to intervention after this time.

F   Unstable patients with infected necrosis should be considered for urgent debridement. However, in stable patients, antibiotics should be given first with consideration for delayed minimally invasive necrosectomy, preferably performed at least 4 weeks after the onset of disease. Delayed intervention is associated with better morbidity and mortality.

F   Systemic effects and multi-organ failure may be equally severe with sterile necrosis and infected pancreatic necrosis.

T   Minimally invasive endoscopic management is superior to open surgical necrosectomy, as it is associated with less morbidity (less multiple organ failure and surgical complications) and cost.

T   Many patients with either sterile pancreatitis or, to a lesser extent, infected necrosis, do not require surgical intervention and recover with supportive therapy alone.

1.   Tenner S, Baillie J, DeWitt J, *et al*. American College of Gastroenterology Guideline: management of acute pancreatitis. *Am J Gastroenterol* 2013; 108(9): 1400-15.

2.   Bakker OJ, van Santvoort HC, van Brunschot S, *et al*. Endoscopic transgastric vs. surgical necrosectomy for infected necrotising pancreatitis, a randomised controlled trial. *JAMA* 2012; 307: 1053-61.

Answer 4: Regarding management of arrhythmias: True b & e

F   The acute management of regular narrow complex tachycardias (QRS <0.12sec), such as SVT, is with vagal manoeuvres, followed by an intravenous bolus of adenosine 6mg. Two further doses of adenosine 12mg may be given for resistant SVT. If adenosine is contraindicated, intravenous verapamil 2.5 to 5mg may be considered.

T   Several agents may be used as an interim measure in severe bradycardia whilst transcutaneous or transvenous pacing is arranged, including atropine, glycopyrrolate, isoprenaline and adrenaline.

F   Intravenous amiodarone 300mg over 20-60 minutes followed by 900mg over 24 hours is recommended in patients with stable, regular broad complex tachycardias such as ventricular tachycardia with a pulse.

F   Verapamil should be avoided in ventricular tachycardia (VT) or hypotensive patients with left ventricular dysfunction, as it may cause profound hypotension.

T   In patients with arrhythmias, it is advisable to target serum potassium of 4 to 5mmol/L to minimise the destabilising effect of hypokalaemia and hyperkalaemia on myocardial cell action potentials.

1.   Beed M, Sherman R, Mahajan R. *Emergencies in Critical Care*, 2nd ed. Oxford, UK: Oxford Medical Publications, 2013.

2.   Resuscitation Council (UK). Advanced life support, 6th ed. London, UK: Resuscitation Council (UK), 2011. www.resus.org.uk.

Answer 5: Hypertonic saline: True a-c

T   7.5% sodium chloride contains 1283mmol/L of Na⁺.

T   Hypertonic saline draws interstitial and intracellular water into the intravascular space.

T   Hypertonic saline can decrease cerebral swelling and ICP.

F   Small volumes of hypertonic fluids, for example, 250ml of 7.5% sodium chloride, may be adequate for initial resuscitation doses.

F   May cause severe hypernatraemia.

1.   Waldmann C, Soni N, Rhodes A. *Oxford Desk Reference Critical Care*. Oxford, UK: Oxford University Press, 2008.

2.   Myburgh JA, Mythen MG. Resuscitation fluids. *New Engl J Med* 2013; 369: 1243-51.

Answer 6: Humidification: True a & b

T   Absolute humidity is defined as the weight of water vapour contained in a given volume of gas.

T   Relative humidity (RH) is the content of water in air at a specific temperature compared to the capacity of water that air can hold at the same temperature.

F   If there is no humidification, the gas arriving to the airway from the ventilator will be cold and dry, with a relative humidity of approximately 2%.

F   The nose can humidify air up to a relative humidity of 80%.

F   Hydrophobic HMEs can filter bacteria.

1.   Wilkes AR. Humidification: its importance and delivery. *Contin Educ Anaesth Crit Care Pain* 2001; 1(2): 40-3.

2.   Waldmann C, Soni N, Rhodes A. *Oxford Desk Reference Critical Care*. Oxford, UK: Oxford University Press, 2008.

3.   Wilkes, AR. Heat and moisture exchangers and breathing systems filters: their use in anaesthesia and intensive care. Part 1 - history, principles and efficiency. *Anaesthesia* 2011; 1: 31-9.

Answer 7: The following are common pathological changes following brainstem death: True a & c

T   Hypotension is the most common physiological change seen after brainstem death and may occur in up to 80% of patients.

F   Hypernatraemia occurs more commonly after brainstem death as a result of diabetes insipidus.

T   Pulmonary oedema is frequently seen, and is often neurogenic in origin.

F   Thrombotic events are uncommon. In patients with brainstem death it is more common for bleeding tendencies to be displayed, due to disseminated intravascular coagulation.

F   Metabolic acidosis may occur in up to 10% of patients, but alkalosis is uncommon.

1.   Waldmann C, Soni N, Rhodes A. *Oxford Desk Reference Critical Care*. Oxford, UK: Oxford University Press, 2008.

Answer 8: When inserting a chest drain, the following statements are true: True a, c & e

T   The 'safe' triangle recommended when inserting a chest drain is bordered by the latissimus dorsi, pectoralis major and a line superior to the horizontal level of the nipple. These landmarks should be used as anatomical markers when preparing the patient.

F   Small-bore chest tubes have been successfully used for pneumothorax, effusions, or loculated empyemas, according to guidance from the British Thoracic Society.

T   A meta-analysis has demonstrated that the use of prophylactic antibiotics in association with chest drain insertion, reduces the absolute risk of empyema and all infectious complications.

F   Chest drain insertion is associated with pain during insertion in survey data. 50% of patients in one study reported pain scores of 9-10 during the procedure.

T   Chest drain suction may be required in cases of non-resolving pneumothorax or following chemical pleurodesis.

1.   Laws D, Neville E, Duffy J. On behalf of the British Thoracic Society Pleural Disease Group, a subgroup of the British Thoracic Society Standards of Care Committee. BTS guidelines for the insertion of a chest drain. *Thorax* 2003; 58(Suppl II): ii53-9.

Answer 9: Heat: True a & c

T   The specific heat capacity is the amount of heat needed to raise the temperature of 1kg of a substance by 1°C.

F   The wet and dry bulb hygrometer consists of two thermometers, one of which is surrounded by a wick placed in water. The difference between the temperatures detected by the two thermometers depends on the rate of evaporation of the water, causing a cooling effect, which in turn depends on the ambient humidity. The relative humidity is worked out using the temperature difference and a set of reference tables.

T   As the molar concentration of a solute increases, there is an increase in osmotic pressure, a decrease in freezing point and a decrease in vapour pressure of the solvent. These are known as colligative properties.

F   Thermocouples utilise the Seebeck effect, where a voltage, which is proportional to the temperature, is generated at the junction of two different conductors.

F   Absolute humidity is the mass of water vapour in a given volume of gas at a given temperature and pressure, and is not expressed as a percentage.

1.   Davis PD, Kenny GNC. *Basic Physics and Measurement in Anaesthesia*, 5th ed. Edinburgh, UK; Butterworth Heinemann, 2003.

Answer 10: Drugs in pregnancy: True a, d & e

T   Ketamine increases intrauterine pressure and can result in foetal asphyxia. This is not apparent during the third trimester.

F   Suxamethonium exhibits a low lipid solubility and does not readily cross the placenta.

F   Chronic exposure to NSAIDs in the third trimester may cause premature closure of the ductus arteriosus, which can lead to persistent pulmonary hypertension of the newborn.

T   Suxamethonium may have a prolonged action in pregnancy. This is due to reduced plasma cholinesterase concentrations in pregnancy.

T   Anti-epileptic drugs affect the metabolism of folate, which can result in major congenital malformation (MCM)

1.   Allman KG, Wilson IH, O'Donnell A. *Oxford Handbook of Anaesthesia*, 3rd ed. Oxford, UK: Oxford University Press, 2011.
2.   Sasada M, Smith S. *Drugs in Anaesthesia and Intensive Care*, 3rd ed. Oxford, UK: Oxford University Press, 2003.

Answer 11: Biological terrorist attacks: True a, b & d

T   Examples of Category A biological weapons which can be easily diseminated include: anthrax, botulism and smallpox. Category B biological weapons are those that are moderately easy to disseminate. This classification system comes from the Centers for Disease Control and Prevention (CDC), Atlanta.

T   A particle size of 0.6-5µm will result in deposition in the alveoli. Smaller particles will be exhaled, whereas larger particles will be filtered by the nose.

F   Anthrax is a bacillus.

T   Post-exposure antimicrobial prophylaxis should be continued for 60 days in unvaccinated exposed persons exposed to anthrax. Before 2001, penicillin was considered the first-line treatment for anthrax infection; however, there is now concern over genetically engineered penicillin-resistant strains.

F   The incubation period may be anywhere between 2-60 days following pulmonary exposure to anthrax.

1.   Bersten AD, Soni N. *Oh's Intensive Care Manual*, 6th ed. Butterworth Heinemann Elsevier, 2009.

Answer 12: Ventilator-associated pneumonia (VAP): True b & e

F   The most common pathogens are usually aerobic Gram-negative bacilli.

T   The Clinical Pulmonary Infection Score utilises a points system with five categories. These are: temperature, leucocyte count, oxygenation, radiography and tracheal secretions.

F   There is no evidence that one diagnostic modality is better than another.

F   Only a few small studies have been performed looking at this, with inconsistent results.

T   Invasive strategies to diagnose VAP do not alter mortality.

1.   Hunter JD. Ventilator-associated pneumonia. *Br Med J* 2012; 344: e3325.

2.   Rea-Neto A, Youssef NCM, Tuche F, *et al*. Diagnosis of ventilator-associated pneumonia - a systematic review of the literature. *Crit Care* 2008; 12: R56.

3.   Shorr AF, Sherner JH, Jackson WL, Kollef MH. Invasive approaches to the diagnosis of ventilator-associated pneumonia: a meta-analysis. *Crit Care Med* 2005; 33(1): 46-53.

Answer 13: Epidural catheters: True b, c & e

F   It is recommended that epidural catheters should not be inserted for 12 hours post-prophylactic LMWH and for 24 hours post-therapeutic doses of LMWH.

T   Epidural catheter removal is deemed safe 4 hours after cessation of systemic unfractionated heparin, due to its short half-life.

T   No additional precautions are required in patients receiving low-dose aspirin with either epidural insertion or removal.

F   The long elimination half-life of fondaparinux results in prolonged anticoagulant effects and bleeding risk. Therefore, it is recommended that fondaparinux should be stopped for 42 hours for epidural removal and 36 hours for epidural insertion.

T   An INR of less than 1.4 is deemed safe for epidural insertion and removal.

1.   The Association of Anaesthetists of Great Britain and Ireland (AAGBI). Regional anaesthesia in patients with abnormalities in coagulation, 2011. http://www.aagbi.org/sites/default/files/RAPAC%20for%20consultation.pdf.

Answer 14: With reference to thromboelastography (TEG): True a, b & d

T   The R value is the time from initiation of TEG to fibrin formation with a normal value of 15-30mm. It is prolonged with anticoagulant use and in haemophilia.

T   The K value is the time measured from clot formation until an amplitude equal to 20mm. The normal value is 6-12mm and it is prolonged with inhibitors of platelet function such as aspirin.

F   Maximum amplitude (MA) reflects clot strength with a normal range of 50-60mm. Rates less than this suggest weak clot formation and may indicate platelet dysfunction/deficiency.

T   LY30 is the rate of amplitude reduction 30 minutes after maximum amplitude. It has a normal value of less than 7.5%. Fibrinolysis is characterised by a continuous reduction in MA resulting in a LY30 time of greater than 7.5%.

F   The α-angle measures acceleration of fibrin build up and cross-linkage. Normal values are 40-50° or 54-67° with celite. Decreased α-angle measures occur with anticoagulation, whereas increased measures are seen with hypercoagulable states.

1.   Curry ANG, Pierce JMT. Conventional and near-patient tests of coagulation. *Contin Educ Anaesth Crit Care Pain* 2002; 7(2): 45-50.

2.   Bersten AD, Soni N. *Oh's Intensive Care Manual*, 6th ed. Butterworth Heinemann Elsevier, 2009.

3.   Srivastava A, Kelleher A. Point-of-care coagulation testing. *Contin Educ Anaesth Crit Care Pain* 2013; 13(1): 12-6.

Answer 15: Non-invasive ventilation (continuous positive airway pressure [CPAP]/bilevel positive airway pressure [BiPAP]) is contraindicated in: True a & b

T   Coma (GCS <8/15) of any cause, the patient is unable to protect their airway and is at risk of aspiration. This is particularly true if non-invasive ventilation is used.

T   Mechanical bowel obstruction poses a significant aspiration risk which may be exacerbated with non-invasive ventilation.

F   There is a hypothetical risk of aspiration and strain of suture lines post-oesophagectomy with non-invasive ventilation. However, there is increasing evidence that CPAP with nasogastric tube decompression is safe and may prevent the need for re-intubation post-oesophagectomy. Further studies are warranted to investigate further.

F   There is a significant mortality benefit with non-invasive ventilation use in cardiogenic pulmonary oedema.

F   Non-invasive ventilation may be beneficial in chest trauma with persistent hypoxaemia, as it may establish and maintain lung recruitment, improving overall gas exchange.

1.   Waldmann C, Soni N, Rhodes A. *Oxford Desk Reference Critical Care*. Oxford, UK: Oxford University Press, 2008.

2.   Michelet P, D'Journo XB, Seinaye F, *et al*. Non-invasive ventilation for the treatment of postoperative respiratory failure after oesophagectomy. *Br J Surg* 2009; 96: 54-60.

Answer 16: Phaeochromocytoma: True d

F   Approximately 10% of cases of phaeochromocytoma are malignant.

F   Phaeochromocytoma is classically associated with multiple endocrine neoplasia (MEN) Type 2 (Table 3.1).

F   24-hour urinary collection for catecholamines and metanephrines has an 87.5% sensitivity and a 99.7% specificity.

T   Hyperglycaemia, hypercalcaemia and erythrocytosis are laboratory features of phaeochromocytoma.

F   β-blocker therapy should only be commenced after adequate α-blockade has been instigated (usually 2 days). If β-blockade is started prior to this, then unopposed α-stimulation can precipitate a hypertensive crisis. Pre-operatively there is no consensus regarding preferred drugs for blood pressure control. Often α-blockade with phenoxybenzamine is started 10-14 days to allow expansion of blood volume.

Table 3.1. Multiple endocrine neoplasia (MEN) types.

MEN 1	Pituitary adenoma, parathyroid hyperplasia and pancreatic tumours
MEN 2A	Parathyroid hyperplasia, medullary thyroid carcinoma and phaeochromocytoma
MEN 2B	Mucosal neuromas, Marfanoid body habitus, medullary thyroid carcinoma and phaeochromocytoma

1.   Sheps SG, Jiang NS, Klee GG, van Heerden JA. Recent developments in the diagnosis and treatment of phaemochromocytoma. *Mayo Clin Proc* 1990; 65(1): 88- 95.

2.   Därr R, Lenders JWM, Hofbauer LC, *et al*. Phaemochromocytoma: update on disease management. *Ther Adv Endo Metab* 2012; 3(1): 11-26.

Answer 17: Acute adrenocortical insufficiency (Addisonian crisis): True a, c & d

T   Acute adrenocortical insufficiency usually causes distributive shock with relative hypovolaemia due to low systemic vascular resistance secondary to vasodilatation.

F   Waterhouse-Friderichsen syndrome is defined as adrenal gland failure due to bleeding into the adrenal glands, and can occur in fulminant meningococcaemia. This is associated with acute adrenocortical insufficiency.

T   Acute steroid withdrawal almost exclusively causes a glucocorticoid deficiency.

T   Therapeutic use of dexamethasone in this situation allows ACTH stimulation testing later without affecting or interfering with the measurement of serum cortisol levels. Otherwise, standard treatment is to administer intravenous hydrocortisone 100mg four times daily.

F   Hypoglycaemia, hyponatraemia and hyperkalaemia are characteristic findings. Hypercalcaemia may be seen in one third of cases.

1.   Hahner S, Allolio B. Therapeutic management of adrenal insufficiency. *Best Pract Res Clin Endocrinol Metab* 2009; 23(2): 167-79.

Answer 18: Antimicrobial resistance (AMR): True a-c

T   This is the World Health Organisation definition.

T   AMR can include all micro-organisms.

T   Daily microbiology ward rounds should address cessation or de-escalation of antimicrobials to prevent this phenomenon.

F   Resistance patterns in Gram-negative bacteria are largely related to an increase in ESBLs in *Klebsiella pneumoniae*, *Escherichia coli* and *Proteus* species. This is in addition to third-generation cephalosporin β-lactamase resistance among *Enterobacter spp.* and *Citrobacter spp.* Multi-drug resistance in *Acinetobacter* species and *Pseudomonas aeruginosa* is also seen.

F   *Candida krusei* has intrinsic fluconazole resistance. *Candida glabrata* has dose-dependent resistance to fluconazole.

1.   Brusselaers N, Vogelaers D, Blot S. The rising problem of antimicrobial resistance in the intensive care unit. *Ann Intensive Care* 2011; 1: 47.

Answer 19: Regarding emergency surgery for ruptured abdominal aortic aneurysm (AAA): True c & e

F   The law of Laplace states: T=PR, where T is wall tension, P is transmural pressure and R is radius. The risk of aneurysmal rupture increases with increasing size — 6.6% annual risk of rupture with 6-7cm aneurysms compared to 0.5-1% risk with aneurysms smaller than 5.5cm — in keeping with the law of Laplace.

F   The physiological and operative severity score for the enumeration of mortality and morbidity (POSSUM) modified for vascular patients is useful for audit and assessment of surgical performance but should not be used to predict outcomes of emergency AAA surgery.

T   There is a risk of severe hypotension on induction of anaesthesia, therefore, induction in theatre with the surgeon and patient fully prepared for incision, is vital to reduce time to aortic cross-clamp and haemorrhage control.

F   Rapid resuscitation with packed red cells, fresh frozen plasma (FFP), platelets and cryoprecipitate to maintain a palpable radial pulse is preferable to massive fluid resuscitation to reduce the risk of worsening haemorrhage through dilutional coagulopathy and relative hypertension.

T   If the aneurysm perforates into the duodenum or colon, massive gastrointestinal haemorrhage may occur.

1.   Ruskin KJ, Rosenbaum SH. *Anaesthesia Emergencies*. Oxford, UK: Oxford University Press, 2011; Chapter 14.

2.   Mosquera D, Chiang N, Gibberd R. Evaluation of surgical performance using V-POSSUM risk-adjusted mortality rates. *ANZ J Surg* 2008; 78(7): 535-9.

Answer 20: Regarding the neonatal circulation: True a, c & e

T   In utero blood leaves the placenta in a single umbilical vein with an oxygen saturation of 80%.

F   The ductus venosus shunts approximately 50% of oxygenated placental blood from the left umbilical vein blood to the IVC, thus bypassing the liver. The ductus arteriosus shunts blood from the pulmonary artery to the aorta to bypass the pulmonary circulation.

T   The majority of blood — approximately two thirds — entering the IVC is directed through the foramen ovale to the left atrium and left ventricle to supply the heart, upper body and brain. The remaining one third passes into the right ventricle.

F   Blood returns to the placenta from the neonatal circulation via two umbilical arteries which arise from the internal iliac arteries. There is a single umbilical vein which transports blood from the placenta.

T   At first breath, pulmonary vascular resistance falls, allowing blood flow into the right ventricle. Placental flow ceases on clamping of the umbilical cord causing systemic vascular resistance to rise and reversal of the right to left shunt through the ductus arteriosus. Exposure to oxygen and reduced prostaglandin E2 levels stimulate ductal constriction and closure in the majority of newborns within 24 hours.

1.   Smith T, Pinnock C, Lin T. *Fundamentals of Anaesthesia*, 3rd ed. Cambridge, UK: Cambridge University Press, 2009.

Answer 21: Pulmonary artery catheters (PAC): True b & e

F   The PAC-man trial found no clear evidence of benefit or harm associated with the use of PAC. The FACCT trial from the ARDSnet group found PAC use did not improve survival and was associated with more complications. In 1996, Connors *et al* published a prospective observational study which found PAC use was associated with higher mortality and healthcare costs.

T   PAC may be used to provide physiological values that can help to differentiate between cardiogenic, hypovolaemic, septic and obstructive shock in critically ill patients.

F   Tricuspid regurgitation, intracranial shunts and injecting the dilutent too slowly may all cause error when using thermodilution techniques to measure cardiac output.

F   The Stewart-Hamilton equation is used in PAC software to calculate cardiac output

T   The area under the thermodilution curve is inversely proportional to the cardiac output. High cardiac output is associated with a large initial change in blood temperature which is short lived; poor cardiac output has a small initial change in blood temperature but change is more prolonged.

1.   Connors AF, Speroff T, Dawson NV, *et al*. The effectiveness of right heart catheterisation in the initial care of critically ill patients. *JAMA* 1996; 276: 889-97.
2.   Waldmann C, Soni N, Rhodes A. *Oxford Desk Reference Critical Care*. Oxford, UK: Oxford University Press, 2008.
3.   Paunovic B, Peter K. Pulmonary artery catheterisation. Medscape reference, 2013. http://emedicine.medscape.com/article/1824547-overview#showall.

Answer 22: Management of acute ST-elevation myocardial infarction (STEMI): True a, c & d

T   Dual antiplatelet therapy following STEMI with aspirin (150-300mg PO/IV) and an ADP-receptor blocker — ideally ticagrelor (180mg loading PO, 90mg bd maintenance) — is recommended. Prasugrel (60mg loading PO, 10mg od maintenance) may be given in clopidogrel-naïve patients with no history of cerebrovascular disease and aged less than 75 years. Ticagrelor and prasugrel have a more rapid onset of action and greater potency with proven superiority to clopidogrel in large outcome trials. Clopidogrel should be given if ticagrelor or prasugrel are unavailable or specifically contraindicated.

F   Primary PCI is recommended within 90 minutes of acute STEMI if initially seen at a PCI-capable hospital or 120 minutes of first medical contact if initially seen at a non-PCI capable hospital, as immediate transfer is required to a PCI-capable centre. PCI is the preferred first-line treatment in STEMI due to the lower rates of mortality, reinfarction and cerebrovascular events compared to fibrinolysis, provided that it is performed in a timely fashion.

T   An injectable anticoagulant must be used in primary PCI. From trial data, bivalirudin is preferred over heparin and a GPIIb/IIIa blocker, with an associated reduction in all-cause and cardiovascular mortality at 30 days, maintained up to 3 years. A bivalirudin 0.75mg/kg IV bolus is followed by an IV infusion of 1.75mg/kg/hr for up to 4 hours after PCI as clinically warranted. After cessation of the 1.75mg/kg/hr infusion, a reduced infusion dose of 0.25mg/kg/hr may be continued for 4-12 hours as clinically necessary. Enoxaparin (0.5mg/kg IV, followed by SC treatment) may be preferred over unfractionated heparin as it may reduce secondary mortality without increasing bleeding risk. Unfractionated heparin (70-100U/kg bolus when no GPIIb/IIIa inhibitors are being used or 50-60U/kg with GPIIb/IIIa inhibitors), is advised in those not receiving either bivalirudin or enoxaparin. The use of fondaparinux in primary PCI for STEMI was associated with potential harm in the Oasis 6 trial and is not recommended.

T   Should primary PCI be unavailable within 120 minutes of first medical contact to patients presenting with acute STEMI, then attempted revascularisation with fibrinolytic therapy is recommended, provided that the patient is presenting within 12 hours of symptom onset and has no contraindications to fibrinolysis.

F   Fibrinolysis is considered to have failed if there is evidence of ongoing ischaemia, evidence of re-occlusion or less than 50% ST-segment resolution at 60 minutes following fibrinolysis. Immediate rescue PCI is indicated if failed fibrinolysis occurs.

1.   http://www.escardio.org/guidelines-surveys/esc-guidelines/GuidelinesDocuments/ Essential_Messages_AMI_STEMI.pdf.

2.   O'Gara PT, Kushner FG, Ascheim DD, *et al*. 2013 ACCF/AHA guideline for the management of ST-elevation myocardial infarction: executive summary: a report of the American College of Cardiology Foundation/American Heart Association Task Force on Practice Guidelines. *Circulation* 2013; 127(4): 529-55.

Answer 23: Complications following obesity surgery include: True a-c & e

T   Dumping syndrome is a common complication after obesity surgery. It occurs when the stomach rapidly empties calorifically dense carbohydrates into the small intestine. Symptoms occur 15 minutes to 2 hours after eating and include tachycardia, dizziness, sweating, nausea, vomiting, bloating, cramping and diarrhoea. It is more common following Roux-en-Y gastric bypass.

T   Gallstone development is a complication related to postoperative weight loss, rather than surgery itself. It occurs in approximately one third of patients who undergo bariatric surgery. Prophylactic cholecystectomy is not recommended as many cases of gallstones resolve spontaneously.

T   Patients undergoing obesity surgery are at a high risk of developing venous thromboembolism in the postoperative period. PE is the leading cause of death following bariatric surgery accounting for 15-32% of deaths.

F   The presence of Type 2 diabetes mellitus in patients with a BMI greater than 35 is an indication for bariatric surgery. The reduction in BMI that follows successful surgery often improves and in some cases reverses problems with glucose control, leading to a reduced incidence of diabetes and its complications postoperatively.

T   Sepsis is a significant complication accounting for about 18% of deaths following bariatric surgery, and may arise from the surgical site or other organ systems such as the lungs or urinary system.

1.   http://journals.lww.com/ajnonline/Fulltext/2012/09000/Outcomes_and_ Complications_After_Bariatric_Surgery.20.aspx.

2.   Gagnon LE, Karwaki Sheff EJ. Outcomes and complications after bariatric surgery. *AJN* 2012; 112(9): 26-36.

Answer 24: Regarding oxygen delivery in adults: True b-d

F   0.0225ml of oxygen for each 1kPa of partial pressure oxygen is carried in every 100ml of blood.

T   Normal resting oxygen delivery is approximately 1000ml/min. Basal oxygen consumption (VO_2) at rest is approximately 250ml/min.

T   Oxygen content is calculated via the following equation: CaO_2=[1.34 x Hb x SaO_2] + [0.02 x PaO_2 kPa] or + [0.003 x PaO_2 mmHg].

T   At an arterial oxygen content of 19.5ml O_2 per 100ml and venous oxygen content of 15ml O_2 per 100ml — which represents normal physiological conditions — then the <u>uptake</u> by tissues is 4.5ml O_2 per 100ml blood delivered.

F   Direct measurement of maximum oxygen content of blood is 1.34ml/g Hb and is called Hufner's constant. 1.39ml/g Hb is the theoretical maximum O_2-carrying capacity of a gram of haemoglobin.

1.   Bersten AD, Soni N. *Oh's Intensive Care Manual*, 6th ed. Butterworth Heinemann Elsevier, 2009.

2.   http://www.frca.co.uk/article.aspx?articleid=100344.

Answer 25: Scoring systems in acute liver disease: True b & d

F   The MELD score is comprised of bilirubin, INR and creatinine only. It has a maximum score of 40 and has been found to be useful in predicting short-term survival in cirrhotic patients and the urgency of need for liver transplantation.

T   The Lille Model was created from a series of patients with alcoholic hepatitis treated with steroids and was found to be more accurate than MELD, Child-Pugh and Maddrey for predicting 6-month survival in alcoholic hepatitis. Patients with a score of above 0.45 had a 6-month mortality rate of 75% while those with a score <0.45 had a mortality rate of only 15%.

F   The Maddrey discriminant function is used in alcoholic hepatitis and stratifies the risk of mortality and use of steroids. A score of >32 indicates severe alcoholic hepatitis, which carries a poor prognosis and suggests steroids should be considered.

T   The Glasgow Alcoholic Hepatitis score is modelled on age, white cell count, urea, INR and bilirubin, with each variable given between 1 and 3 points according to severity. An overall score of 9 or above has been shown to predict 28-day mortality.

F   The Child-Pugh score is used predominantly in chronic liver failure to prognosticate in patients with cirrhosis. The Child-Pugh score comprises five variables — encephalopathy, ascites, bilirubin, albumin, prothrombin time — with ranking of severity A to C predicting mortality at 1 year.

1.   Jackson P, Gleeson D. Alcoholic liver disease. *Contin Educ Anaesth Crit Care Pain* 2010; 10(3): 66-71.

2.   Flood S, Bodenham A, Jackson P. Mortality of patients with alcoholic liver disease admitted to critical care: a systematic review. *J Intensive Care Soc* 2012; 13(2): 130-5.

3.   Durand F, Valla D. Assessment of prognosis of cirrhosis. *Semin Liver Dis* 2008; 28(1): 110-22

Answer 26: Dexmedetomidine: True e

F   Dexmedetomidine and clonidine are α2-adrenoceptor agonists.

F   Clonidine is 200 times more specific for α2-adrenoceptors compared to α1-adrenoceptors. Dexmedetomidine is 1600 times more specific.

F   Both agents have analgesic properties, although the mechanism by which this is achieved remains controversial. α2-receptors are located in the dorsal region of the spinal cord and in supraspinal sites. These may be the sites of action for analgesia.

F   Dexmedetomidine undergoes almost complete metabolism in the liver. The products of metabolism are excreted by the kidneys.

T   A biphasic blood pressure response may be seen. Hypertension is followed by dose-dependent hypotension. The heart rate decreases due to a direct effect on the sinus and AV node.

1.   Roberts M, Stuart G. Dexmedetomidine in paediatric anaesthesia and intensive care. Anaesthesia Tutorial of the Week 293, 2013. www.aagbi.org/education/educational-resources/tutorial-week.

2.   Barr J, Puntillo K, Ely EW, *et al.* Clinical practice guidelines for the management of pain, agitation, and delirium in adult patients in the intensive care unit. *Crit Care Med* 2013; 41(1): 263-306.

Answer 27: Management of acute aneurysmal subarachnoid haemorrhage (SAH): True: a, c-e

T   Acute management of hypertension in an unprotected recently ruptured aneurysm should be undertaken to prevent rebleeding and secondary brain injury. Systolic blood pressure should be maintained below 160mmHg (and MAP 110mmHg) to reduce the risk of rebleeding. It is also vital to avoid hypotension and reduced cerebral perfusion pressure (CPP).

F   Triple H therapy aims to improve cerebral blood flow and oxygen delivery, and prevent delayed cerebral ischaemia and vasospasm post-SAH. However, a recent systematic review found no controlled studies demonstrating a beneficial effect from any triple H therapy component.

T   Nimodipine has been found to be safe and cost-effective at preventing delayed cerebral ischaemia, due to vasospasm, and improves outcome after SAH. It can be given enterally or intravenously and is started on diagnosis and continued for 21 days.

T   The International Subarachnoid Aneurysm Trial (ISAT) found that endovascular coiling compared to surgical clipping for acute ruptured intracranial aneurysm was associated with better outcomes and as such surgical clipping is reserved for aneurysms unsuitable for coiling only. Since ISAT, there are some concerns that aneurysm coiling may not be as durable as surgical clipping in the long term, leading many neurosurgeons to continue clipping. Also, the majority of aneurysms in ISAT were good grade, small (<10mm) anterior circulation aneurysms. Often the superiority of coiling is extrapolated to patients not studied (e.g. different grade or aneurysm location) in the original trial or treated with new devices not available at the time. The ISAT2 multi-centre trial is now recruiting non-ISAT patients allocated to coiling or clipping, to investigate clinical outcomes further.

T   Overall mortality from SAH is around 50%, with up to 25% of patients dying before reaching hospital. Up to 33% of patients will be dependent on care and up to 50% will have cognitive impairment sufficient to affect quality of life.

1.   Luoma A, Reddy U. Acute management of aneurysmal subarachnoid haemorrhage. *Contin Educ Anaesth Crit Care Pain* 2013; 13(2): 52-8.

2.   http://clinicaltrialsfeeds.org/clinical-trials/show/NCT01668563.

Answer 28: Regarding severe acute adult meningitis: True a, b & d

T   Bacterial seeding of the meninges via the bloodstream from a colonised or established source of localised infection (such as nasopharyngeal, respiratory or ear) is the most common mode of spread of infection in acute meningitis.

T   The classic triad presentation of fever, headache and neck stiffness is consistent with meningitis. Other symptoms and signs include nausea, vomiting, photalgia (photophobia), sleepiness, confusion, irritability, delirium and coma. Viral meningitis usually has preceding systemic symptoms of myalgia, fatigue and anorexia.

F   Dexamethasone significantly reduces hearing loss and neurological sequelae in adult acute bacterial meningitis, but has been found not to reduce mortality. Subgroup analysis of a 2013 Cochrane review suggested that there may be a reduction in mortality with dexamethasone use in meningitis due to *Streptococcus pneumoniae*, but no effect with *Haemophilus influenzae* and *Neisseria meningitidis*.

T   Large patient registry data from the Netherlands have suggested that adjunctive dexamethasone therapy may predispose patients with bacterial meningitis to delayed cerebral thrombosis at days 7 to

42 post-initial infection. The incidence of thrombosis is higher in patients with *Streptococcus pneumoniae* meningitis and is associated with poor neurological outcomes.

F   Induced hypothermia may be harmful in acute meningitis and not currently recommended — mortality from acute meningitis was increased in one study where therapeutic hypothermia was used during initial treatment.

1.   Hasburn R, Bronze MS, Biliciler S, *et al*. Meningitis. Medscape reference, 2014. http://emedicine.medscape.com/article/232915-overview#showall.

2.   Brouwer MC, McIntyre P, Prasad K, van de Beek D. Corticosteroids for acute bacterial meningitis. *Cochrane Database Syst Rev* 2013; 6: CD004405.

3.   NHS British National Formulary link: http://www.evidence.nhs.uk/formulary/bnf/current/6-endocrine-system/63-corticosteroids/632-glucocorticoid-therapy/dexamethasone.

4.   Lucas MJ, Brouwer MC, van de Beek D. Delayed cerebral thrombosis in bacterial meningitis: a prospective cohort study. *Intensive Care Med* 2013; 39: 866-71.

5.   Mourvillier B, Tubach F, van de Beek, *et al*. Induced hypothermia in severe bacterial meningitis a randomised controlled trial. *JAMA* 2013; 310(20): 2174-83.

Answer 29: Regarding pain: True b, c & e

F   C fibre endings are unmyelinated and responsible for slow pain sensation.

T   C fibres synapse with cells in laminae II and III of the spinal cord (substantia gelatinosa), whilst Aδ fibres synapse with cells in laminae I and V.

T   This relates to the gate control theory of pain, where stimulation of large (Aβ) fibres closes the gate, preventing pain, whilst stimulation of small (C) fibres opens the gate, causing pain. The gate is thought to be located in the substantia gelatinosa and laminae II and III of the dorsal horn.

F   Ketamine is a non-competitive antagonist of the NMDA receptor calcium channel pore and inhibits NMDA receptor activity by interaction with the phencyclidine binding site.

T   Activation is thought to result in increased potassium and/or decreased calcium conductance across the cell membrane, decreasing excitability.

1. Smith T, Pinnock C, Lin T. *Fundamentals of Anaesthesia*, 3rd ed. Cambridge, UK: Cambridge University Press, 2009.

Answer 30: During adult cardiopulmonary resuscitation: True b & c

F   If intravenous access is not immediately available during cardiopulmonary resuscitation, then intraosseous access should be obtained. Drug delivery via the tracheal route is no longer recommended.

T   Blood products can be delivered by the intraosseous route; application of pressure (for example, with a pressure bag) will usually be required to deliver reasonable flow rates.

T   According to resuscitation guidelines, in a shockable rhythm amiodarone 300mg IV should be delivered after the third shock.

F   Atropine is no longer included as part of the advanced life support algorithm.

F   Current flow is inversely proportional to transthoracic impedance, which is influenced by electrode to skin contact, electrode size and phase of ventilation.

1. Resuscitation Council (UK). Advanced life support, 6th ed. London, UK: Resuscitation Council (UK), 2011. www.resus.org.uk
2. Resuscitation Council (UK). Use of intraosseous access during cardiac arrest. London, UK: Resuscitation Council (UK), 2011. www.resus.org.uk.

Answer 31: Pathophysiology of sepsis: True b-e

F   Lipopolysaccharide is a component of the outer membrane of Gram-negative organisms, which binds to the CD14 receptor in the surface of monocytes.

T   Interleukin 4 and 10 have anti-inflammatory properties.

T   Cytokines lead to increased production of nitric oxide and decreased systemic vascular resistance.

T   Tumour necrosis factor causes cardiovascular insufficiency through direct myocardial depression and due to vasodilation and capillary leak.

T   A thromboelastogram in a patient with severe sepsis may show a reduced maximum amplitude during the hypocoagulable state.

1.   Bersten AD, Soni N. *Oh's Intensive Care Manual*, 6th ed. Butterworth Heinemann Elsevier, 2009.

Answer 32: Haematological malignancies and critical care: True b, c & e

F   GCSF is a glycoprotein that stimulates bone marrow production of granulocytes, stem cells and neutrophils and is used in neutropaenic patients to promote neutrophil recovery. It has no effect on lymphocyte recovery.

T   There are a number of factors which increase the risk of GVHD, including increased donor and recipient age, HLA incompatibility, unrelated rather than related donor and donor-recipient sex mismatch.

T   GVHD is graded from I to IV according to disease severity and degree of body system involvement. Morbidity and mortality increase with higher grades of disease. The 100-day survival for Grade I is 78-90%; Grade II 66-92%; Grade III 29-62% and Grade IV 23-25%.

F   GVHD occurs due to recognition of host cells by immune cells contained within the 'graft' (transplanted cells from a non-identical donor) and the subsequent immune reaction that occurs. As such, cytokines play a central role in mediating many of the manifestations of GVHD via their role in the immune response.

T   Respiratory failure may affect up to 10-15% of patients following bone marrow transplantation and is the commonest cause of death in patients undergoing bone marrow transplant.

1.   Beed M, Levitt M, Bokhari SW. Intensive care management of patients with haematological malignancy. *Contin Educ Anaesth Crit Care Pain* 2010; 10(6): 167-71.

2.   Bersten AD, Soni N. *Oh's Intensive Care Manual*, 6th ed. Butterworth Heinemann Elsevier, 2009.

Answer 33: Following burn injury: True a, b & e

T   Systemic and pulmonary vascular resistance is increased with the development of hypovolaemia and increased blood viscosity, reducing cardiac output initially.

T   The greatest rate of oedema formation occurs in the first few hours with further fluid extravasation continuing up to 24 hours post-burn.

F   Hypermetabolism tends to occur from day 3 onwards and is a manifestation of the systemic inflammatory response syndrome.

F   Renal blood flow and creatinine clearance increase at around 48 hours post-burn injury.

T   Serum albumin levels drop, therefore benzodiazepines, which normally bind to albumin, will show an increased free fraction.

1.   Bersten AD, Soni N. *Oh's Intensive Care Manual*, 6th ed. Butterworth Heinemann Elsevier, 2009.

Answer 34: *Clostridium difficile*: True a, d & e

T   *Clostridium difficile* is often due to antibiotic usage, especially cephalosporins and quinolones. Underlying malignancy, renal or pulmonary disease, albumin level <25mg/ml and previous treatment with proton pump inhibitors are also risk factors.

F   Intravenous vancomycin is not effective. It should be given orally.

F   It is diagnosed through testing for the toxin produced by the organism.

T   There is evidence for the use of probiotics to prevent *Clostridium difficile*-associated diarrhoea.

T   It produces two toxins: toxin A, an enterotoxin, and toxin B, a cytotoxin.

1.   Waldmann C, Soni N, Rhodes A. *Oxford Desk Reference Critical Care*. Oxford, UK: Oxford University Press, 2008.

2.   Yentis SM, Hirsch NP, Smith GB. *Anaesthesia and Intensive Care A-Z. An Encyclopaedia of Principles and Practice*, 3rd ed. Edinburgh, UK: Elsevier Butterworth Heinemann, 2004.

3.   Goldenberg JZ, Ma SS, Saxton JD, *et al*. Probiotics for the prevention of *Clostridium difficile*-associated diarrhoea in adults and children. *Cochrane Database Syst Rev* 2013; doi: 10.1002/14651858.CD006095.pub3.

Answer 35: Peripartum cardiomyopathy (PPCM): True a, b, d & e

T   The European Society of Cardiology and the American Heart Association describe PPCM as a form of dilated cardiomyopathy, although it is accepted that PPCM is distinct from other types of heart failure.

T   The ejection fraction is often less than 45% in PPCM.

F   There are various definitions of PPCM. However, the time frame stated by the National Heart Lung and Blood Institute and the Office of Rare Diseases (2000) is that PPCM occurs within the last month of pregnancy or within 5 months postpartum.

T   Oxygen and non-invasive ventilation (NIV) should be used to achieve an arterial oxygen saturation of ≥95%, with intravenous diuretics given where there is evidence of congestion or overload. Intravenous nitrate is recommended where the systolic blood pressure is >110mmHg and can be used with caution with a systolic pressure between 90-110mmHg. Morphine should also be considered, especially where there is anxiety, dyspnoea, restlessness or chest pain.

T   In this situation, left ventricular assist device (LVAD) implantation or cardiac transplantation should be considered, although the optimum strategy is not known.

1.   Sliwa K, Hilfiker-Kleiner D, Petrie MC, *et al*. Current state of knowledge on aetiology, diagnosis, management, and therapy of peripartum cardiomyopathy: a position statement from the Heart Failure Association of the European Society of Cardiology Working Group on Peripartum Cardiomyopathy. *Eur J Heart Failure* 2010; 12: 767-78.

2.   Dickstein K, Cohen-Salal A, Filipattos G, *et al*. ESC guidelines for the diagnosis and treatment of acute and chronic heart failure 2008. The Task Force for the Diagnosis and Management of Acute and Chronic Heart Failure 2008 of the European Society of Cardiology. Developed in collaboration with the Heart Failure Association of the ESC (HFA) and endorsed by the European Society of Intensive Care Medicine. *Eur Heart J* 2008; 29: 2388-442.

Answer 36: In relation to medical statistics, and Type II errors: True a, c & d

T   Type II errors occur when a study erroneously concludes that an intervention has no effect.

F   Type II errors may also be referred to as β-errors or false negatives.

T   See above.

T   Type II errors frequently arise due to underpowering of studies and the inclusion of an insufficient number of subjects, to demonstrate a significant effect.

F   A Type I or α-error occurs when a study concludes that an intervention has a significant effect when, in fact, it occurs due to chance. This may also be referred to as a false positive.

1.   Altman D. *Practical Statistics for Medical Research*. London, UK: Chapman and Hall, 1990.

2.   McCluskey A, Ghaaliq Lalkhen A. Statistics I: data and correlations. *Contin Educ Anaesth Crit Care Pain* 2007; 7(3): 95-9.

Answer 37: In relation to extracorporeal membrane oxygenation (ECMO): True b-d

F   Veno-arterial ECMO (VA ECMO) drains deoxygenated blood from the right atrium or a central vein, and returns it to a central artery.

T   Veno-venous ECMO (VV ECMO) is preferred to VA ECMO in the treatment of respiratory failure as normal pulmonary blood flow is maintained. In VV ECMO, venous cannulae are usually placed in the right femoral vein for drainage and right internal jugular vein for infusion. An alternative arrangement is for a dual-lumen catheter to be sited into the right internal jugular vein. Blood is drained from the vena cavae and returned into the right atrium.

T   An ECMO circuit consists of a drainage cannula, pump, oxygenator, and an arterial-return cannula.

T   Blood products are often needed daily during ECMO, requiring a well-resourced blood transfusion service. This includes the need for packed red cells, platelets, fresh frozen plasma and cryoprecipitate.

F   The CESAR trial (published in 2009) included 180 patients with severe but potentially reversible respiratory failure, who had a

Murray score of >3 or uncompensated hypercapnia (pH <7.2). 63% who received ECMO survived to 6 months without disability compared to only 47% who received conventional ventilation and management. ECMO was recommended in such patients and found to be cost-effective (NNT=6). Of note, of 90 patients referred to the ECMO centres, only 75% ultimately received ECMO.

1. Martinez G, Vuylsteke A. Extracorporeal membrane oxygenation in adults. *Contin Educ Anaesth Crit Care Pain* 2011; 12(2): 57-61.

2. Peek GJ, Mugford M, Tiruvoipati R, *et al*. Efficacy and economic assessment of conventional ventilatory support versus extracorporeal membrane oxygenation for severe adult respiratory failure (CESAR): a multicentre randomised controlled trial. *Lancet* 2009; 374(9698): 1351-63.

Answer 38: Following liver transplantation: True a, d-e

T   'Small for size syndrome' comprises hyperbilirubinaemia, graft dysfunction, ascites and portal hypertension with associated end-organ dysfunction. It is thought to be a result of portal hyperaemia, with portal flow passing into a small liver remnant/graft with associated pathophysiological consequences. It can also occur after liver resection.

F   This is not universally true. Some patient groups may be prothrombotic, for example, those with pre-operative portal or hepatic venous thrombosis, primary biliary cirrhosis or primary sclerosing cholangitis. Such patients may require anticoagulation in the early postoperative period.

F   Patients can be woken and weaned from mechanical ventilation immediately if, the procedure has been straightforward, they are stable and there is evidence of good graft function.

T   The porto-pulmonary syndrome, resulting in elevated right-sided pressures, necessitates management in order to prevent liver congestion and graft dysfunction. Treatment strategies include inhaled nitric oxide and intravenous prostacyclin.

T   Normal IAP is 5-7mmHg. Intra-abdominal hypertension is defined as a sustained or repeated pathological elevation of IAP ≥12mmHg.

1. Bersten AD, Soni N. *Oh's Intensive Care Manual*, 6th ed. Butterworth Heinemann Elsevier, 2009.

2.   Kirkpatrick AW, Roberts DJ, De Waele J, *et al.* Intra-abdominal hypertension and the abdominal compartment syndrome: updated consensus definitions and clinical practice guidelines from the World Society of the Abdominal Compartment Syndrome. *Intensive Care Med* 2013; 39(7): 1190-206.

Answer 39: Appropriate treatments in the management of poisoning are: True a, c-e

T   An overdose of an SSRI may cause serotonin syndrome, which can be managed with cooling and benzodiazepine administration.

F   Iron is poorly absorbed by activated charcoal.

T   Hyperinsulinaemia and euglycaemia therapy (HIET) can be used in the management of β-blocker and calcium channel blocker overdose.

T   Haemodialysis can be used to remove drugs which have a low molecular weight, low volume of distribution, low water-solubility and low protein binding. It is recommended in the treatment of lithium overdose. In patients with an absolute level of 4mEq/L in acute toxicity and a level of 2.5mEq/L in chronic toxicity, renal replacement therapy should be considered, although treatment based on only levels is subject to debate.

T   Atropine blocks the muscarinic effects seen in organophosphate overdose. An initial suggested regimen is a dose of 20-50μg/kg every 15 minutes, though expert guidance should be sought.

1.   Ward C, Sair M. Oral poisoning: an update. *Contin Educ Anaesth Crit Care Pain* 2010; 10(1): 6-11.

2.   Lheureux PER, Zahir S, Gris M, *et al.* Bench-to-bedside review: hyperinsulinaemia/euglycamia therapy in the management of overdose of calcium-channel blockers. *Crit Care* 2006; 10: 212.

Answer 40: In the management of traumatic brain injury (TBI): True b-e

F   The Brain Trauma Foundation guidelines suggest a general threshold for mean arterial pressure, in the realm of 60mmHg. Adjustment of this target should be titrated to the individual patient, based on monitoring and assessment. The routine use of volume expansion and vasopressor therapy to maintain a CPP >70mmHg is not supported in the guidance, based on perceived benefit and systemic complications that can potentially occur.

T   Recommendations from the Brain Trauma Foundation are that intracranial pressure should be monitored in all salvageable patients, with a severe TBI and abnormal CT scan.

T   The Brain Trauma Foundation recommends the use of mannitol at a dose of 0.25g to 1g per kg body weight, in patients with TBI. 175ml of 20% mannitol would be equal to a dose of 35g, or 0.5g/kg in a 70kg patient.

T   Both hypokalaemia and hyperkalaemia are associated with induction and cessation of thiopentone barbiturate coma. Regular monitoring of potassium concentrations in the blood is mandatory in patients receiving infusions of thiopentone.

T   Hypothermia represents an area of much debate and research in patients with traumatic brain injury. Although it has not been shown that therapeutic hypothermia in TBI patients reduces mortality, it has been shown that patients treated with hypothermia were more likely to have favourable neurological outcomes, although the evidence is conflicting. The Eurotherm 3235 trial, which is currently recruiting patients, will examine the relationship between therapeutic hypothermia for ICP reduction after traumatic brain injury and patient outcome.

1.   Brain Trauma Foundation. Guidelines for the management of severe traumatic brain injury. 3rd ed. A joint project of the Brain Trauma Foundation, American Association of Neurological Surgeons (AANS), Congress of Neurological Surgeons (CNS) and AANS/CNS Joint Section on Neurotrauma and Critical Care. *J Neurotrauma* 2007; 24(1): 1-116.

Answer 41: The following may cause a raised mean corpuscular volume (MCV) without anaemia on full blood count analysis (FBC): All True

T   Raised MCV without anaemia is termed macrocytosis. The amount of haemoglobin increases proportionately with the increase in cell size. This can occur with several conditions including alcohol excess, COPD, hypothyroidism and treatment with several drugs including phenytoin, zidovudine (AZT), the oral contraceptive pill and both purine and pyrimidine antagonists.

T   Raised MCV with a megaloblastic anaemia results in anaemia due to impaired red cell DNA synthesis and is the most common cause of a macrocytic anaemia. This commonly occurs due to B12 and folate deficiency, pregnancy and treatment with drugs such as hydroxyurea.

T   Drug-induced macrocytosis is the most common cause in non-alcoholic patients. Folate antagonists such as methotrexate can cause macrocytosis. Several myelodysplastic syndromes including aplastic anaemia may also cause macrocytosis.

T   Phenytoin therapy can cause macrocytosis.

T   Hypothyroidism is a recognised cause of macrocytosis.

1.   Kumar P, Clarke M. *Clinical Medicine*, 8th ed. Saunders Ltd, 2012.

Answer 42: Human albumin solution (HAS): True c & e

F   Is derived from multiple donors (1000s).

F   4.5% HAS is iso-oncotic. 20% HAS is hyperoncotic.

T   20% HAS is hyperoncotic but salt poor, so it is mildly hypotonic.

F   The SAFE study found no difference in outcomes, and a worse mortality association with HAS in traumatic brain injury patients. The Albios study (2014) found that albumin replacement in addition to crystalloids as compared with crystalloids alone did not improve survival at 28 or 90 days in septic shock.

T   HAS may have an outcome benefit when used post-ascitic drainage.

1.   Waldmann C, Soni N, Rhodes A. *Oxford Desk Reference Critical Care*. Oxford, UK: Oxford University Press, 2008.

2.   Myburgh JA, Mythen MG. Resuscitation fluids. *New Engl J Med* 2013; 369: 1243-51.

3.   Caironi P, Tognoni G, Masson S, *et al*. Albumin replacement in patients with severe sepsis or septic shock. *New Engl J Med* 2014; 370(15): 1412-21.

Answer 43: In relation to an empyema, the following statements are true: True a & b

T   Over 75% of empyemas are thought to be caused by anaerobic bacteria, often *Streptococcus*.

T   Empyemas tend to form 7 to 14 days after the onset of pneumonia.

F   Pleural aspirate with a pH greater than 7.2 should be managed conservatively in the first instance; pH <7.2 is an indication for drainage and chest drain insertion.

F   Organised and loculated pleural collections usually require surgical decortication.

F   Lactate dehydrogenase (LDH) is raised in empyematous pleural collections and a level of >1000IU/L is often seen. See Table 3.2 below for guidance in relation to pleural aspirate.

Table 3.2. Parapneumonic effusions and empyema characteristics.

Group	Appearance	Characteristics	Comments
Uncomplicated parapneumonic effusions	Clear-fluid Slightly cloudy	No organisms on Gram stain or culture pH >7.2, LDH <1000IU/L Glucose >2.2mmol/L	Inflammatory neutrophilic effusion Resolve with appropriate antibiotic treatment If required: chest drain for symptom relief only
Complicated parapneumonic effusions	Cloudy/turbid	Increased neutrophils Decreased glucose levels Pleural fluid Acidosis pH <7.2 Elevated LDH >1000IU/L May be positive culture or Gram stain	Occur due to bacterial invasion of pleural space Effusions often sterile as bacteria often rapidly cleared Requires chest tube drainage for resolution
Empyema thoracis	Frank pus	Thick, viscous and opaque pus May be positive culture or Gram stain	Frank pus accumulates in pleural space Requires chest tube drainage and antibiotics Video-assisted thoracoscopic surgery (VATS) may be required for resolution

1. Walters J, Foley N, Molyneux M. Pus in the thorax: management of empyema and lung abscess. *Contin Educ Anaesth Crit Care Pain* 2011; 11(6): 229-33.

2. Davies CW, Gleeson FV, Davies RJ. Pleural Diseases Group, Standards of Care Committee, British Thoracic Society. BTS guidelines for the management of pleural infection. *Thorax* 2003; 58(Suppl2): ii18-28.

3. Limsukon A, Soo Hoo GW, Byrd RP, *et al.* Parapneumonic pleural effusions and empyema thoracis. Medscape reference, 2014. http://emedicine.medscape.com/article/298485-overview#1.

Answer 44: Acute tubulo-interstitial nephritis: True a, b & e

T   Although any drug can induce a hypersensitivity reaction, commonly associated agents are as follows: rifampicin, NSAIDs, antibiotics, allopurinol, phenytoin, proton pump inhibitors and interferon-α.

T   Rifampicin is amongst the frequently implicated agents.

F   ACE-inhibitors are not frequently implicated.

F   A rash may be supportive of an allergic cause of interstitial nephritis. However, absence of rash does not exclude the diagnosis.

T   Oedema, significant proteinuria and hypoalbuminamia may be seen with acute tubulo-interstitial nephritis. Renal biopsy findings may, in addition to the usual findings of interstitial nephritis, show minimal change histology.

1. Perazella MA, Glen S, Markowitz GS. Drug-induced acute interstitial nephritis: review. *Nature Rev Nephrol* 2010; 6: 461-70.

Answer 45: Sodium: True b-e

F   Sodium is the principal cation of the ECF, accounting for 86% of its osmolality.

T   Total extracellular sodium equates to approximately 35mmol/kg.

T   Osmotic demyelination syndrome (pontine and extra-pontine myelinolysis) and congestive cardiac failure are reported complications with 3% saline therapy.

T   Hypernatraemia is always associated with hyperosmolality.

T   Hyperlipidaemia and hyperproteinaemia are associated with 'spurious' isotonic hyponatraemia. Hyperglycaemia is associated with spurious hypertonic hyponatraemia, as the ECF sodium is diluted by movement of water into the hypertonic ECF. Serum sodium is reduced by 1mmol/L for every 3mmol/L rise in glucose.

1.   Bersten AD, Soni N. *Oh's Intensive Care Manual*, 6th ed. Butterworth Heinemann Elsevier, 2009.

2.   Weisberg LS. Pseudohyponatraemia: a reappraisal. *Am J Med* 1989; 86: 315-8.

Answer 46: Regarding suxamethonium apnoea: True b

F   Plasma cholinesterase hydrolyses suxamethonium to succinyl choline and choline.

T   Suxamethonium apnoea has a number of acquired causes, which occur due to either decreased plasma cholinesterase concentration — as is seen in pregnancy, chronic renal failure, haemodialysis and hypothyroidism — or decreased plasma cholinesterase activity, which may be caused by several drugs including: etomidate, ketamine, ester local anaesthetics and anticholinesterases.

F   Inheritance of abnormal cholinesterase is linked to several autosomal recessive genes with 25 possible gene variants described.

F   Dantrolene is used in the management of malignant hyperpyrexia, which may occur following administration of suxamethonium, but not for the treatment of suxamethonium apnoea.

F   Dibucaine and fluoride inhibition testing is used in the investigation and diagnosis of suxamethonium apnoea. Halothane and caffeine are used in the diagnosis of malignant hyperpyrexia on muscle biopsy testing.

1.   Allman KG, Wilson IH. *Oxford Handbook of Anaesthesia*, 3rd ed. Oxford, UK: Oxford University Press, 2011.

2.   Smith T, Pinnock C, Lin T. *Fundamentals of Anaesthesia*, 3rd ed. Cambridge, UK: Cambridge University Press, 2009.

Answer 47: Regarding the diaphragmatic foramina: True c

F The IVC passes through the caval opening in the central tendon of the diaphragm at the level of T8.

F The right phrenic nerve also passes through the caval opening of the diaphragm, along with the IVC, at the level of T8. The left phrenic nerve pierces the left dome of the diaphragm.

T The thoracic duct passes through the aortic hiatus of the diaphragm, which is in the posterior part of the diaphragm between the left and right crus at the level of T12. The aorta and azygos vein also pass through the aortic hiatus.

F The azygos vein passes through the diaphragm via the aortic hiatus at the level of T12. The vagi pass through the oesophageal hiatus at the level of T10 with the oesophagus.

F The oesophagus passes through the posterior part of the diaphragm slightly to the left of the midline at the level of T10.

1. Smith T, Pinnock C, Lin T. *Fundamentals of Anaesthesia*, 3rd ed. Cambridge, UK: Cambridge University Press, 2009.

Answer 48: Macrophage activation syndrome (MAS): True a-d

T Macrophage activation syndrome (MAS) is a potentially life-threatening complication of rheumatic disease with multisystem involvement including: pancytopenia, liver failure, coagulopathy and neurological disturbance.

T MAS belongs to the histiocytic group of disorders, sometimes referred to as haemophagocytic lymphohistiocytosis (HLH). It is thought to occur as a result of uncontrolled proliferation of T-lymphocytes and well-differentiated macrophages causing widespread haemophagocytosis and cytokine overproduction.

T MAS is frequently associated with hyperferritinaemia. Ferritin levels should be checked in all patients in whom a diagnosis of MAS is suspected.

T Symptoms attributable to a cytokine storm are frequently seen with MAS. Differentiation from a clinical picture of sepsis may at times be difficult.

F Immunosuppression is the mainstay of treatment for MAS, with high-dose corticosteroids being the usual first-line treatment. Other agents such as cyclophosphamide, cyclosporin A and tumour necrosis factor (TNF) inhibitors may be considered in steroid-resistant cases.

1. Kuppe C, Westphal S, Bucher E, *et al*. Macrophage activation syndrome in a patient with pulmonary inflammatory myofibrolastic tumour. *Allergy Asthma Clin Immunol* 2012; 8: 6.

2. Rosario C, Zandman-Goddard G, Meyron-Holtz EG, *et al*. The hyperferritinemic syndrome: macrophage activation syndrome, Still's disease, septic shock and catastrophic antiphospholipid syndrome. *BMC Med* 2013; 11: 185.

Answer 49: Acute pancreatitis: True b & d

F The Atlanta criteria of 1993 described two categories of severity for acute pancreatitis (mild and severe); however, the revised criteria of 2013 introduced a third category — moderately-severe — which is characterised by the presence of transient organ failure or local and systemic complications in the absence of persistent organ failure.

T A serum triglyceride should be obtained in the absence of gallstones or a history of significant alcohol use as a diagnostic test. Hypertriglyceridaemia should be considered as the cause of acute pancreatitis if serum levels are greater than 1000mg/dL.

F The diagnosis of acute pancreatitis is most established by the presence of two out of three of the following criteria: abdominal pain consistent with acute pancreatitis, serum amylase or lipase greater than three times the upper limit of normal, characteristic findings on CT abdomen. Serum amylase usually rises within a few hours of the onset of acute pancreatitis and returns to normal within 3-5 days but may remain normal in alcohol-induced and hypertriglyceridaemia-induced pancreatitis.

T Predictive scoring systems for acute pancreatitis are of limited value clinically. Most are cumbersome, lack accuracy if measured in the first 48 hours following admission, and in severe disease, the gravity of the patient's condition is often obvious regardless of the score.

F Steroids are a potential cause of acute pancreatitis, and thus should be avoided in acute pancreatitis unless specifically indicated by other conditions that may also be present.

1.   Tenner S, Baillie J, DeWitt J, *et al.* American College of Gastroenterology Guideline: management of acute pancreatitis. *Am J Gastroenterol* 2013; 108(9): 1400-15.

2.   Bersten AD, Soni N. *Oh's Intensive Care Manual*, 6th ed. Butterworth Heinemann Elsevier, 2009.

Answer 50: The following are normal right heart pressures on pulmonary artery catheter (PAC) insertion: True a, b & d

T   Right atrial pressure has a mean value of 0-7mmHg in healthy adults.

T   Right ventricular pressure in healthy adults is 15-25mmHg systolic and 0-8mmHg diastolic.

F   Mean pulmonary artery pressure in health tends to be between 10-20mmHg. A mean pulmonary artery pressure of 25-35mmHg is suggestive of the presence of pulmonary arterial hypertension.

T   Pulmonary artery wedge or pulmonary capillary wedge pressure (PCWP) is the pressure generated when the inflated balloon of the PAC creates an uninterrupted column of blood between the balloon in the pulmonary artery and the left atrium. PCWP is taken as a marker of left ventricular preload and in health is 6-12mmHg. Conditions which elevate left atrial pressure (LAP) also elevate PCWP and include: left ventricular failure, mitral valve stenosis, mitral valve regurgitation, aortic valve stenosis and aortic regurgitation. PCWP can be used to evaluate patients with primary pulmonary hypertension. When PCWP exceeds 20mmHg, pulmonary oedema is likely to be present. PCWP may guide diuretic therapy.

F   A pulmonary artery systolic pressure of 35-45mmHg would be suggestive of pulmonary hypertension.

1.   Waldmann C, Soni N, Rhodes A. *Oxford Desk Reference Critical Care*. Oxford, UK: Oxford University Press, 2008.

Answer 51: Considering jaundice: True b, d & e

F   Although the normal upper reference limit for serum bilirubin levels is often quoted as being 20µmol/L, jaundice is usually only clinically detectable when serum bilirubin exceeds 50µmol/L.

T   Prehepatic jaundice occurs when the liver's capacity to process bilirubin is exceeded, usually due to excessive breakdown of haem subunits or haemolysis. Causes of haemolysis include: haemoglobinopathies, drugs, sepsis, red cell defects (such as heriditary spherocytosis) and microangiopathic haemolytic anaemia.

F   Unconjugated bilirubin, which is elevated in prehepatic jaundice, does not present in the urine as it is not water-soluble. In contrast, conjugated bilirubin is water-soluble and may lead to urinary discolouration if high levels are present.

T   Hepatocellular jaundice may occur on critical care due to liver ischaemic injury following hypotension due to any cause, and is usually seen in association with a marked elevation of transaminase enzymes, such as aspartate aminotransferase (AST) and alanine aminotransferase (ALT).

T   Post-hepatic jaundice caused by biliary obstruction results in pale stools and dark urine secondary to conjugated bilirubin, which is water-soluble, being excreted in the urine and causing dark discolouration.

1.   Waldmann C, Soni N, Rhodes A. *Oxford Desk Reference Critical Care*. Oxford, UK: Oxford University Press, 2008.

Answer 52: Oesophageal Doppler: True: a & c

T   Peak velocity of blood flow in the aorta is measured via the oesophageal Doppler and is considered to provide a good estimate of myocardial contractility.

F   Peak velocity declines with age, with normal values of 90-120cm/s at the age of 20, falling to 50-80cm/s by the age of 70.

T   Stroke distance (SD) is the area under the velocity-time waveform. It is multiplied by the aortic diameter to provide an estimate of stroke volume.

F   An increase in stroke volume of less than 5-10% following a fluid bolus suggests that a plateau in the Starling curve for that patient has been reached and they have adequate intravascular fluid volume.

F   Corrected flow time (FTc) is the duration of forward flow of blood in the aorta corrected for the patient's heart rate. Normal FTc is 330-360ms. The FTc may be shortened by reduced left ventricular filling, as is seen with hypovolaemia, and prolonged by vasodilatation.

1.   Waldmann C, Soni N, Rhodes A. *Oxford Desk Reference Critical Care*. Oxford, UK: Oxford University Press, 2008.

Answer 53: Calcium channel blocker overdose: True a, d & e

T   Gastric decontamination with activated charcoal (50g) is advocated within 1 hour of overdose of calcium channel blockers to reduce drug absorption. However, if sustained release preparations have been taken, then activated charcoal may be of benefit many hours after overdose.

F   Hypocalcaemia is caused by calcium channel blocker overdose. Metabolic acidosis, hyperkalaemia, severe hypotension, bradycardia, seizures, pancreatitis, hyperglycaemia, hepatotoxicity and cardiac arrest may all occur.

F   Atropine at a dose of 0.5-1.2mg is the first-line therapy for symptomatic bradycardia following calcium channel blocker overdose. Isoprenaline, dobutamine, adrenaline and temporary transvenous pacing may be required in resistant cases.

T   Severe hypotension associated with calcium channel blocker overdose may require treatment with 10% calcium chloride (0.2ml/kg), an insulin and dextrose infusion or intravenous glucagon (5-10mg). In rare cases, cardiac bypass and an intra-aortic balloon pump have been used successfully to manage refractory hypotension.

T   In the presence of unresponsive cardiotoxicity due to calcium channel blocker overdose, Intralipid® 20% (1.5ml/kg) has been used effectively.

1.   www.toxbase.org.

Answer 54: The following are recognised effects of medication toxicity: True a & b

T   Lithium in plasma levels greater than 3mmol/L produces toxicity. Signs and symptoms include: nausea and vomiting, abdominal pain, diarrhoea, blurred vision, ataxia and tremor, dysrhythmias, nystagmus, hyperreflexia, convulsions, coma and death.

T   Metoclopramide may cause methaemoglobinaemia which can cause
     a slight gray-blue discoloration of skin (3-15% fraction), cyanosis
     (15-20%), headache, dyspnoea, delirium (25-50%), profound
     acidosis, coma and death (above 50%).

F   The precise action of nefopam hydrochloride is unclear, but it does
     exhibit central anticholinergic and sympathomimetic activity. It also
     inhibits serotonin reuptake, but development of serotonin syndrome
     has never been reported following overdose.

F   Certain tyramine-containing foods (red wine, cheese, yeast extracts)
     may precipitate a hyperadrenergic crisis within 2 weeks of taking
     monoamine oxidase inhibitors (MAOIs) and reversible monoamine
     oxidase inhibitors (such as moclobemide).

F   Metformin overdose is rarely associated with hypoglycaemia.
     Severe lactic acidosis occurs in overdose which can be fatal. Other
     signs include: nausea, vomiting, sweating, hyperventilation,
     tachycardia, hypotension, drowsiness, coma, hyperreflexia and
     convulsions.

1.   Flood S, Bodenham A. Lithium: mimicry, mania, and muscle relaxants. *Contin Educ Anaesth Crit Care Pain* 2010; 10(3): 77-80.

2.   Denshaw-Burke M. Methemoglobinemia. Medscape reference, 2013; http://emedicine.medscape.com /article/204178-overview.

3.   http://www.evidence.nhs.uk/formulary/bnf/current/4-central-nervous-system/46-drugs-used-in-nausea-and-vertigo/domperidone-and-metoclopramide/metoclopramide-hydrochloride.

4.   www.toxbase.org.

5.   http://www.evidence.nhs.uk/formulary/bnf/current/4-central-nervous-system/43-antidepressant-drugs/432-monoamine-oxidase-inhibitors/reversible-maois#PHP2409.

Answer 55: Management of a donation after brainstem death (DBD) organ donor: True a, d & e

T   Donation after brainstem death (DBD) donors are more likely than
     donation after cardiac death (DCD) donors to donate multiple
     organs. The mean numbers of organs donated are 3.9 organs from
     DBD and 2.5 organs from DCD donors in the UK.

F   Physiological derangements which can occur in DBD donors
     include hypothermia, hypotension, diabetes insipidus, disseminated

intravascular coagulation, arrhythmias and pulmonary oedema. Hypothermia is the most commonly occurring derangement. Diabetes insipidus occurs in 46-78% of DBD donors.

F   The incidence of donor loss prior to retrieval may be as high as 25%. Catecholamine storm and associated acute and transient cardiovascular changes are often to blame and need to be managed with active resuscitation, arterial monitoring and vasoactive drugs to reduce this incidence. Donor centres should have a policy on practice in the event of cardiovascular instability in a DBD donor. Vasopressin (0-2.4 units/hr) may reduce catecholamine requirements. High doses of noradrenaline (>0.05µg/kg/min) should be avoided. Triiodothryonine bolus and infusion may be indicated and modified according to local policy or retrieval team advice.

T   The incidence of pulmonary emboli is high at retrieval, therefore, thromboprophylaxis should be maintained.

T   Methylprednisolone use in DBD donors is associated with increased organ retrieval rates and should be given as soon as possible. This may be due to modulation and reduction of the inflammatory response to brainstem death.

1.   McKeown DW, Bonser RS, Kellum JA. Management of the heartbeating brain-dead organ donor. *Br J Anaesth* 2012; 108(Supp1): i96-107.

2.   Gordon JK, McKinlay J. Physiological changes after brain stem death and management of the heart-beating donor. *Contin Educ Anaesth Crit Care Pain* 2012; 12(5): 225-9.

Answer 56: Neonatal and paediatric intensive care: True b, d & e

F   Children with septic shock may present with a low cardiac output state and high systemic vascular resistance (cold shock), high cardiac output state with low systemic vascular resistance (warm shock), or low cardiac output state and low systemic vascular resistance. A child may move from one state to the other, requiring vasopressor and inotropic therapy to be used and tailored accordingly. In cold septic shock, dopamine (up to 10µg/kg/min), or if resistant/refractory shock, adrenaline (0.05 to 0.3µg/kg/min), is recommended first-line. If warm septic shock is present, noradrenaline is recommended. Where vasopressors are required in children, inotropes are often also required to maintain cardiac output.

T   In persistent catecholamine-resistant shock, hydrocortisone should be added. It is important to rule out or correct pericardial effusion, pneumothorax and intra-abdominal pressures >12mmHg. Cardiac output monitoring devices are recommended at this point, with a goal of maintaining a cardiac index >3.3 and <6.0L/min/m². If shock is not reversed, extracorporeal membrane oxygenation (ECMO)/life-support techniques are recommended.

F   Tight glycaemic control in critically ill children was found to have no significant effect on major outcomes. There was a higher incidence of hypoglycaemia in the tight glucose control group.

T   A restrictive blood transfusion policy was found to be safe with associated lower transfusion volumes and a reduced hospital length of stay in patients with non-cyanotic congenital heart defects undergoing elective cardiac surgery.

T   Lower O_2 saturation targets in infants are associated with reduced rates of retinopathy of prematurity. However, when target O_2 saturations of 85-89% were compared to saturations of 91-95% in preterm infants (born before 28 weeks), an increased rate of death at 36 weeks was found in the lower O_2 saturation group. The study group recommend targeting O_2 saturations >90% in this preterm infant group.

1.   Dellinger RP, Levy MM, Rhodes A, et al. Surving Sepsis Campaign: international guidelines for management of severe sepsis and septic shock: 2012. Crit Care Med 2013; 41: 580-637.

2.   Dibb-Fuller E, Liversedge T. Management of paediatric sepsis. Anaesthesia Tutorial of the Week 278, 2013. www.aagbi.org/education/educational-resources/tutorial-week.

3.   Macrae D, Grieve R, Allen E, et al. A randomised trial of hyperglycaemic control in pediatric intensive care. New Engl J Med 2014; 370: 107-18.

4.   de Gast-Bakker DH, de Wilde RBP, Hazekamp MG, et al. Safety and effects of two red blood cell transfusion strategies in pediatric cardiac surgery patients: a randomised controlled trial. Intensive Care Med 2013; 39(11): 2011-9.

5.   The BOOST II United Kingdon, Australia and New Zealand Collaborative Groups. Oxygen saturations and outcomes in preterm infants. New Engl J Med 2013; 368: 2094-104.

Answer 57: Signs of spinal cord injury (SCI) in the unconscious patient include: True a, b & d

T   Flaccid areflexia in the arms or legs, which may be elicited by physical examination in the unconscious patient, is suggestive of a SCI. Flaccid paralysis is a sign of early SCI and occurs below the level of injury.

T   Elbow flexion with the inability to extend may occur due to the development of upper limb spasticity which develops after resolution of spinal shock following SCI. Limb spasticity follows the initial flaccidity that is seen in SCI and is suggestive of injury at the cervical spine level.

F   Unexplained bradycardia and hypotension, with marked vasodilatation, may be seen in the first 2 weeks following SCI due to interruption of the sympathetic outflow from the cord. Tachycardias only occur very rarely in the early phase post-SCI.

T   Priapism (erection of the penis which does not return to its flaccid state) is seen in SCI due to the peripheral pooling of the blood that occurs secondary to loss of arteriolar tone.

F   Following SCI it may be possible to elicit a response to pain above, but not below the suspected spinal cord level of injury in the unconscious patient. There is also likely to be loss of anal tone and deep tendon reflexes below the level of injury.

1.   Bersten AD, Soni N. *Oh's Intensive Care Manual*, 6th ed. Butterworth Heinemann Elsevier, 2009.

Answer 58: Regarding pulmonary artery catheter (PAC) insertion via the internal jugular vein: True a, d & e

T   Typically the right atrial waveform will become evident once the PAC has been advanced 15-20cm from its point of insertion into the internal jugular vein.

F   The PAC balloon is inflated in the right atrium to aid passage into the pulmonary tree. It is vital that the balloon is deflated once in position in the pulmonary artery to reduce the risk of vessel rupture or pulmonary infarction. The catheter should never be withdrawn with the balloon inflated as it may cause serious damage to pulmonary vasculature.

F   A right ventricular (RV) pressure trace is seen at 25-30cm from internal jugular insertion of the PAC. An RV pressure trace may be seen at 40cm from the insertion point if femoral vein access is used to insert the PAC.

T   The pulmonary artery waveform is usually seen at 35-50cm from insertion via the internal jugular route.

T   The balloon of the PAC should always be deflated to reduce the risk of damage to the pulmonary artery, pulmonary valve and tricuspid valve during withdrawal of the PAC.

1.   Waldmann C, Soni N, Rhodes A. *Oxford Desk Reference Critical Care*. Oxford, UK: Oxford University Press, 2008.

2.   Paunovic B, Peter K. Pulmonary artery catheterisation. Medscape reference, 2013. http://emedicine.medscape.com/article/1824547-overview#showall.

Answer 59: Regarding the mechanism of action of anticoagulant drugs: True c & d

F   Warfarin antagonises vitamin K and hence synthesis of vitamin K-dependent clotting factors, which in turn leads to inhibition of clotting activation and anticoagulation.

F   Heparin activates the protease inhibitor anti-thrombin III, and also acts on thrombin (IIa), prothrombin (II) and Factor X, with thrombin activity in particular being very sensitive to heparin.

T   LMWHs have their main anticoagulant effect through inhibition of activated Factor X, and thus monitoring of their clinical activity should be via anti-Xa level assays and not the activated partial thromboplastin time (APTT) ratio.

T   Danaparoid is used as an alternative anticoagulant to heparin in patients with heparin intolerance or heparin-induced thrombocytopenia. It works via inhibition of Factors Xa and IIa and exhibits a higher degree of inhibition of these factors than heparin.

F   Rivaroxaban acts via inhibition of activated Factor X. Other activated Factor X inhibitors are apixaban and edoxaban. Direct thrombin inhibitors include dabigatran and etexilate.

1.   Anaesthesia UK. http://www.frca.co.uk.

2.   Riva N, Lip GYH. A new era for anticoagulation in atrial fibrillation. *Pol Arch Med Wewn* 2012; 122(1-2): 45-53

Answer 60: Regarding gastrointestinal (GI) perforation: True a, c & e

T   Boerhaave syndrome is rupture of the oesophagus that usually occurs at the left posterior-lateral aspect of the distal oesophagus and is a recognised cause of GI perforation. It occurs due to increased intraluminal oesophageal pressures due to vomiting.

F   Free air beneath the diaphragm will be visible on erect chest X-ray (CXR) in approximately 80% of cases of intraperitoneal perforation, making an erect CXR a useful diagnostic tool in suspected GI perforation.

T   Peritonism may be absent in patients with GI perforation who are receiving corticosteroids, large doses of sedative agents and are obese or elderly.

F   There is no evidence for treating the colonic distension seen in pseudomembranous colitis with colonoscopy. Pseudomembranous colitis is normally treated successfully with conservative measures alone, but toxic megacolon development may require surgery to prevent perforation or achieve sepsis source control.

T   The degree of sepsis varies with the site of perforation, as stomach and duodenal fluid is fairly sterile but caustic, compared to the high bacterial load that occurs in faecal peritonitis associated with distal small bowel and large bowel perforation.

1.   Salo J, Sihvo E, Kauppi J, Rasanen J. Boerhaave's syndrome: lessons learned from 83 cases over three decades. *Scand J Surg* 2013; 102: 271-3.

2.   Waldmann C, Soni N, Rhodes A. *Oxford Desk Reference Critical Care*. Oxford, UK: Oxford University Press, 2008.

Answer 61: Regarding the storage of blood products: True c & e

F   Saline, adenine, glucose and mannitol — otherwise known as SAGM — allows red cells to be stored for 35 days. The phosphate-based additive ACPD — which contains adenine, citrate, phosphate and dextrose — allows packed cells to be stored for up to 42 days.

F   Platelets may be stored at 20-24°C for a maximum of 5 days due to the risk of bacterial contamination after this time. They must be continually agitated during storage to prevent platelet clumping.

T   Use of ABO-identical or -compatible platelets is preferable; however, ABO-incompatible platelets may be used in emergency situations as the amount of plasma contained is too small to be of clinical significance and thus full cross-matching is not required.

F   FFP is stored at -20°C and must be used immediately after thawing. It contains clotting factors, fibrinogen and plasma proteins and must be ABO-compatible. Cryoprecipitate is stored at -30°C.

T   Cryoprecipitate is produced from a single donation, and is precipitated from thawing FFP. It is stored at -30°C and may be stored for up to 12 months. It contains high levels of Factor VIII and fibrinogen, and only ABO-compatible units should be used.

1.   Anaesthesia UK. Blood storage. http://www.frca.co.uk.

Answer 62: Spinal cord anatomy: True c-e

F   The posterior columns transmit fine touch, sensation and proprioception. Pain and temperature sensation are transmitted via the spinothalamic tract which is located in the lateral column of the spinal cord.

F   The spinothalamic tract, located in the lateral column of the spinal cord, conveys pain and temperature sensation. The cell bodies lie in the posterior horn of the opposite side and fibres cross in the anterior white commissure to ascend to the thalamus. Proprioception is transmitted in the posterior column.

T   Although the solid spinal cord effectively terminates at the L1/L2 level in adults, the fibres of the filum terminale are attached to the coccyx.

T   The solid spinal cord usually ends at L1/L2 in adults, although the loose nerve fibres of the filum terminale extend below this level suspended in cerebrospinal fluid.

T   The arteria radicularis magna or artery of Adamkiewicz is the largest anterior segmental medullary artery. It typically arises from a left posterior intercostal artery, which branches from the aorta, and supplies the lower two thirds of the spinal cord via the anterior spinal artery.

1.   Smith T, Pinnock C, Lin T. *Fundamentals of Anaesthesia*, 3rd ed. Cambridge, UK: Cambridge University Press, 2009.

Answer 63: Causes of right ventricle (RV) failure include: All True

T Causes of RV failure can be divided into: intrinsic RV failure in the absence of pulmonary hypertension, usually due to RV infarction; RV failure secondary to increased RV afterload and pulmonary hypertension; and RV failure due to volume overload. Acute pulmonary emboli may cause an increase in pulmonary vascular resistance and thus RV afterload and therefore may cause RV failure.

T Protamine is used to reverse the effects of heparin and results in the production of protamine-heparin complexes. The complexes stimulate complement activation and the production of thromboxane, which can in turn lead to pulmonary arterial vasoconstriction, increased pulmonary afterload and RV failure.

T Extensive lung resection may result in increased pulmonary artery pressures — due to several different mechanisms — and this can potentially result in increased RV afterload and RV failure.

T The extensive alveolar and capillary lesions seen in acute respiratory distress syndrome (ARDS) have deleterious effects on pulmonary circulation and may result in increased pulmonary vascular resistance, increased RV afterload and RV failure.

T Obstructive sleep apnoea may cause raised pulmonary artery pressures and subsequently RV failure.

1. Kevin LG, Barnard M. Right ventricular failure. *Contin Educ Anaesth Crit Care Pain* 2007; 7(3): 89-94.

Answer 64: Liver function test abnormalities: True d & e

F Albumin is a negative acute phase marker and thus falls in critical illness regardless of synthetic liver function. However, in chronic liver disease a low serum albumin is a marker of poor synthetic liver function.

F The cytoplasmic hepatic enzyme ALT is more specific for liver injury than AST. The enzyme AST is present in skeletal muscle and myocardium to a greater degree than ALT and, therefore, AST may be raised due to non-hepatic pathology including renal and bowel infarction, pancreatitis and hypothyroidism.

F   Alkaline phosphatase (ALP) is the primary enzyme raised in cholestatic liver disease. Raised transaminases such as AST and ALT are more suggestive of hepatocellular liver disease.

T   The liver detoxifies ammonia to urea via the urea cycle prior to its renal excretion. Raised ammonia levels reflect reduced synthetic liver function and may contribute to hepatic encephalopathy. The normal serum range for ammonia is 15-45µg/dL.

T   The PT is indirectly a sensitive test of liver synthetic function in the absence of vitamin K deficiency. PT is sensitive to — and prolonged by — the low levels of Factor VII that is seen with reduced liver function. Prolongation of PT is associated with increased mortality in acute and chronic liver failure.

1.   Waldmann C, Soni N, Rhodes A. *Oxford Desk Reference Critical Care*. Oxford, UK: Oxford University Press, 2008.

Answer 65: Regarding noradrenaline (norepinephrine): True b-d

F   The usual dosage range of noradrenaline is between 0.1µg/kg/min to 2.0µg/kg/min.

T   Noradrenaline predominantly acts via α1-adrenoceptors, which in vascular smooth muscle promotes vasoconstriction and increased systolic and diastolic blood pressure. At higher doses there may be stimulation of β-adrenoceptors resulting in tachycardia.

T   Noradrenaline is recommended in the Surviving Sepsis Campaign Guidelines 2012, as the first-line vasopressor in septic shock.

T   Unlike adrenaline and dopamine, up to 25% of noradrenaline is taken up and metabolised as it passes through the pulmonary circulation.

F   The VASST study found that intravenous low-dose vasopressin (0.02-0.03U/min) alone did not reduce mortality compared to noradrenaline (5-15µg/min) in patients with septic shock. However, the addition of vasopressin to noradrenaline is currently recommended in fluid and vasopressor-resistant septic shock.

1.   Vincent JL, De Backer D. Circulatory shock. *New Engl J Med* 2013; 369: 1726-34.

2.   Peck TE, Hill SA, Williams M. *Pharmacology for Anaesthesia and Intensive Care*, 3rd ed. Cambridge, UK: Cambridge University Press, 2008.

3.   Dellinger RP, Levy MM, Rhodes A, *et al.* Surviving Sepsis Campaign: international guidelines for management of severe sepsis and septic shock: 2012. *Crit Care Med* 2012; 41(2): 580-637.

4.   Russell JA, Walley KR, Singer J, *et al.* Vasopressin versus norepinephrine infusion in patients with septic shock. *New Engl J Med* 2008; 358(9): 877-87.

Answer 66: Acute intracerebral haemorrhage (ICH): True a, b & d

T   Acute ICH is an acute spontaneous bleed into the brain parenchyma. It accounts for 10-30% of all strokes, but is associated with poor outcomes such as major disability and death.

T   The haematoma may expand for several hours after the initial bleed in ICH and reach greater than 33% of its original size. Haematoma expansion and perihaematoma oedema may both result in clinical deterioration following initial presentation.

F   Blood pressure should not be treated unless greater than 180/105mmHg in an attempt to balance risks of further bleeding against adequate cerebral perfusion. Systolic blood pressure should be maintained above 90mmHg to prevent secondary hypotensive cerebral injury.

T   Warfarin anticoagulation doubles the risk of progressive bleeding and clinical deterioration in ICH. Human prothrombin complex (e.g. Beriplex®) is indicated for immediate reversal to minimise this risk.

F   The benefits of early surgery in patients with superficial ICH without intraventricular haemorrhage are uncertain and determined by surgical preference. Conflicting evidence from the literature means that uncertainty remains as to which patients benefit from surgical intervention.

1.   Waldmann C, Soni N, Rhodes A. *Oxford Desk Reference Critical Care.* Oxford, UK: Oxford University Press, 2008.

2.   Anderson CS, Heeley E, Huang Y, *et al.* Rapid blood-pressure lowering in patients with acute intracerebral haemorrhage. *New Engl J Med* 2013; 368: 2355-65.

3.   CSL Behring UK. Beriplex P/N. http://www.cslbehring.co.uk.

4. Mendelow AD, Gregson BA, Rowan EN, *et al.* Early surgery versus initial conservative treatment in patients with spontaneous supratentorial lobar intracerebral haematomas (STICH II): a randomised trial. *Lancet* 2013; 382: 397-408.

5. Broderick JP. The STICH trial: what does it tell us and where do we go from here? *Stroke* 2005; 36: 1619-20.

Answer 67: Considering salicylate poisoning: True d & e

F   Gastric lavage should be considered within 1 hour of ingestion should expertise and patient condition allow. However, after this time the clinical benefits are negligible and associated with a risk of pulmonary aspiration.

F   Urinary alkalisation increases renal salicylate excretion and therefore sodium bicarbonate solution may be used to attain a urinary pH of 7.5-8.5 and promote renal excretion of salicylates following poisoning.

F   In severe overdose, the anion gap may appear normal due to a falsely high chloride concentration, although the classic metabolic picture following salicylate overdose is of a high anion gap acidosis.

T   A 'bezoar' is a mass found trapped in the gastrointestinal system. Tablet bezoars of aspirin may significantly delay absorption, giving falsely low levels on initial blood tests and result in late toxicity occurring.

T   A target of treatment in severe poisoning is to keep the arterial pH 7.5-7.6. Loss of the usual hyperventilatory drive due to intubation, may result in relative hypoventilation and profound acidosis, cardiovascular instability and loss of sympathetic discharge.

1. www.toxbase.org.

Answer 68: Physiology of pregnancy: True a-c

T   Plasma volume increases by 45% through the activation of the aldosterone-renin-angiotensin system.

T   At term, vena caval occlusion occurs in about 90% of supine pregnant patients and can reduce the stroke volume to approximately 30% of normal.

T   Uterine blood flow at term is great with potential for massive blood loss.

F   Cardiac output is increased by 50% by the third trimester.

F   FRC generally reduces by approximately 20% but may decrease more than this when supine. Pre-oxygenation is less effective and desaturation occurs much faster than in the non-pregnant patient.

1.   Heidemann BH, McClure JH. Changes in maternal physiology during pregnancy. *Contin Educ Anaesth Crit Care Pain* 2003; 3(3): 65-8.

2.   Rucklidge M, Hinton C. Difficult and failed intubation in obstetrics. *Contin Educ Anaesth Crit Care Pain* 2012; 12(2): 86-91.

Answer 69: In relation to the transplanted heart: True a, b & e

T   Following a heart transplant, there is no autonomic innervation. Only drugs or manoeuvres that act directly on the heart will therefore have an effect.

T   Intrinsic control mechanisms are not affected in the transplanted heart, and thus a normal response to volume loading will occur.

F   The response to hypovolaemia and hypotension may be delayed due to denervation.

F   Adenosine may cause severe hypotension and even asystole in the transplanted heart; this is due to an increased response of the donor sinus and atrioventricular nodes.

T   Amiodarone and lidocaine are effective for the treatment of ventricular arrhythmias in the transplanted heart.

1.   Bersten AD, Soni N. *Oh's Intensive Care Manual*, 6th ed. Butterworth Heinemann Elsevier, 2009.

2.   Thajudeen A, Stecker EC, Shehata M, *et al.* Arrhythmias after heart transplantation: mechanisms and management. *J Am Heart Ass* 2012; 1: e001461.

Answer 70: The focused assessment with sonography in trauma (FAST): True b, d & e

F   The FAST scan is a four-view scan — subcostal, right upper quadrant, left upper quadrant and suprapubic views are obtained.

Trauma patients may have injuries that are not immediately apparent on clinical examination. Significant bleeding into the peritoneal, pleural, or pericardial spaces may not be accompanied by initial signs of shock, thus can be missed. The purpose of bedside ultrasound in trauma is to rapidly identify free fluid (usually blood) and hence guide appropriate management.

T   Volumes of free fluid greater than 100-250ml can be detected by a FAST scan.

F   A FAST scan is not considered sensitive enough to reliably detect retroperitoneal haematoma.

T   FAST scanning is capable of detecting gross injury to solid organs, but it is not as sensitive as CT scanning at identifying solid organ injury. Certain injuries may not be seen, for example, pancreatic trauma and renal pedicle injury.

T   Increasing the frequency improves image resolution but reduces the degree and accuracy of tissue penetration.

1.   Geeraerts T, Chhor V, Cheisson G, *et al*. Clinical review: initial management of blunt pelvic trauma patients with haemodynamic instability. *Crit Care* 2007; 11(1): 204.

Answer 71: High-frequency ventilation (HFV): True a & b

T   Tidal volume must exceed dead space for effective ventilation during conventional ventilation: VA=f(VT-VD).

T   Tidal volumes are near to or less than anatomical dead space during HFV.

F   Pendelluft is the exchange of gas between adjacent lung units due to their differing time constants. Gas flows from fast- to slow-filling units at the end of inspiration and the reverse occurs at the end of expiration.

F   Taylor dispersion is the interplay between convective forces and molecular diffusion causing laminar and radial gas dispersion.

F   Molecular diffusion is the principal mechanism of gas transport in the terminal airways.

1.   Waldmann C, Soni N, Rhodes A. *Oxford Desk Reference Critical Care*. Oxford, UK: Oxford University Press, 2008.

Answer 72: Indications for extracorporeal membrane oxygenation (ECMO) include: True a, c-e

T   Cardiac failure and acute cardiogenic shock are indications for ECMO.

F   Patients with advanced chronic lung disease and irreversible conditions such as pulmonary fibrosis are usually excluded from the use of ECMO, unless it is being used as a bridge to transplant.

T   Resuscitation/cardiorespiratory arrest is an indication.

T   Primary graft failure following heart or lung transplant is an indication.

T   ECMO-assisted organ donation has been used to facilitate organ retrieval from DCD donors and is therefore an indication.

1.   Martinez G, Vuylsteke A. Extracorporeal membrane oxygenation in adults. *Contin Educ Anaesth Crit Care Pain* 2011; 12(2): 57-61.

2.   Waldmann C, Soni N, Rhodes A. *Oxford Desk Reference Critical Care.* Oxford, UK: Oxford University Press, 2008.

Answer 73: 0.9% saline: True b & e

F   0.9% saline does not contain the same amount of sodium as plasma. The Na^+ concentration of 0.9% saline is 154mmol/L and of plasma is approximately 144mmol/L.

T   Administration of 0.9% NaCl does not cause the intravascular space to gain or lose water by osmosis. It contains equal concentrations of sodium and chloride as compared with extracellular fluid, making it isotonic.

F   A small number of recent studies have shown that normal saline use compared to chloride-restrictive fluids (PlasmaLyte®, Hartmann's) is associated with worse postoperative outcomes and an increased incidence of acute kidney injury and a need for renal replacement therapy. Further studies are warranted to assess the safety and efficacy of saline as compared to balanced salt solutions/chloride-restrictive fluids.

F   Hyperchloraemic metabolic acidosis can result from a decreased strong ion difference due to hyperchloraemia or dilution of bicarbonate.

T   Excessive 0.9% NaCl may cause abdominal discomfort.

1.   Waldmann C, Soni N, Rhodes A. *Oxford Desk Reference Critical Care*. Oxford, UK: Oxford University Press, 2008.

2.   Myburgh JA, Mythen MG. Resuscitation fluids. *New Engl J Med* 2013; 369: 1243-51.

Answer 74: Potassium: True a, d & e

T   Greater than 98% of total body potassium is found in the intracellular fluid.

F   Hyperkalaemia is exacerbated in the acidotic state by increasing potassium efflux from the cell.

F   The figure is closer to 90%.

T   This is true and is achieved by binding to cell surface receptors.

T   This maintains the transcellular gradient of potassium and sodium concentrations.

1.   Manoj Parikh M, Webb ST. Cations: potassium, calcium, and magnesium. *Contin Educ Anaesth Crit Care Pain* 2012; 12(4): 195-8.

Answer 75: Contrast-induced nephropathy (CIN): True a, c-e

T   A 2005 study (Weisbord *et al*) showed CIN to be responsible for 12.5% of all hospital-acquired acute renal failure.

F   Risk factors for the development of CIN include chronic kidney disease, the type and volume of contrast medium used, as well as other patient-related factors such as age, diabetes, congestive heart failure, sex, anaemia and reduced circulating volume.

T   Bicarbonate solutions may be more effective than saline for CIN prophylaxis. This was demonstrated by the trials referenced below.

T   The mechanism of action is likely to be via inhibition of adenosine A1 receptor-mediated afferent renal vasoconstriction.

T   This has been demonstrated in patients with chronic renal failure undergoing coronary angiography

1.   Weisbord SD, Palevsky PM. Radiocontrast-induced acute renal failure. *J Intensive Care Med* 2005; 20: 63-75.

2.   Merten GJ, Burgess WP, Gray LV, *et al*. Prevention of contrast-induced nephropathy with sodium bicarbonate: a randomised controlled trial. *JAMA* 2004; 291: 2328-34.

3.   Briguori C, Airoldi F, Davide DA, *et al*. Renal insufficiency following contrast media administration trial (REMEDIAL): a comparison of 3 preventative strategies. *Circulation* 2007; 115(10): 1211-7.

4.   From A, Bartholmai B, Williams A, *et al*. Sodium bicarbonate is associated with an increased incidence of contrast nephropathy: a retrospective cohort study of 7977 patients at Mayo Clinic. *Clin J Am Soc Nephrol* 2008; 3: 10-8.

5.   Brar S, Shen AA, Jorgensen MB, *et al*. Sodium bicarbonate vs. sodium chloride for the prevention of contrast medium-induced nephropathy in patients undergoing coronary angiography. *JAMA* 2008; 300(9): 1038-46.

6.   Hogan SE, L'Allier P, Chetcuti S, *et al*. Current role of sodium bicarbonate-based preprocedural hydration for the prevention of contrast-induced acute kidney injury: a meta-analysis. *Am Heart J* 2008; 156(3): 414-21.

7.   KDIGO. Kidney Disease Improving Global Outcomes (KDIGO): KDIGO clinical practice guideline for acute kidney injury. *Kidney Int Suppl* 2012; 2: 2.

Answer 76: Heart-lung interactions: True a, c-e

T   Lung underinflation and hyperinflation increase pulmonary vascular resistance.

F   Spontaneous inspiration decreases intrathoracic pressure.

T   Artificial ventilatory inspiration increases intrathoracic pressure.

T   Lung inflation does alter autonomic tone.

T   Spontaneous effort against resistive (bronchospasm) or elastic (acute lung injury) load, can decrease left ventricular stroke volume and manifest as pulsus paradoxus.

1.   Waldmann C, Soni N, Rhodes A. *Oxford Desk Reference Critical Care*. Oxford, UK: Oxford University Press, 2008.

Answer 77: Regarding the cranial nerves (CN): All False

F   The trochlear nerve (CN IV) supplies motor supply to the superior oblique muscle. The superior rectus muscle is supplied by the oculomotor nerve (CN III) which supplies all of the other muscles of eye movement other than lateral rectus which is supplied by the abducent nerve (CN VI).

F Sensory nerve supply of the nose, face and mouth is supplied by the trigeminal nerve (CN V), which also provides motor supply to the muscles of mastication. The facial nerve (CN VII) provides motor supply to the muscles of facial expression.

F The abducent (CN VI) nucleus resides in the lower pons. It travels through the cavernous sinus lying lateral to the internal carotid artery. Aneurysms or tumours in this region may compress the abducent nerve causing VIth nerve palsy and loss of lateral eye movement.

F Sensation to the posterior third of the tongue is supplied by the glossopharyngeal nerve (CN IX). Sensation is supplied to the anterior two thirds of the tongue via the cordae tympani, which is a branch of the facial nerve (CN VII).

F The occulomotor nerve (CN III) has parasympathetic fibres, which synapse within the ciliary ganglion supplying the sphincter pupillae and ciliary muscles. The optic nerve (CN II) innervates the retina and transmits visual information.

1. Smith T, Pinnock C, Lin T. *Fundamentals of Anaesthesia*, 3rd ed. Cambridge, UK: Cambridge University Press, 2009.

Answer 78: Considering atrial fibrillation (AF): True a, c-e

T Within the developed world the prevalence of AF is approximately 1.5-2% of the general population. It is most commonly seen in patients aged 75 to 85 years of age.

F AF is associated with a five-fold increase in the risk of stroke and three-fold increase in the incidence of congestive heart failure. Mortality from heart failure is also higher in patients with AF compared to those in sinus rhythm.

T The drug vernakalant has a rapid antiarrhythmic effect and is effective in the cardioversion of patients with acute AF of short duration. It has been demonstrated in meta-analyses to be superior to amiodarone in stable patients but should be avoided in patients with heart failure, hypotension, acute coronary syndrome, severe aortic stenosis and prolonged QTc.

T   Catheter ablation is reasonable for first-line therapy in patients with paroxysmal AF and no structural heart disease. It may be used as an alternative to antiarrhythmic drug therapy for patients with symptomatic recurrent paroxysmal AF on antiarrhythmic drug therapy (i.e second-line).

T   ESC guidelines recommend that dronedarone not be given to patients in AF who have moderate or severe heart failure. It should be avoided in patients with less severe heart failure if an appropriate alternative exists. Dronedarone is appropriate for maintaining sinus rhythm in patients with paroxysmal or persistent AF.

1.   Camm AJ, Lip GYH, De Caterina R, *et al*. Focused update of the ESC guidelines for the management of atrial fibrillation. An update of the 2010 ESC guidelines for the management of atrial fibrillation. *Eur Heart J* 2012; 33: 2719-47.

Answer 79: Acute acalculous cholecystitis (AAC): True c

F   Acute acalculous cholecystitis is a relatively uncommon but well-recognised cause of inflammation of the gallbladder in the absence of gallstones. It may occur secondary to opportunist infections, gallbladder ischaemia and hypoperfusion, and in the immunocompromised.

F   AAC is less common in adults than in children, but in the adult population it tends to affect men and is frequently seen following surgery or trauma. Its incidence in the mixed critical care population is generally low (less than 1%) but this figure rises sharply in trauma patients.

T   Trauma patients with a high Injury Severity Score >12, who are tachycardic and have received blood resuscitation, are at risk of developing AAC and therefore should be monitored by ultrasound.

F   AAC may be caused by microvascular changes associated with several vasculitides including primary antiphospholipid syndrome, which should be managed with anticoagulation rather than cholecystectomy. In SLE, Henoch-Schönlein purpura and other vasculitides, steroid treatment may be sufficient treatment provided there is no intestinal perforation.

F   Mortality is up to 50-85% without treatment. Clinical presentation is often non-specific, resulting in late diagnosis with severe complications such as gangrene of the gallbladder, gallbladder perforation, abscess formation, ascending cholangitis, peritonitis and sepsis present.

1.   Waldmann C, Soni N, Rhodes A. *Oxford Desk Reference Critical Care*. Oxford, UK: Oxford University Press, 2008.
2.   Huffman JL, Schenker S. Acute acalculous cholecystitis: a review. *Clin Gastroenterol Hepatol* 2010; 8: 15-22.

Answer 80: Renal replacement therapy (RRT) may be used in the overdose management of: True b, c & e

F   RRT is of no value following tricyclic antidepressant overdose due to the large volume of distribution of these drugs following their ingestion.

T   RRT is very effective at removing salicylates from the systemic circulation and also may reverse the profound acidosis that occurs with salicylate poisoning and is therefore the treatment of choice for severe salicylate overdose.

T   Due to its high solubility in plasma and predominant renal excretion, lithium is readily removed by RRT. Due to the relatively low levels of lithium that are required to produce toxicity, rapid removal of lithium via RRT is considered the treatment of choice for lithium overdose.

F   Diltiazem, like all calcium channel antagonists, has a very large volume of distribution following ingestion and therefore RRT is relatively ineffective as a treatment for overdose.

T   Metformin is a highly soluble drug in plasma that is readily removed by RRT. Should overdose result in a severe lactic acidosis, renal replacement therapy is the treatment of choice.

1.   Flood S, Bodenham A. Lithium: mimicry, mania, and muscle relaxants. *Contin Educ Anaesth Crit Care Pain* 2010; 10(3): 77-80.
2.   www.toxbase.org.

Answer 81: Concerning corrected flow time (FTc) measured by oesophageal Doppler: True a, b & e

T   An FTc <330ms can be caused by vasoconstriction giving rise to increased systemic vascular resistance (SVR) and afterload, which can be seen following excessive use of vasopressors such as metaraminol.

T   FTc is prolonged by vasodilatation, and therefore an FTc of up to 400ms may be considered normal in anaesthetised patients, in particular, in those with a working epidural *in situ*, due to the vasodilatation that is encountered.

F   FTc is the duration of forward flow of blood in the aorta corrected for the patient's heart rate and is expressed in milliseconds (ms). The normal range for FTc in healthy adults is 330-360ms.

F   Increased afterload may result in a low peak velocity and low FTc. This should be countered with patient warming, a reduction in vasopressors, serial fluid challenges and consideration of vasodilators such as glyceryl trinitrate (GTN) depending on the clinical picture.

T   Goal-directed fluid therapy using the oesophageal Doppler has been associated with improved outcomes and reduced length of stay in high-risk surgical patients, although there is some conflict from trial data.

1.   Waldmann C, Soni N, Rhodes A. *Oxford Desk Reference Critical Care*. Oxford, UK: Oxford University Press, 2008.

2.   http://guidance.nice.org.uk/MTG3.

Answer 82: Acute ischaemic stroke (AIS): True c & d

F   In AIS, aspirin 300mg (PO, PR, NG) should be given as soon as possible, but should be held for 24 hours after thrombolysis. The addition of clopidogrel is thought to be superior to aspirin alone in preventing further stroke events in the first 90 days with no increased risk of haemorrhage.

F   Controversy surrounds the immediate use of statins post-AIS, as increased rates of haemorrhagic transformation have been reported. It is recommended that statins are started 48 hours post-AIS as there is clear evidence of long-term benefit.

T   It is recommended that patients with AIS should receive thrombolysis with tPA should they present within 4.5 hours of onset. Earlier thrombolytic treatment of AIS is associated with reduced mortality and symptomatic intracranial haemorrhage, and higher rates of independent ambulation at hospital discharge and number of patients discharged home.

T   Malignant MCA infarction describes rapid neurological deterioration due to the development of cerebral oedema following a middle cerebral artery (MCA) territory ischaemic stroke. Performing decompressive craniectomy within 48 hours is suggested to produce more favourable outcomes, with a significant difference in survival between those treated surgically compared to those managed medically in patients below the age of 60.

F   Tight glycaemic control is not indicated post-AIS. However, both the National Institute for Health and Care Excellence (NICE) and American Heart Association/American Stroke Association (AHA/ASA) do recommend that hyperglycaemia should be avoided at all times and suggest controlling blood glucose levels to between 4-11mmol/L or 140-180mg/dL.

1.   Wang Y, Wang Y, Zhao X, et al. Clopidogrel with aspirin in acute minor stroke or ischaemic attack. New Engl J Med 2013; 369: 11-9.

2.   Raithatha A, Pratt G, Rash A. Developments in the management of acute ischaemic stroke: implications for anaesthetic and critical care management. Contin Educ Anaesth Crit Care Pain 2013; 13(3): 80-6.

3.   Saver JL, Fonarow GC, Smith EE, et al. Time to treatment with intravenous tissue plasminogen activator and outcome from acute ischaemic stroke. JAMA 2013; 309(23): 2480-8.

4.   Wijdicks EFM, Sheth KN, Carter BS, et al. Recommendations for the management of cerebral and cerebellar infarction with swelling: a statement for healthcare professionals from the American Heart Association/American Stroke Association. Stroke 2014; 45(4): 1222-38.

Answer 83: Regarding spinal cord syndromes: True b & e

F   The arteria radicularis magna or artery of Adamkiewicz is the largest anterior segmental medullary artery. Damage or obstruction to this artery results in motor function impairment with extensive bilateral paralysis and loss of pain and temperature sensation, but preservation of posterior white column-mediated fine touch and proprioception, also known as an anterior spinal cord syndrome.

T   Conus medullaris syndrome occurs due to injury at the T12/L1 level with damage to lumbar and sacral cord segments. This leads to extensive paralysis in the legs of both upper and lower motor neurone type.

F   The central cord syndrome affects the upper limbs more than the lower limbs, has greater distal than proximal involvement and a larger motor impairment than sensory. Bladder dysfunction and disproportionate paralysis of the arms are frequently seen. The Brown-Sequard syndrome is caused by damage to one side of the spinal cord with loss of ipsilateral motor and proprioceptic function and contralateral loss of pain and temperature sensation, but usually affects both limbs equally on the affected side.

F   Complete cord transection — which may occur due to trauma, infarction, transverse myelitis, abscess or tumours — presents with complete loss of sensation and motor function below the level of the injury.

T   The cauda equina syndrome is caused by injuries below the level of L1 with damage to the lumbosacral nerve roots resulting in lower motor neurone paralysis, saddle anaesthesia, bladder and bowel dysfunction, areflexia and sexual dysfunction.

1.   Bersten AD, Soni N. *Oh's Intensive Care Manual*, 6th ed. Butterworth Heinemann Elsevier, 2009.

2.   http://lifeinthefastlane.com/education/ccc/spinal-cord-syndromes.

Answer 84: Starch-based intravenous fluids: True: d & e

F   Starch-based intravenous fluids are derived from hydrolysed maize.

F   With albumin as the reference colloid, the incidence rate ratio for anaphylactoid reactions was 4.51 after hydroxyethyl starch (HES), 2.32 after dextran and 12.4 after gelatin.

F   Starch use has recently been found to be associated with an increased incidence of acute kidney injury and the need for renal replacement therapy in critically ill patients, in particular in sepsis.

This may impact on overall mortality. Starch use in critical care patients is not recommended.

T Starch use is associated with an increased need for dialysis in the critically ill.

T Itch occurs in up to 13% of patients who have received starch intravenous fluids.

1. Waldmann C, Soni N, Rhodes A. Oxford Desk Reference Critical Care. Oxford, UK: Oxford University Press, 2008.

2. Reinhart K, Perner A, Sprung CL, et al. Consensus statement of the ESICM task force on colloid volume therapy in critically ill patients. Intensive Care Med 2012; 38: 368-83.

3. Perel P, Roberts I, Ker K. Colloids versus crystalloids for fluid resuscitation in critically ill patients. Cochrane Database Syst Rev 2013; 2: CD000567.

4. Myburgh JA, Mythen MG. Resuscitation fluids. New Engl J Med 2013; 369: 1243-51.

5. Barron ME, Wilkes MM, Navickis RJ. A systematic review of the comparative safety of colloids. Arch Surg 2004; 139(5): 552-63.

Answer 85: Regarding postoperative management following liver resection: True a & b

T Up to 30% of liver resection patients are estimated to have a major complication including: bleeding, liver dysfunction, respiratory failure, sepsis, intra-abdominal infection following surgery.

T Self-limiting ascites may occur within the first 48 hours following surgery, which may result in intravascular fluid depletion and hypovolaemia. This may be attenuated to some degree by the administration of human albumin solution in the immediate postoperative period.

F A transient rise in hepatic transaminases and alkaline phosphatase as a result of hepatocellular damage and ischaemia following resection is common. However, persistent elevation is an uncommon and sinister finding suggestive of ongoing hepatic ischaemia.

F Paracetamol is generally avoided in the immediate postoperative period due to the risk of causing hepatocellular toxicity. However, it may be used once postoperative liver function tests have returned to normal.

F   Hypophosphataemia may indicate liver regeneration, as phosphate is rapidly consumed via increased hepatic ATP production during periods of tissue regeneration.

1.   Hartog A, Mills G. Anaesthesia for hepatic resection surgery. *Contin Educ Anaesth Crit Care Pain* 2009; 9(1): 1-5.

2.   Wang DW, Yin YM, Yao YM. Advances in the management of acute liver failure. *World J Gastroenterol* 2013; 19(41): 7069-77.

Answer 86: Ventilator-induced lung injury (VILI): True a, d & e

T   Gross barotrauma manifesting as pneumothorax is a frequent complication of mechanical ventilation. Other complications include: pulmonary interstitial emphysema or subcutaneous emphysema, progression of pneumothorax to tension pneumothorax and cardiac arrest.

F   Direct injury to alveoli from over-distension is volutrauma.

F   Atelectrauma occurs due to the repetitive collapse and opening during mechanical ventilation causing shearing injury to alveoli. Biotrauma results from inflammatory mediators in the airspace and circulation.

T   Development of extra-alveolar air due to perivascular alveoli disruption is thought to be an initial mechanism of barotrauma.

T   Biotrauma in the lung increases leucocytes, TNF, Il-6 and Il-8 release.

1.   Waldmann C, Soni N, Rhodes A. *Oxford Desk Reference Critical Care.* Oxford, UK: Oxford University Press, 2008.

Answer 87: Regarding hepatic encephalopathy: True a, c & d

T   The West Haven system is used to stage hepatic encephalopathy from 0 to IV: Grade 0 is when no abnormality is detected; Grade I is lack of awareness, euphoria, agitation, reduced attention span; Grade II is intermittent disorientation, drowsiness, inappropriate behaviour; Grade III is marked, confusion, incoherent speech, reduced conscious level but rousable to voice; Grade IV is comatose with or without response to painful stimuli.

F Hepatic encephalopathy may occur in acute liver failure, acute on chronic liver failure or become a long-term problem complicating cirrhosis. Hepatic encephalopathy may complicate any acute exacerbation of chronic liver disease including sepsis, GI bleeding, electrolyte disturbances, constipation, drug effects and following transjugular intrahepatic portosystemic shunt (TIPS) insertion.

T Hyperammonaemia is central to the pathogenesis of hepatic encephalopathy and cerebral oedema. Serum ammonia levels correlate poorly with clinical outcome but levels above 100g/dL increase the risk of encephalopathy and levels >200g/dL are associated with cerebral oedema and herniation risk.

T Reduction in the nitrogenous load of the gut by maintaining 3-4 soft stools daily is thought to reduce levels of serum ammonia and encephalopathy risk. Lactulose reduces colonic pH, alters gut flora in favour of lactobacillus species and helps to sequester ammonia.

F Rifaximin is a semi-synthetic derivative of the antibiotic rifamycin, which decreases intestinal production and absorption of ammonia and potentially the neurocognitive symptoms of hepatic encephalopathy. However, its use as prophylaxis against hepatic encephalopathy is not currently recommended by the National Institute for Health and Care Excellence (NICE).

1. Patton H, Misel M, Gish RG. Acute liver failure in adults: an evidence-based management protocol for clinicians. *Gastroenterol Hepatol* 2012; 8(3): 151-212.

2. Waldmann C, Soni N, Rhodes A. *Oxford Desk Reference Critical Care.* Oxford, UK: Oxford University Press, 2008.

3. http://www.nice.org.uk/guidance/index.jsp?action=article&o=65844.

Answer 88: A pneumothorax: True d & e

F Pneumothoraces have a male predominance, being up to five times more common than in females.

F Smaller asymptomatic pneumothoraces may be treated conservatively or by percutaneous needle drainage.

F   A tension pneumothorax may cause tracheal deviation away from the affected side, whereas a simple pneumothorax may cause tracheal deviation towards the affected side.

T   A pneumothorax is a recognised early complication of tracheostomy insertion; it may be revealed on a post-insertion chest radiograph.

T   A pneumothorax has a significantly higher incidence in smokers, as compared to non-smokers.

1.   Paramasivam E, Bodenham A. Air leaks, pneumothorax, and chest drains. *Contin Educ Anaesth Crit Care Pain* 2008; 8(6): 204-9.

2.   Waldmann C, Soni N, Rhodes A. *Oxford Desk Reference Critical Care*. Oxford, UK: Oxford University Press, 2008.

Answer 89: Electrocution and radiation injuries: True b, d & e

F   Tetanic contractions occur with currents in excess of 15-20mA.

T   A current flow across the chest of 100mA can cause ventricular fibrillation.

F   Small currents are potentially lethal in patients with ventral venous catheters, because a high current density is produced at the heart.

T   One gray is the absorption of one joule of energy in the form of ionising radiation per kilogram of matter.

T   An exposure dose of one gray will result in a change in blood count. It may also result in nausea, vomiting, fatigue and loss of appetite.

1.   Bersten AD, Soni N. *Oh's Intensive Care Manual*, 6th ed. Butterworth Heinemann Elsevier, 2009.

2.   Taylor J, Chandramohan M, Simpson KH. Radiation safety for anaesthetists. *Contin Educ Anaesth Crit Care Pain* 2012; 13(2): 67-70.

Answer 90: In relation to tracheostomy: All False

F   Haemorrhage from the innominate vessels is a late complication of tracheostomy insertion, secondary to vessel erosion.

F   In order to allow the tracheostomy stoma to establish initially, the first tracheostomy change should not occur sooner than 72 hours following a surgical tracheostomy and not before 3-5 days (ideally 7-10 days) after a percutaneous tracheostomy.

F Ultrasound scanning of the neck prior to percutaneous tracheostomy is not mandatory, but is recommended by the Intensive Care Society (ICS) as it may improve safety, avoid potential overlying blood vessels and help with risk-benefit analysis for surgical or percutaneous intervention.

F The TRACMAN study (UK) was published in 2013, and included data on 909 patients. It examined the timing of tracheostomy, early (within 4 days) versus late (after 10 days if still indicated). There was no significant difference in mortality at 30 days or 2 years, intensive care length of stay, hospital length of stay or antibiotic use. Patients in the early group had fewer days of sedation (6.6 versus 9.3 days) and the early group had more tracheostomies. In relation to tracheostomy-related complications there were 5.5% in the early group and 7.8% in the late group. It is important to note that whilst 91.9% of patients assigned to the early group received a tracheostomy, only 44.9% of patients in the late group received a tracheostomy.

F Meta-analyses have found that percutaneous tracheostomies are more cost-effective and result in fewer complications compared to an open surgical technique.

1. Bhandary R, Niranjan N. Tracheostomy. Anaesthesia Tutorial of the Week 241, 2011. www.aagbi.org/education/educational-resources/tutorial-week.

2. Young D, Harrison DA, Cuthbertson BH, et al. Effect of early vs late tracheostomy placement on survival in patients receiving mechanical ventilation. The TracMan Randomised Trial. JAMA 2013; 309(20): 2121-9.

3. Delaney A, Bagshaw SM, Nalos M. Percutaneous dilatational tracheostomy versus surgical tracheostomy in critically ill patients: a systemic review and meta-analysis. Crit Care 2006; 10: R55.

4 MCQ Paper 4: Questions

Question 1: Malignant hyperpyrexia (MH):

a   Is inherited as an autosomal recessive condition.

b   A defect involving the dihydropyridine receptor and ryanodine receptor predisposes to this condition.

c   Signs include bradycardia, hypotension, increased end-tidal carbon dioxide production and muscle flaccidity.

d   A previous uneventful anaesthetic using a potential triggering agent excludes MH.

e   An immediate intravenous bolus of dantrolene 4mg/kg is recommended.

Question 2: Approximate cerebrospinal fluid (CSF) composition includes:

a   Osmolality 265mOsm/kg.

b   Specific gravity 1.001.

c   Glucose 3.0mmol/L.

d   Chloride 90mmol/L.

e   Protein 0.2g/L.

Question 3: The thoracic inlet:

a   Is bound posteriorly by the first thoracic vertebra.

b   The subclavian vein lies inferior to the subclavian artery when passing over the first rib.

c   Transmits the thoracic duct.

d   The inferior surface of the first rib lies on the pleura.

e   The brachial plexus lies anterior to scalenus anterior.

Question 4: The cricothyroid membrane:

a   Lies between the thyroid cartilage and the cricoid cartilage.

b   Is normally felt in the first midline space, moving caudad from the thyroid cartilage.

c   A 9mm space exists between the overlying cricothryoid muscles.

d   The space between the hyoid bone and thyroid cartilage is the cricothyroid membrane.

e   Is avascular.

Question 5: Blood products and Jehovah's Witnesses:

a   Autologous pre-donation of blood is acceptable prior to a major operation.

b   Recombinant erythropoietin is not acceptable.

c   Intra-operative cell salvage may be acceptable.

d   If the Jehovah's Witness status is unknown, blood may be administered in an emergency.

e   In an emergency, it is acceptable to give blood to a known, unconscious Jehovah's Witness to save their life.

Question 6: Renal replacement therapy (RRT):

a   Fluid overload is an indication for RRT.

b   A serum creatinine >500µmol/L is an indication for RRT.

c   Hybrid therapies offer improved cardiovascular stability as compared to intermittent haemodialysis (IHD).

d   Haemofiltration utilises the physical principle of convection for clearance of small- and middle-sized molecules.

e   Haemodialysis utilises the physical principle of convection for clearance of small- and middle-sized molecules.

Question 7: Sickle cell disease (SCD):

a   Normal adult haemoglobin consists of two α and two γ subunits.

b   Is caused by underproduction of the β-globin subunit.

c   The heterozygous state results in sickle cell disease.

d   Is characterised by haemolytic anaemia and recurrent painful intermittent vascular occlusion.

e   Oxygenation, analgesia and rehydration are important in an acute crisis.

Question 8: Abnormalities of coagulation:

a   A prolonged prothrombin time (PT) is seen in haemophilia.

b   In von Willebrand's disease (VWD) the platelet count is unaffected.

c   Vitamin K deficiency results in a prolonged bleeding time.

d   Aspirin prolongs PT and activated partial thromboplastin time (APTT).

e   Uraemia prolongs the APTT.

Question 9: Infective endocarditis (IE):

a   Is more common in females.

b   The majority of cases are caused by Gram-negative bacteria.

c   *Chlamydia* species must be considered whenever blood-culture-negative IE is suspected.

d   The diagnosis is confirmed in the presence of one major and two minor Duke criteria.

e   Antimicrobial therapy is curative in over 80% of patients.

Question 10: Hepatorenal syndrome (HRS):

a   Is defined as a serum creatinine >133µmol/L (1.5mg/dL) in a patient with advanced liver disease in the absence of an identifiable cause of renal failure.

b   Portal hypertension is the initiating factor.

c   Type II HRS has a more acute rise in serum creatinine and poorer prognosis.

d   Renal replacement therapy may improve short-term survival.

e   Liver transplantation offers little benefit.

Question 11: Valvular heart disease and surgery:

a   In aortic regurgitation, pathology of the aortic root is uncommon.

b   Aortic stenosis surgery should only be considered in symptomatic patients.

c   Most patients with severe mitral regurgitation undergo percutaneous mitral commissurotomy.

d   Aspirin is favoured for 6 months postoperatively following aortic bioprothesis.

e   Transcatheter aortic valve implantation (TAVI) is indicated in severe symptomatic aortic stenosis, in patients who are unsuitable for surgery but have sufficient life expectancy.

Question 12: Hypertensive crisis:

a   Is defined by the National Institute for Health and Care Excellence (NICE) as a blood pressure >140/90mmHg.

b   May present with encephalopathy.

c   Immediate management aims to reduce systolic blood pressure by 20%.

d   Glyceryl trinitrate (GTN) may be considered acutely if pulmonary oedema is evident.

e   Labetalol hydrochloride acts through β-blockade only.

Question 13: Acute transfusion reactions:

a   May be defined as immediate or delayed according to the Serious Hazards of Transfusion (SHOT) UK group.

b   Urticaria and/or hypotension may be the only signs in an anaesthetised patient.

c   During transfusion an increase of 2°C is diagnostic, if other causes of pyrexia are excluded.

d   May be confirmed with a positive Coombs' test.

e   Platelets have the lowest risk of bacterial contamination.

Question 14: Electrocardiography:

a   The PR interval is usually ≤0.2 seconds.

b   Bazett's formula can be used to measure the QT interval.

c   A normal QTc is <0.44 seconds.

d   The QT interval is measured from the start of the Q-wave to the start of the T-wave.

e   A normal QRS duration is 0.2 seconds.

Question 15: Pulmonary artery occlusion pressure (PAOP) will not accurately reflect left ventricular end-diastolic pressure in the presence of:

a   Mitral valve stenosis.

b   Mitral valve regurgitation.

c   Pulmonary fibrosis.

d   When the tip of the pulmonary artery catheter is lying outside West zone 3.

e   Ventricular septal defect (VSD).

Question 16: Which of the following are recognised causes of hypocalcaemia?:

a   Hypermagnesaemia.

b   Acute hypophosphataemia.

c   Vitamin D deficiency.

d   Tumour lysis syndrome.

e   Rhabdomyolysis.

Question 17: Coronary artery revascularisation:

a   Percutaneous coronary intervention (PCI) is indicated in non-ST elevation myocardial infarction with ongoing chest pain.

b   Thrombolysis is the treatment of choice in acute ST elevation myocardial infarction.

c   PCI confers a mortality benefit in chronic stable angina (one- or two-vessel disease).

d   Immediate PCI is associated with a 3% absolute reduction in mortality from ST-elevation myocardial infarction (STEMI) compared to thrombolysis.

e   Coronary artery bypass grafting (CABG) is not superior to PCI in left main stem or three vessel coronary artery disease.

Question 18: Beriplex® (human prothrombin complex concentrate):

a   Contains clotting Factors II, V, VII and X.

b   Is indicated for the emergency treatment of any life-threatening bleeding.

c   The recommended dose is 30 units/kg body weight.

d   Has a long half-life.

e   Vitamin K (5-10mg IV) should also be administered.

Question 19: Causes of raised cardiac troponins include:

a   Myocarditis.

b   Subarachnoid haemorrhage.

c   Renal dysfunction.

d   Pulmonary embolism.

e   Sepsis.

Question 20: Intestinal obstruction:

a   Large bowel obstruction typically presents with vomiting.

b   Fluid and electrolyte replacement with nasogastric tube decompression may be effective at treating adhesional obstruction.

c   A history of appendicectomy may be associated with severe and extensive adhesions.

d   Neostigmine may be beneficial in pseudo-obstruction.

e   Small bowel loops are dilated if >3cm wide.

Question 21: Intra-abdominal sepsis:

a   Raised inflammatory markers and persistent organ failure may be the only sign.

b   CT should be undertaken before laparotomy in acute generalised peritonitis.

c   Laparotomy is frequently the investigation and treatment of choice.

d   Abscess and fistula formation may develop following laparotomy if infection persists.

e   Abdominal compartment syndrome in the closed septic abdomen is uncommon.

Question 22: Variant Creutzfeldt-Jakob disease (vCJD):

a   The prion protein gene (PRNP) is located on chromosome 20.

b   Is caused by the accumulation of the scrapie isoform of prion protein (PrP^Sc).

c   Bovine spongiform encephalopathy is caused by the same prion strain.

d   Early diagnosis is possible with a blood test.

e   Prion protein is destroyed by autoclaving.

Question 23: Gastroparesis:

a   Is characterised by delayed gastric emptying in the presence of mechanical obstruction.

b   Vomiting may cause hyponatraemia.

c   In females it is commonly idiopathic.

d   Secondary gastroparesis may present in Type I diabetes mellitus.

e   Management is often ineffective.

Question 24: The Child-Pugh score:

a   Consists of four clinical features used to assess the prognosis of chronic liver disease and cirrhosis.

b   Hypoalbuminaemia (<35g/L) scores 3 points.

c   Class A has a poor 1-year survival.

d   Is more accurate in predicting prognosis in the critically ill with chronic liver disease than the Acute Physiology and Chronic Health Evaluation II (APACHE II) or Sequential Organ Failure Assessment (SOFA) score.

e   A score of 10 has a 45% predicted 1-year survival.

Question 25: Industrial chemical poisoning:

a   Moderate to severe poisoning with paraquat always results in pulmonary fibrosis.

b   Strychnine used in rat poison is a competitive agonist of the inhibitory neurotransmitter glycine.

c   Laryngeal oedema may be a significant problem in chlorine gas exposure.

d   Anhydrous ammonia reacts with tissue water to form an acidic solution causing an exothermic thermal injury.

e   Patients with organophosphate poisoning should be given fomepizole immediately.

Question 26: Causes of hyperlactaemia include:

a   Pancreatitis.

b   Short bowel syndrome.

c   Metformin.

d   Linezolid.

e   Thiamine deficiency.

Question 27: Baclofen toxicity:

a   Constricted pupils which react to light are commonly seen.

b   Intubation and ventilation are rarely required in intrathecal overdose.

c   Prognosis is usually poor.

d   Baclofen withdrawal signs include hypotension and hypothermia.

e   Haemodialysis is not effective.

Question 28: Risk factors for cerebral oedema in acute liver failure include:

a   Encephalopathy (Grade III or IV).

b   An ammonia level of 70µmol/l for 3 days since admission.

c   Acute onset.

d   Requirement for renal replacement therapy.

e   Vasopressor support.

Question 29: Hyperthermia:

a   Describes a situation where the set point for temperature is raised.

b   Antipyretics are indicated in heat stroke.

c   Malignant hyperthermia does not occur with sevoflurane.

d   Central release of dopamine causing parasympathetic overactivity is associated with ecstasy (MDMA) use.

e   Neuroleptic malignant syndrome is caused by potentiation of dopamine (D2) receptors by antipsychotic drugs.

Question 30: Status epilepticus (SE):

a   Any seizure lasting more than 5 minutes should be considered as SE.

b   Lorazepam (0.1mg/kg) has been shown to result in a higher rate of seizure control compared to phenytoin.

c   Phenobarbital extravasation can result in extensive tissue necrosis.

d   Ketamine can be effective in cases of refractory SE.

e   Levetiracetam acts on voltage-dependent Na^+ channels and may be useful in refractory SE.

Question 31: Regarding pathophysiological mechanisms of diarrhoea:

a   An 'osmotic' mechanism results in increased loss or reduced absorption of salts and water across the gastrointestinal mucosa.

b   A 'secretory' mechanism results in loss of mucosal integrity and colitis.

c   An 'inflammatory' mechanism results in loss of mucosal integrity often leading to bloody diarrhoea if the colorectum is involved.

d   A 'dysmotility' mechanism results in impaired gut motility causing retention of fluid and electrolytes within the small bowel.

e   An 'infective' mechanism results in failure of the gut to absorb osmotically active solutes.

Question 32: Acute adult encephalitis:

a   Is associated with a history of febrile illness and altered behaviour.

b   Most cases of *Herpes simplex* virus (HSV) encephalitis are caused by HSV-2.

c   Autonomic dysfunction, myoclonus and cranial neuropathies may indicate thalamic or basal ganglia involvement.

d   Aciclovir (10-15mg/kg IV tds) is recommended for *Varicella zoster* viral (VZV) encephalitis.

e   Antibodies to the voltage-gated potassium channel (VGKC) complex and the N-methyl-D-aspartic acid (NMDA) receptor may account for up to 8% of encephalitides.

Question 33: Delirium in the intensive care unit:

a   May be defined as a sudden severe confusion with rapid changes in brain function that occurs with physical or mental illness.

b   Is associated with increased mortality.

c   Regular haloperidol reduces duration of delirium.

d   Minimising sedation and early mobility does not influence delirium development.

e   Patients with hyperactive delirium are least likely to survive compared to those with hypoactive delirium.

Question 34: Vaughan-Williams classification:

a   Lidocaine shortens the refractory period of cardiac muscle.

b   Propanolol prevents peripheral conversion of thyroxine (T4) to triiodothyronine (T3).

c   Amiodarone demonstrates potassium channel blockade only.

d   Flecainide prolongs the refractory period of cardiac muscle through Na+ channel blockade.

e   Verapamil is a Class III antiarrhythmic.

Question 35: Regarding sedatives used in critical care:

a   Midazolam is a GABA-B antagonist.

b   Lorazepam has a faster onset of action than midazolam.

c   Dexmedetomidine has no effect on intracranial or cerebral perfusion pressure.

d   Isoflurane sedation can be easily controlled using the AnaConDa® system.

e   Hypertriglyceridaemia may be seen with propofol use.

Question 36: Drugs which may cause drug-induced liver injury include:

a   Co-amoxiclav.

b   Nitrofurantoin.

c   Propylthiouracil.

d   Simvastatin.

e   3,4,-methylenedioxy-N-methylamphetamine.

Question 37: Drug pharmacokinetics:

a   Glucuronidation is a phase 2 reaction.

b   In zero-order kinetics, the rate of elimination is proportional to the amount of drug in the body.

c   With regards to compartmental models, plotting concentration versus time can lead to calculation of half-life and clearance.

d   The volume of distribution of a drug is inversely proportional to protein binding.

e   A weak base is more ionized when the ambient pH is less than the pKa.

Question 38: Donation after cardiac death (DCD):

a   Functional warm ischaemic time begins at asystole and ends with cold perfusion.

b   The decision to withdraw cardiorespiratory support should always be independent and made before any consideration of DCD organ donation.

c   Cardiopulmonary resuscitation (CPR) is an acceptable intervention to maintain life whilst the retrieval team is being mobilised.

d   It is acceptable for the donor transplant coordinator to care for the potential donor whilst they are still alive.

e   Kidneys retrieved from DCD donors have worse long-term outcomes compared to those from DBD donors.

Question 39: Do not attempt resuscitation (DNAR) orders:

a   There are two options for managing a DNAR order peri-operatively: to withdraw or keep.

b   If a DNAR order is withdrawn peri-operatively, it should be reinstated when the patient returns to the ward unless in exceptional circumstances.

c   The first time a DNAR decision is considered is often at first contact with the critical care team.

d   If a patient is admitted acutely unwell, a DNAR order should be withheld until after the acute event.

e   In an emergency where there is insufficient information and insufficient time to properly assess a patient, the default is that cardiopulmonary resuscitation should be started.

Question 40: Caustic ingestion:

a   Acids cause liquefactive necrosis and extensive deep burns.

b   Alkali ingestion causes more damage to the oesophagus than the stomach.

c   Full personal protective equipment should be worn by medical staff during resuscitation and intubation.

d   Repeated endoscopies are not recommended in asymptomatic patients.
e   Following caustic injury, there is an increased risk of oesophageal cancer (up to 1000x higher than the general population).

Question 41: Paediatric trauma:
a   Cervical spine injury is common in paediatric trauma.
b   >80% of injuries are caused by blunt trauma.
c   Orotracheal intubation with manual in-line immobilisation and rapid sequence induction should be used to secure the airway in children with blunt trauma and an uncleared C-spine.
d   Isotonic crystalloid (20ml/kg IV bolus) should be given as initial fluid resuscitation in hypovolaemic shock.
e   Non-accidental injury is the most common cause of head injury in the first year of life.

Question 42: Regarding *Plasmodium falciparum* malaria:
a   Most deaths due to malaria are caused by *P. falciparum*.
b   The initial development of the parasite after transmission occurs in the spleen.
c   The incubation period is typically <7 days.
d   Thick and thin blood films remain the gold standard for diagnosis.
e   Monotherapy is recommended by the World Health Organisation (WHO) for treatment.

Question 43: Tuberculosis (TB):
a   Causes one million deaths worldwide annually.
b   Secondary TB is responsible for 90% of TB cases in patients not infected with the human immunodeficiency virus (HIV).
c   Chest radiography is the most sensitive radiographic examination.
d   Diagnosis is aided by thick and thin blood films.
e   Lumbar puncture findings in tuberculous meningitis include raised protein and lymphocytosis.

Question 44: Regarding botulism and tetanus:

a   Botulism causes an acute descending motor paralysis.

b   In botulism, a toxin irreversibly blocks acetylcholinesterase at the presynaptic junction.

c   Diagnosis of botulism is through serum endotoxin measurement.

d   Tetanus results in skeletal muscle flaccidity and autonomic instability.

e   High-dose benzodiazepine therapy is an appropriate management strategy in tetanus.

Question 45: *Clostridium difficile*:

a   Is a Gram-positive aerobic bacillus.

b   It is named 'difficile' because it is difficult to eradicate.

c   Duodenal infusion with donor faeces is significantly more effective for the treatment of recurrent infection than vancomycin use.

d   *Clostridium difficile* toxins (A and B) affect intracellular levels of cyclic adenosine monophosphate (cAMP).

e   Infection risk may be increased by chemotherapy for cancer.

Question 46: Multi-drug-resistant (MDR) bacteria:

a   A large number of agents have been developed against Gram-negative rods in the past 15 years, but few have been developed against Gram-positive cocci.

b   Vancomycin-resistant enterococci (VRE) have evolved mutated penicillin-binding proteins, conferring resistance to β-lactam antibiotics.

c   The genes for extended spectrum β-lactamase (ESBL) enzymes are transferrable between bacteria via chromosomes or plasmids.

d   *Pseudomonas aeruginosa* and *Acinetobacter* species are Gram-positive, have minimal nutritional requirements and pose a great risk to critically ill patients.

e   There is a lack of evidence and wide variation in strategies to prevent infection and spread of MDR organisms.

Question 47: Electrical safety:

a The risk of ventricular fibrillation is greater if electrical current passes through the heart during repolarization.

b An earth wire is required for Class II equipment.

c Type CF equipment should have a leakage current under 100µA.

d Type B equipment should have a leakage current under 500µA.

e Wet skin may have up to half the resistance of dry skin.

Question 48: Venous thromboembolism in pregnancy:

a Plasma concentration of all clotting factors increases.

b Platelet function remains normal in pregnancy.

c Thromboembolic risk increases 10x in the postpartum period.

d Obesity is the most important risk factor for thromboembolism in pregnancy.

e In the management of acute pulmonary embolus, thrombolysis is contraindicated during pregnancy.

Question 49: Intubation of the pregnant patient:

a Pregnant patients have an increased risk of bleeding from airway manipulation.

b A poor view at laryngoscopy can be due to airway oedema, caused by increased total body water and increased colloid oncotic pressure.

c Pregnant women have an increased barrier pressure, increasing the risk of pulmonary aspiration.

d When pulmonary aspiration occurs following antacid administration, Mendelson's syndrome will not occur.

e Pregnant patients have an increased risk of pulmonary oedema.

Question 50: Sepsis in pregnancy:

a   In the United Kingdom, deaths as a result of infection of the genital tract are falling.

b   Quinolones should not be used in pregnancy.

c   Gram-negative organisms are frequently the causative organism in maternal septic shock.

d   Goals to achieve in the initial resuscitation of the pregnant patient with sepsis-induced tissue hypoperfusion include a mean arterial pressure of ≥ 65mmHg and a urine output of ≥ 0.5ml/kg/hour.

e   Empiric combination antimicrobial therapy can be used for up to 7 days.

Question 51: Pulse oximetry and oxygen measurement:

a   In the pulse oximeter, a photodetector compares absorption of red light and infrared light at 590nm and 805nm, respectively.

b   Beer's law states that each layer of equal thickness of a sample or solution absorbs an equal fraction of radiation which passes through it.

c   Methaemoglobinaemia causes a falsely low SpO_2.

d   The Clark electrode contains a platinum cathode and a silver/silver chloride anode.

e   Oxygen is attracted into a magnetic field.

Question 52: Endocrine physiology:

a   Growth hormone is secreted by the anterior lobe of the pituitary gland.

b   Phaeochromocytoma may be diagnosed by measuring plasma catecholamines.

c   Glucocorticoids are secreted by the zona glomerulosa of the adrenal medulla.

d   Glucagon acts via the second messenger, cyclic adenosine monophosphate (cAMP).

e   Iodine reacts with tyrosine to form diiodotyrosine (DIT).

Question 53: During resuscitation of a full-term neonate:

a   Evaluation consists of checking colour, tone, respiratory rate and oxygen saturation.

b   A compression: ventilation ratio of 3:1 is appropriate.

c   A size 3.5mm endotracheal tube is appropriate.

d   There are two umbilical veins available for vascular access.

e   A neonate requiring resuscitation post-delivery usually needs circulatory support.

Question 54: Indications for synchronised DC cardioversion include:

a   Sinus tachycardia with syncope.

b   Atrial fibrillation with a systolic blood pressure of 75mmHg.

c   Atrial flutter with ischaemic chest pain.

d   Pulseless ventricular tachycardia.

e   Mobitz II atrioventricular block.

Question 55: Following liver transplantation:

a   Graft dysfunction is always caused by rejection.

b   Pulsed methylprednisolone is an appropriate management regime for an episode of acute rejection.

c   *Cytomegalovirus* (CMV) infection is the most common opportunistic infection after solid organ transplantation.

d   A calcineurin inhibitor or steroids should be used for immunosuppression in the postoperative period.

e   Following critical care discharge, there are no predictors of readmission.

Question 56: A 70kg male presents to the emergency department having fallen into a running bath. He has sustained scalds to his head, torso and both arms:

a   He has sustained approximately 50% body surface area (BSA) burns.

b   He should receive approximately 18L of crystalloid over the next 24 hours, starting from the time of admission.

c   He should receive an intravenous broad-spectrum antibiotic.

d   The main cause of mortality in burn injuries is hypovolaemia.

e   Traditional indicators of sepsis are sensitive for diagnosing infection in burns patients.

Question 57: Spinal and neurogenic shock:

a   Cord injury above the level of T1 will remove intercostal function.

b   There is one anterior spinal artery and two posterior spinal arteries.

c   Approximately 5% of vertebral column fractures result in damage to the spinal cord.

d   Spinal shock is the interruption of autonomic pathways leading to hypotension and bradycardia.

e   10% of patients with spinal cord injury (SCI) will develop deep vein thrombosis (DVT).

Question 58: Postoperative care of the cardiac transplant patient:

a   Milrinone is an appropriate therapeutic strategy in the management of low cardiac output.

b   Insertion of an intra-aortic balloon pump (IABP) is contraindicated in the immediate postoperative period.

c   Ciclosporin is well absorbed from the gastrointestinal tract.

d   Routine surveillance cardiac biopsies can be graded using the Billingham classification of mild, moderate, severe and resolving rejection.

e   Signs of cardiac tamponade include arterial hypotension, low central venous pressure, muffled heart sounds and reduced drain volumes.

Question 59: In the adult trauma patient:

a   Loss of 15-30% blood volume would suggest Class III haemorrhagic shock as per Advanced Trauma Life Support guidelines.

b   Pulse pressure increases with haemorrhage severity.

c   Appropriate sites of intraosseous (IO) access include the sternum, proximal and distal tibia, and proximal humerus.

d   IO access can be placed in a bone which has sustained a fracture.

e   All resuscitation drugs can be given via the IO route.

Question 60: The following are recognised causes of a raised anion gap acidosis:

a   Ethylene glycol poisoning.

b   Renal tubular acidosis.

c   Carbonic anhydrase inhibitor therapy.

d   Diabetic ketoacidosis.

e   Salicylate poisoning.

Question 61: Consent and confidentiality:

a   Treatment must not be given to critical care patients without their prior written consent.

b   Competent intensive care patients can refuse treatment that may be in their best interests, even if this were to result in their death.

c   An enduring power of attorney may make decisions regarding treatment on behalf of an incompetent adult.

d   Individual patient consent is required for use of anonymised patient data for quality improvement purposes.

e   Individual patient consent is required for the disclosure of information to third parties.

Question 62: The following are recognised tests for analysis of non-parametric data:

a   Unpaired t-test.

b   Mann-Whitney U test.

c   Pearson's test.

d   Wilcoxon matched pairs test.

e   Spearman's rank correlation coefficient test.

Question 63: Complications of extracorporeal membrane oxygenation (ECMO):

a   Up to 33% of patients on ECMO suffer an acute stroke event.
b   Clots in the circuit are a terminal event.
c   Bleeding is the most common complication.
d   Pump failure is not an issue, as a second back-up pump is usually on the circuit.
e   Cannula migration, although rare, is a catastrophic event.

Question 64: The following are included in Well's criteria for the risk of pulmonary embolism (PE):

a   Recent immobilisation or surgery.
b   Pleuritic chest pain.
c   Haemoptysis.
d   Right axis deviation on ECG.
e   Tachycardia >100/min.

Question 65: Tracheostomy:

a   High-volume low-pressure cuffs reduce the incidence of cuff-related mucosal damage.
b   Cuff pressure should not exceed 18cmH$_2$O.
c   The inner cannula of a tracheostomy should be removed for cleaning every 7-14 days.
d   Decannulation should be considered when the patient has a satisfactory respiratory drive and effective cough.
e   Tracheal stenosis is a common long-term complication following tracheostomy.

Question 66: Physiotherapy:

a   Ventilator-associated pneumonia (VAP) rates are less in patients treated with physiotherapy.

b   A pressure of 50cmH$_2$O is recommended as the upper limit for hyperinflation techniques.

c   Mucociliary clearance is not altered by sedation.

d   Cough assist may be indicated for patients with inspiratory muscle weakness.

e   Intrapulmonary percussive ventilation is a technique that has no effect on sputum weight or mucociliary transport.

Question 67: When assessing a pleural effusion, it is deemed exudative if:

a   Pleural fluid protein/serum protein ratio is greater than 0.5.

b   Pleural fluid lactate dehydrogenase (LDH)/serum LDH ratio is greater than 0.6.

c   Pleural fluid LDH is more than two thirds the upper limit of normal serum LDH.

d   Pleural fluid protein is >30g/L.

e   Pleural fluid pH is <7.2.

Question 68: Regarding irregularities in serum potassium:

a   Thiazide and loop diuretics are common causes of hypokalaemia.

b   Hypokalaemia with high serum bicarbonate is seen in Bartter's syndrome.

c   In the correction of hypokalaemia, infusions of potassium with a concentration >10mEq/100ml should always be given via a central venous line.

d   In severe hyperkalaemia, electrocardiography changes include prolongation of the PR interval, loss of the P-wave and widening of the QRS complex.

e   In severe hyperkalaemia, membrane stabilisation with insulin-dextrose therapy is a key component of management.

Question 69: Pulmonary function tests:

a   The Fowler method can be used to determine functional residual capacity (FRC).

b   Vital capacity (VC) monitoring is useful in all critically ill patients when predicting the need for intubation.

c   The ratio of respiratory frequency to tidal volume (f/VT) is not a reliable predictor of weaning outcome.

d   Intrinsic positive end-expiratory pressure (PEEPi) may develop during mechanical ventilation if the expiratory time is too short or expiratory resistance is increased.

e   Respiratory drive can be assessed by measuring airway pressure 0.1 sec after occluding the airway against inspiratory effort.

Question 70: End-tidal carbon dioxide (CO_2) monitoring:

a   Is an Association of Anaesthetists of Great Britain and Ireland (AAGBI) standard of monitoring.

b   Raman spectroscopy is the principle that is employed in bedside capnography monitors.

c CO_2 selectively absorbs infra-red light at a wavelength of 4.6μm.

d   Is the gold standard for confirmation of correct placement of an endotracheal tube.

e   The difference between arterial ($PaCO_2$) and end-tidal ($PetCO_2$) carbon dioxide is 0.2-0.6kPa (2-5mmHg).

Question 71: Calcium:

a   Approximately 75% of total body calcium is contained within the bones.

b   ECG abnormalities in hypercalcaemia include a widened T-wave and prolonged QT interval.

c   Hypercalcaemia may be seen in secondary hyperparathyroidism.

d   Use of loop diuretics is associated with hypercalcaemia.

e   Mithramycin, calcitonin, bisphosphonates and glucocorticoids are all recognised treatments in the management of hypercalcaemia.

Question 72: Propofol infusion syndrome (PRIS):

a   Studies have suggested an incidence of 3-4% in adult intensive care patients.

b   New-onset metabolic acidosis is a common presenting feature.

c   Electrocardiogram (ECG) changes include Brugada syndrome-like changes with ST elevation in the pre-cordial leads.

d   Severe head injury is a risk factor for developing PRIS.

e   In high-risk patients, monitoring of triglyceride and creatine phosphokinase (CK) levels may stop PRIS from progressing.

Question 73: Magnesium:

a   Two grams of magnesium sulphate is equivalent to 10mmol of magnesium ions.

b   ACE inhibitors are associated with hypomagnesaemia.

c   Intravenous administration of magnesium is associated with loss of deep tendon reflexes, hypotension and bradycardia.

d   Characteristic ECG findings in hypomagnesaemia include prolongation of the PR interval, QRS complex and QT interval.

e   Magnesium potentiates the effects of non-depolarising neuromuscular blockers.

Question 74: Infection control and critical care:

a   Ward patients have the same likelihood of developing a nosocomial infection as patients admitted to intensive care units.

b   Increasing distance between bed spaces may reduce nosocomial infection.

c   Arterial and/or venous pressure transducer sets should be changed at least every 72 hours.

d   Use of biomarkers such as pro-calcitonin (PCT) has consistently been shown to reduce mortality as part of an infection control strategy.

e   When assessing the risk of invasive candidiasis, the Ostrosky-Zeichner clinical prediction rule has a high positive predictive value.

Question 75: Renal replacement therapy (RRT) is indicated in overdose of the following drugs:

a   Lithium.

b   Digoxin.

c   Phenytoin.

d   Barbiturates.

e   Warfarin.

Question 76: Colitis:

a   Fever, anorexia and weight loss are associated with infective colitis.

b   Bloody diarrhoea is a common presenting complaint.

c   Can occur following abdominal aortic aneurysm surgery.

d   Antidiarrhoeal drugs should be used in severe acute colitis.

e   Immunosuppressant drugs (ciclosporin/azathioprine) may reduce the need for colectomy in severe ulcerative colitis.

Question 77: Kidney structure and function:

a   Each kidney contains approximately 1 million nephrons.

b   Cortical nephrons tend to have shorter loops of Henle than juxtamedullary nephrons.

c   Renal blood flow equates to approximately 10% of the cardiac output.

d   The glomerular filtration rate (GFR) for an average human is approximately 100L/day.

e   Approximately 99% of the glomerular filtrate returns to the extracellular compartment during tubular reabsorption.

Question 78: 5mg of prednisolone is equivalent to:

a   Hydrocortisone 50mg.

b   Prednisone 3mg.

c   Methylprednisolone 4mg.

d   Dexamethasone 2mg.

e   Betamethasone 20mg.

Question 79: In relation to patients with HIV and critical care:

a   *Pneumocystis jiroveci* is responsible for >50% of acute respiratory failure.

b   Anti-retroviral therapy (ART) should be continued during severe illness.

c   Sepsis is a common cause of critical care admission.

d   In HIV-positive patients with lower GI bleeding, <50% of cases are related directly to the HIV infection.

e   *Neisseria meningitidis* is the commonest cause of meningitis in HIV-positive patients.

Question 80: Concerning the confirmation of brainstem death in the UK:

a   It may be confirmed after 2 hours of apnoeic coma.

b   The tests must be performed by two qualified practitioners at least 6 hours apart.

c   Time of death is recorded as the time at which the second set of tests were completed.

d   It is not necessary to correct hypernatraemia (>160mmol/L) prior to confirming brainstem death.

e   One set of the tests may be performed by a member of the transplant team.

Question 81: Critical care and haematological malignancies:

a   Patients with neutropenic sepsis have similar rates of acute respiratory distress syndrome (ARDS) to other critically ill patients.

b   A temperature greater than 38°C is necessary for the diagnosis of neutropenic sepsis.

c   Catheter-related bacteraemia always necessitates removal of the indwelling intravenous catheter.

d   Steroids are an appropriate initial therapy for graft versus host disease (GVHD).

e   Allopurinol inhibits xanthine oxidase.

Question 82: Anti-neutrophil cytoplasmic antibody (ANCA):

a   There are three forms of ANCA.
b   If ANCA is positive, two target antigens should be checked (myeloperoxidase [MPO] and serine proteinase-3 [PR3]).
c   A positive perinuclear-ANCA (p-ANCA) may be seen in cystic fibrosis.
d   Microscopic polyarteritis is not associated with positive cytoplasmic-ANCA (c-ANCA).
e   Minocycline use may cause positive ANCA vasculitis.

Question 83: In relation to pregnancy and critical care the following are true:

a   Alveolar ventilation is increased during pregnancy.
b   There is increased glomerular filtration in pregnancy.
c   Major obstetric haemorrhage is the leading cause of maternal mortality worldwide and is the most frequent indication for pregnancy-related critical care admission.
d   Anaemia seen in the HELLP syndrome is non-haemolytic in nature.
e   The majority of survivors of amniotic fluid embolus syndrome suffer chronic neurological deficits.

Question 84: Considering propofol:

a   Propofol is a phenol derivative.
b   Vasodilation occurs secondary to production and release of nitric oxide.
c   The 1% preparation has a calorific value of 0.1 calorie per ml.
d   Propofol may produce seizure activity on electroencephalogram (EEG) recordings.
e   Hepatic disease has no clinically significant effect on the metabolism of propofol.

Question 85: Inotropes and vasopressors:

a   In septic shock dopamine is associated with an increased 28-day mortality compared to noradrenaline in adults.

b   Low-dose vasopressin as a single agent reduces mortality in septic shock compared to noradrenaline.

c   An intravenous dobutamine dose greater than 20μg/kg/min is beneficial in septic shock.

d   Low-dose dopamine exhibits a protective effect on renal function.

e   Adrenaline has predominant α-adrenergic effects at low doses.

Question 86: Ultrasound in critical care:

a   Focused echocardiography can be useful during fluid resuscitation.

b   During cardiopulmonary resuscitation, focused echocardiography has been shown to improve outcome.

c   In the supine critically ill patient, loss of comet tail artefacts and lung sliding is suggestive of pneumothorax.

d   On an echocardiogram, right ventricular dilatation and impairment with circulatory collapse is potentially an indication for thrombolysis.

e   Central venous access should be performed using ultrasound guidance.

Question 87: Indications for intubation and ventilation after traumatic brain injury prior to transfer include:

a   Glasgow Coma Scale (GCS) score <12.

b   Decrease in motor response score >2 points.

c   Bilateral mandibular fractures.

d   Spontaneous hyperventilation.

e   Seizures.

Question 88: Anaphylaxis:

a   Occurs due to an antigen-cell surface IgA antibody interaction.

b   An appropriate intravenous dose of epinephrine (adrenaline) is 100µg.

c   Epinephrine acts by inhibiting further release of histamine through increasing intracellular levels of cyclic guanosine monophosphate (cGMP).

d   Risk factors for latex anaphylaxis include being a healthcare worker, a history of spina bifida and an allergy to kiwi fruit.

e   Neuromuscular blocking agents account for 60% of drug-related anaphylaxis.

Question 89: Diagnostic criteria for sepsis, severe sepsis and septic shock include:

a   Decreased plasma procalcitonin levels.

b   Normal white cell count with >10% immature forms.

c   Elevated mixed venous oxygen saturations (>70%).

d   Severe sepsis is sepsis plus organ dysfunction.

e   Septic shock is sepsis plus either hypotension refractory to fluid therapy or hyperlactaemia (>1mmol/L).

Question 90: Drowning:

a   Protective hypothermia usually occurs.

b   The diving reflex is characterised by apnoea, vasoconstriction and bradycardia.

c   If hypothermic, the arrested drowned patient should be kept cool during resuscitation, as this may improve neurological outcome.

d   Five rescue breaths should be delivered when commencing cardiopulmonary resuscitation (CPR).

e   Immersion time should be considered in the decision whether to continue or cease resuscitation.

Answer overview: Paper 4

Question:	a	b	c	d	e	Question:	a	b	c	d	e
1	F	T	F	F	F	46	F	T	T	F	T
2	F	F	T	F	T	47	T	F	F	T	F
3	T	F	T	T	F	48	F	T	F	T	F
4	T	T	T	F	F	49	T	F	F	F	T
5	F	F	T	T	F	50	F	T	T	T	F
6	T	F	T	T	F	51	F	F	T	T	T
7	F	F	F	T	T	52	T	F	F	T	F
8	F	T	F	F	F	53	F	T	T	F	F
9	F	F	T	F	F	54	F	T	T	F	F
10	T	T	F	T	F	55	F	T	T	F	F
11	F	F	F	F	T	56	F	F	F	F	F
12	F	T	F	T	F	57	T	T	F	F	F
13	F	T	T	T	F	58	T	F	F	T	F
14	T	F	T	F	F	59	F	F	T	F	T
15	T	T	T	T	F	60	T	F	F	T	T
16	T	F	T	T	T	61	F	T	F	F	T
17	T	F	F	T	F	62	F	T	F	T	T
18	F	F	T	F	T	63	T	F	T	F	T
19	T	T	T	T	T	64	T	F	T	F	T
20	F	T	T	T	T	65	T	F	T	T	F
21	T	F	T	T	F	66	T	F	F	F	T
22	T	T	T	T	F	67	T	T	T	T	F
23	F	T	T	T	T	68	T	T	T	T	F
24	F	F	F	F	T	69	F	F	F	T	T
25	T	F	T	F	F	70	T	F	F	T	T
26	T	T	T	T	T	71	F	F	T	F	T
27	F	F	F	F	F	72	F	T	T	T	T
28	T	F	T	T	T	73	F	T	T	F	T
29	F	F	F	F	F	74	F	T	F	F	F
30	T	T	T	T	F	75	T	F	F	T	F
31	F	F	T	T	T	76	F	T	T	F	T
32	T	F	F	T	T	77	T	T	F	F	T
33	T	T	F	F	F	78	F	F	T	F	F
34	T	T	F	F	F	79	F	F	T	F	F
35	F	F	T	T	T	80	F	F	F	F	F
36	T	T	T	T	T	81	F	F	F	T	T
37	T	F	F	T	T	82	F	T	T	F	T
38	F	T	F	F	F	83	T	T	T	F	T
39	F	T	T	F	T	84	T	T	F	F	T
40	F	T	T	F	T	85	T	F	F	F	F
41	F	T	T	T	T	86	T	F	T	T	T
42	T	F	F	T	F	87	T	T	T	T	T
43	F	T	F	F	T	88	F	T	F	T	T
44	T	F	F	F	T	89	F	T	T	T	T
45	F	F	T	F	T	90	F	T	F	T	T

4 MCQ Paper 4: Answers

Answer 1: Malignant hyperpyrexia (MH): True b

F   Malignant hyperpyrexia is an autosomal dominant condition affecting skeletal muscle.

T   Loss of normal calcium homeostasis on exposure to triggering agents results in MH. The dihydropyridine receptor and ryanodine receptor (a calcium efflux channel) on the sarcoplasmic reticulum are involved.

F   MH can present with tachycardia, hypertension, hypercapnia, muscle rigidity and hyperthermia. This may progress to cause severe acidaemia, hyperkalaemia, arrhythmias, cardiac arrest, renal failure, rhabdomyolysis and disseminated intravascular coagulation.

F   Previous uneventful anaesthesia using potential triggering agents does not preclude MH development in subsequent anaesthetics using these agents.

F   The Association of Anaesthetists of Great Britain and Ireland (AAGBI) recommends a dose of 2.5mg/kg of dantrolene as an initial intravenous bolus, followed by 1mg/kg boluses as required up to a maximum dose of 10mg/kg.

1.   Halsall PJ, Hopkins PM. Malignant hyperthermia. *Contin Educ Anaesth Crit Care Pain* 2003; 3(1): 5-9.

2.   Allman KG, Wilson IH, O'Donnell A. *Oxford Handbook of Anaesthesia*, 3rd ed. Oxford, UK: Oxford University Press, 2011.

3.   http://www.aagbi.org/sites/default/files/MH%20guideline%20for%20web%20v2.pdf.

Answer 2: Approximate cerebrospinal fluid (CSF) composition includes: True c & e

F   The osmolality of CSF is approximately 280mOsm/kg.

F   The specific gravity of CSF is around 1.005, although a range of values are documented.

T   Glucose 1.5-4.0mmol/L.

F   Chloride 120-130mmol/L. Bicarbonate 25-30mmol/L.

T   Protein 0.15-0.3g/L.

1.   Erdmann AG. *Concise Anatomy for Anaesthesia*. Cambridge, UK: Cambridge University Press, 2002.

Answer 3: The thoracic inlet: True a, c & d

T   The thoracic inlet is bound posteriorly by the first thoracic vertebra, anteriorly by the manubrium and first rib, and laterally by costal cartilage.

F   The subclavian vein lies anterior to the subclavian artery. They are separated by scalenus anterior.

T   The thoracic inlet transmits the trachea, oesophagus, large vascular trunks, vagi, thoracic duct, phrenic nerves and cervical sympathetic chain.

T   The inferior surface of the first rib lies on the pleura.

F   The brachial plexus lies posterior to scalenus anterior.

1.   Smith T, Pinnock C, Lin T. *Fundamentals of Anaesthesia*, 3rd ed. Cambridge, UK: Cambridge University Press, 2009.

Answer 4: The cricothyroid membrane: True a-c

T   The cricothyroid membrane lies between the thyroid cartilage and the cricoid cartilage.

T   The cricothryoid membrane lies about 2cm caudad (towards the feet) to the cranial aspect of the thyroid cartilage.

T   A 9mm space exists between the overlying cricothyroid muscles.

F   This is not the criocothyroid membrane. Making an incision here between the hyoid bone and thyroid cartilage will potentially cause damage to the pharynx and vocal cords.

F   The cricothyroid membrane is not completely avascular. The cricothyroid arteries branch from the superior thyroid arteries and may form a small anastomotic arch traversing the superior aspect of the cricothyroid membrane. A variable number of veins may also cross the membrane.

1.   Popat M. The unanticipated difficult airway: the can't intubate, can't ventilate scenario. Johnston I, Harrop-Griffiths W, Gemmell L, Eds. In: *AAGBI Core Topics in Anaesthesia* 2012; 4: 44-55.

Answer 5: Blood products and Jehovah's Witnesses: True c & d

F   It is unacceptable to Jehovah's Witnesses to receive whole blood, packed red cells and plasma. Procedures that involve the removal and storage of the patient's own blood are not acceptable to most.

F   Cardiopulmonary bypass and renal dialysis are acceptable. Techniques using acute hypervolaemic haemodilution, recombinant erythropoietin, recombinant factor VIIa, iron supplementation and anti-fibrinolytics are deemed acceptable and may be useful in reducing peri-operative blood loss.

T   Areas of controversy include: administration of platelets, clotting factors, albumin, immunoglobulins, epidural blood patches and cell salvage techniques. These need to be discussed with each individual patient to determine acceptability or not.

T   If the Jehovah's Witness status is unknown, the medical team is expected to offer life-saving treatment, which may include blood transfusion.

F   If the unconscious patient is a known Jehovah's Witness and they have a signed, valid advanced directive, the medical team is obliged to respect the patient's competently held views about blood transfusion and products. These views must be respected even if refusal results in the patient's death, regardless of whether this is an emergency or not.

1. Milligan LJ, Bellamy MC. Anaesthesia and critical care of Jehovah's Witnesses. *Contin Educ Anaesth Crit Care Pain* 2004; 4(2): 35-9.

Answer 6: Renal replacement therapy (RRT): True a, c & d

T   Indications for RRT can be remembered by the mnemonic AEIOU. A: acidosis; E: electrolyte imbalance typically hyperkalaemia; I: ingestion of drugs and toxins; O: fluid overload especially in the context of anuria; U: uraemia and uraemic complications (encephalopathy, pericarditis, pericardial effusion and occasionally bleeding complications related to uraemic platelet dysfunction). Temperature regulation may also be an indication for RRT.

F   A high serum creatinine is not an indication in itself for urgent RRT.

T   Both continuous haemofiltration techniques and hybrid therapies tend to be better tolerated from a cardiovascular point of view. This is primarily due to slower rates of fluid removal and less solute disequilibrium.

T   Haemofiltration utilises the physical principle of convection for clearance of small- and middle-sized molecules.

F   Haemodialysis relies principally on the process of diffusion for removal of waste solute. The process involves solute movement across a semi-permeable membrane driven by a concentration gradient.

1. Baker A, Green R. Renal replacement therapy in critical care. Tutorial of the Week 194, 2010. www.aagbi.org/education/educational-resources/tutorial-week.

2. Waldmann C, Soni N, Rhodes A. *Oxford Desk Reference Critical Care*. Oxford, UK: Oxford University Press, 2008.

Answer 7: Sickle cell disease (SCD): True d & e

F   Normal adult haemoglobin, or HbA, consists of two α and two β subunits.

F   Sickle cell disease (SCD) is due to a mutation on chromosome 11 resulting in an amino acid substitution on the β-globin subunit. HbS is unstable and can precipitate out of solution when in a deoxygenated state. Thalassaemias are caused by defective synthesis of α or β chains.

F   The heterozygous state results in sickle cell trait with production of both HbA and HbS. Sickling only occurs under extreme conditions. The homozygous state results in SCD (near 100% HbS).

T   SCD is characterised by haemolytic anaemia, intermittent vascular occlusion, severe pain and end-organ damage, and may result in the following: cardiomegaly, heart failure, pulmonary hypertension secondary to pulmonary infarcts, dyspnoea, cough, chest pain, marrow hyperplasia, renal impairment, splenic infarction, immune compromise, hepatomegaly, gallstones, leg ulcers, skeletal deformities, frontal bossing, transient ischaemic attacks, stroke, severe anaemia, bone marrow failure, splenic sequestration and infection-induced myelosuppression.

T   Oxygenation, fluids, warming, avoiding venous stasis, blood transfusion and analgesia, form the mainstay of management in an acute sickle crisis. Prompt cultures and antibiotics, if infection is suspected as a trigger, are also important.

1.   Wilson M, Forsyth P, Whiteside J. Haemoglobinopathy and sickle cell disease. *Contin Educ Anaesth Crit Care Pain* 2010; 10(1): 24-2.

Answer 8: Abnormalities of coagulation: True b

F   Prolongation of the activated partial thromboplastin time (APTT), not the PT, is seen in haemophilia.

T   Von Willebrand's disease results in a prolonged or normal APTT and prolonged bleeding time. The platelet count is not affected.

F   Vitamin K deficiency results in a prolonged PT and an abnormal or mildly prolonged APTT. It does not affect the bleeding time or platelet count.

F   Aspirin prolongs the bleeding time only.

F   Uraemia prolongs the bleeding time only.

1.   http://www.aacc.org/publications/cln/2012/January/Pages/CoagulationTests.aspx#.
2.   http://www.ncbi.nlm.nih.gov/books/NBK265.
3.   http://www.frca.co.uk/article.aspx?articleid=100101.

Answer 9: Infective endocarditis (IE): True c

F   IE is more common in males, at a ratio of 2:1.

F   The majority of IE is caused by Gram-positive bacteria such as *Staphylococcus aureus* and *Streptococci* (31-54%). Gram-negative organisms (HACEK: *Haemophilus*, *Aggregatibacter aphrophilus*, *Cardiobacterium hominis*, *Eikenella corrodens* and *Kingella kingae*) and fungi (*Candida*/*Aspergillus*) are less common causes (1-3%).

T   *Coxiella burnettii*, *Legionella*, *Brucella*, *Bartonella* and *Chlamydia* species must be considered whenever blood-culture-negative IE is suspected.

F   Using the modified Duke criteria, the diagnosis of infective endocarditis is <u>confirmed</u> in the presence of two major criteria, one major and three minor, or five minor criteria.

F   Antimicrobial therapy is curative in only 50% of cases of IE. The remaining 50% require surgery (valve repair/valve replacement). Early valve surgery may be beneficial.

1.   Martinez G, Valchanov K. Infective endocarditis. *Contin Educ Anaesth Crit Care Pain* 2012; 12(3): 134-8.

Answer 10: Hepatorenal syndrome (HRS): True a, b & d

T   HRS is defined as serum creatinine >133µmol/L in a patient with cirrhosis and ascites when all other pathologies are excluded or treated. The diagnostic criteria for HRS, is based on the 2007 International Ascites Club criteria.

T   Portal hypertension in liver failure is thought to be the initiating factor for HRS, resulting in the production of systemic vasodilators (e.g. nitric oxide, NO). Activation of the sympathetic nervous system and renin-angiotensin-aldosterone system (RAAS) occurs with release of arginine vasopressin to counteract vasodilatation and increased sodium and water retention. Renal autoregulation is altered making renal perfusion more sensitive to changes in mean arterial pressure. As cirrhosis worsens, further renal vasoconstriction and sodium retention occurs to offset increasing systemic vasodilatation leading to functional renal failure.

F   Patients with Type I HRS have a more acute rise in serum creatinine (doubling of creatinine to a value >2.5mg/dL) in a period of less than

2 weeks. Type I HRS usually develops as a result of acute deterioration in hepatic function triggered by bacterial infection and severe alcoholic hepatitis and has a poor prognosis (median untreated survival of 2 weeks). Type II HRS occurs in patients with refractory ascites and involves renal dysfunction (serum creatinine >1.5mg/dL or >133µmol/L) which progresses more slowly than in Type I HRS.

T   Renal replacement therapy may improve short-term survival for patients with HRS, as a bridge to transplant or until an acute reversible cause of hepatic decompensation is treated.

F   The only definitive treatment is liver transplantation for suitable patients with HRS.

1.   Lynch G. Hepatorenal syndrome. Anaesthesia Tutorial of the Week 240, 2011. www.aagbi.org/education/educational-resources/tutorial-week.

2.   Kiser TH. Hepatorenal syndrome. *Int J Clin Med* 2014; 5: 102-10.

Answer 11: Valvular heart disease and surgery: True e

F   In aortic regurgitation, pathology of the aortic root is frequent. Surgery is indicated in Marfan syndrome/bicuspid aortic valve when the maximal ascending aortic diameter is equal to or greater than 50mm and lower for patients with risk factors of disease progression.

F   Surgery should be considered in asymptomatic patients with low operative risk with very severe aortic stenosis or progressive disease.

F   Most patients with severe mitral stenosis and favourable valve anatomy undergo percutaneous mitral commissurotomy.

F   Aspirin is favoured for 3 months postoperatively following aortic bioprosthesis.

T   Transcatheter aortic valve implantation (TAVI) is indicated in patients with severe aortic stenosis who are unsuitable/unfit for surgery, but are deemed to have sufficient life expectancy.

1.   ESC/EACTS. Guidelines on the management of valvular heart disease. *Eur Heart J* 2012; 33: 2451-96.

Answer 12: Hypertensive crisis: True b & d

F   Accelerated hypertension/acute hypertension is defined by the National Institute for Health and Care Excellence (NICE) UK, as a blood pressure >180/110mmHg with end-organ dysfunction. A blood pressure >140/90mmHg is defined as hypertension.

T   A hypertensive crisis occurs when hypertension causes acute end-organ dysfunction. For example, neurological dysfunction (headache, blurred vision, papilloedema, fundal haemorrhages, encephalopathy, limb weakness), cardiovascular dysfunction (acute coronary syndrome, myocardial infarction, pulmonary oedema, aortic dissection) and renal dysfunction (acute kidney injury).

F   Management of an acute hypertensive crisis aims to reduce the mean arterial pressure (MAP) by no more than 10-20%, as greater reductions may cause complications such as ischaemia, in the presence of cerebrovascular or carotid disease.

T   GTN 0.5-20mg/hr intravenously titrated to effect, may be considered for immediate management. At higher doses, GTN only affects arterial tone, causing hypotension. Generally GTN is not recommended for use in an acute hypertensive crisis. However, low-dose GTN may be used in patients with hypertensive emergencies associated with acute coronary syndromes or acute pulmonary oedema. Sodium nitroprusside is an arterial and venous vasodilator and may be used in patients with acute hypertensive emergencies associated with aortic dissection or left ventricular dysfunction.

F   Labetalol hydrochloride may be used in the acute period: 20mg intravenously over 2 minutes followed by an infusion of 2mg/min until there is a satisfactory response (maximum dose 300mg). Labetalol acts on both α1-adrenergic receptors and non-selective β-adrenergic receptors. Other agents considered in the immediate management of hypertensive crisis include: esmolol, sodium nitroprusside and hydralazine.

1.   http://www.nice.org.uk/nicemedia/pdf/CG034NICEguideline.pdf.

2.   Beed M, Sherman R, Mahajan R. *Emergencies in Critical Care*, 2nd ed. Oxford, UK: Oxford Medical Publications, 2013.

Answer 13: Acute transfusion reactions: True b, c and d

F   According to the Serious Hazards of Transfusion (SHOT) UK group, 'acute' reactions by definition occur within 24 hours. Haemolytic transfusion reactions can be acute (within 24 hours) or delayed (occur 3-10 days post-transfusion).

T   The following signs and symptoms are all associated with acute transfusion reactions: fever, chills, pain at injection site, rigors, flushing, urticaria, angio-oedema, hypotension or hypertension, bone/muscle/chest/abdominal pain, tachypnoea, bronchospasm, nausea, vomiting, oliguria, haemoglobinuria, diffuse bleeding and feelings of impending doom. Urticaria and hypotension may be the only signs in anaesthetised patients.

T   A non-haemolytic febrile transfusion reaction is very common and often mild, requiring minor intervention, for example, slowing the transfusion and giving paracetamol. An increase in temperature of 2°C is diagnostic if other causes of pyrexia are excluded. In a severe reaction the blood transfusion must be stopped immediately.

T   Most haemolytic transfusion reactions involve the ABO and Rhesus (Rh) systems. Other common groups are Duffy, Kidd and Kell. Acute haemolytic transfusion reactions can be confirmed by haemoglobin reduction, a positive Coombs' test (a positive direct antiglobulin test), a positive cross-match test and raised lactate dehydrogenase.

F   Platelets have the highest risk of bacterial contamination (1:2000) as they are stored at room temperature. The risk from red cells is much lower (1:500,000). Major bacterial contaminations causing acute transfusion reactions are often due to donor skin organisms. All blood components should be examined for clumps, discoloration and damage to the bag before administration.

1.   Clevenger B, Kelleher A. Hazards of blood transfusion in adults and children. *Contin Educ Anaesth Crit Care Pain* 2014; 14(3): 112-8.

Answer 14: Electrocardiography: True a & c

T   The PR interval is usually 0.12-0.2s.

F   The QT interval is corrected for heart rate using Bazett's formula: $QTc = QT / \sqrt{(RR\ interval)}$.

T   A normal QTc is 0.30-0.44s. >0.44s is considered prolonged.

F   The QT interval is measured from the start of the Q-wave to the end of the T-wave and represents the time taken for ventricular depolarisation and repolarisation.

F   The QRS duration is normally 0.12s or less.

1.   Waldmann C, Soni N, Rhodes A. *Oxford Desk Reference Critical Care*. Oxford, UK: Oxford University Press, 2008.

2.   Hunter JD, Sharma P, Rathi S. Long QT syndrome. *Contin Educ Anaesth Crit Care Pain* 2008; 8(2): 67-70.

Answer 15: Pulmonary artery occlusion pressure (PAOP) will not accurately reflect left ventricular end-diastolic pressure in the presence of: True a-d

T   See explanation below.

T

T

T

F   PAOP is not affected by a ventricular septal defect (VSD).

Pulmonary artery occlusion pressure (PAOP) will not accurately reflect left ventricular end-diastolic pressure (LVEDP) in: mitral valve (MV) stenosis, MV incompetence/regurgitation, pulmonary venous obstruction (pulmonary fibrosis) and if the tip of the pulmonary artery catheter is lying outside West zone 3 — where the pulmonary capillary bed is compressed by the pressure within the alveoli causing inaccurate PAOP estimation.

1.   Waldmann C, Soni N, Rhodes A. *Oxford Desk Reference Critical Care*. Oxford, UK: Oxford University Press, 2008.

Answer 16: Which of the following are recognised causes of hypocalcaemia?: True a, c-e

T

F

T

T

T

Causes of hypocalcaemia are numerous and include: hypoparathyroidism (absence of parathyroid hormone [PTH] secretion), postoperative parathyroid/thyroid surgery, autoimmune (isolated or part of polyglandular autoimmune syndrome), congenital (mutations of CaSR, PTH, and parathyroid aplasia), pseudohypoparathyroidism (Types 1a, 1b and 2), magnesium depletion, severe hypermagnesaemia, deficiency of vitamin D, hyperphosphataemia, renal failure, rhabdomyolysis, tumour lysis, phosphate administration, acute pancreatitis, hungry bone syndrome, chelation (citrate, EDTA, lactate, foscarnet), osteoblastic metastases, malignancy (prostate, breast), sepsis, fluoride administration, surgery, chemotherapy (cisplatin, 5-fluorouracil, leucovorin).

1.   Tohme JF, Bilezekian JP. Hypocalcemic emergencies. *Endocrinol Metab Clin North Am* 1993; 22: 363-5.

Answer 17: Coronary artery revascularisation: True a & d

T   Angiography and percutaneous coronary intervention (PCI) such as angioplasty and stenting is recommended within 72 hours of non-ST elevation myocardial infarction or immediately if high-risk features are present (e.g. arrhythmias, ongoing chest pain).

F   Evidence suggests that immediate PCI is beneficial in ST-elevation myocardial infarction (STEMI). However, if delay in PCI is greater than 90-120 minutes from chest pain onset, thrombolysis is indicated with early PCI within 24 hours.

F   There is no mortality benefit by performing PCI in chronic stable angina. However, PCI is associated with improved symptom control.

T   Immediate PCI in patients with STEMI is associated with an absolute risk reduction in short- and long-term mortality from 8% to 5% (3% reduction) compared with thrombolysis.

F   Coronary artery bypass grafting (CABG) is superior in most patients with chronic stable angina (left main stem or three-vessel disease), with an associated mortality benefit compared to PCI.

1.   http://www.ucl.ac.uk/nicor/audits/adultcardiacintervention/publicreports/documents/pcireport2012.

2.   D'Souza SP, Mamas MA, Fraser DG, *et al.* Routine early coronary angioplasty versus ischaemia-guided angioplasty after thrombolysis in acute ST-elevation myocardial infarction: a meta-analysis. *Eur Heart J* 2011; 32: 972-82.

3.   Moore C, Leslie S. Coronary artery stents: management in patients undergoing non-cardiac surgery. Johnston I, Harrop-Griffiths W, Gemmell L, Eds. In: *AAGBI Core Topics in Anaesthesia* 2012; 2: 17-27.

Answer 18: Beriplex® (human prothrombin complex concentrate): True c & e

F   Beriplex® contains the vitamin K-dependent coagulation Factors: II, VII, IX and X; not V.

F   Beriplex® is indicated only for the treatment of life-threatening bleeding in patients who have an acquired deficiency of the prothrombin complex coagulation factors, such as those receiving vitamin K antagonists (e.g. warfarin) or congenital deficiency of vitamin K-dependent coagulation factors. Beriplex® rapidly corrects the prothombin complex deficiency and may slow or stop bleeding.

T   The dose of Beriplex® is based on Factor IX content, which is 500IU per vial. The dose is 30 units/kg body weight, irrespective of the international normalised ratio (INR), with a maximum single dose of 3000 units (120ml).

F   Beriplex® has a short half-life and temporary effect on INR, which may rise again once the concentrates have been consumed.

T   Due to the temporary effect of Beriplex® on INR, vitamin K (5mg) by slow intravenous injection should also be given. This will reduce the risk of a rebound rise in INR.

1.   CSL Behring UK. Beriplex P/N. http://www.cslbehring.co.uk.

Answer 19: Causes of raised cardiac troponins: All True

Causes of raised cardiac troponins other than acute coronary syndrome include: severe tachyarrhythmias or bradyarrhythmias, myocarditis, dissecting aortic aneurysm, pulmonary embolism, chronic or acute renal dysfunction, stroke and subarachnoid haemorrhage. Raised troponins may be seen in any critically ill patient, especially those with sepsis.

1.   http://www.escardio.org/guidelines-surveys/esc-guidelines/GuidelinesDocuments/Essential%20Messages%20NSTE.pdf.

Answer 20: Intestinal obstruction: True b-e

F   Small bowel obstruction tends to present more frequently with vomiting. Large bowel obstruction tends to present with diarrhoea if subacute obstruction, or constipation in total obstruction.

T   Fluid and electrolyte replacement with nasogastric tube decompression may be effective at managing adhesional bowel obstruction.

T   Appendicectomy and pouch surgery may result in severe and extensive adhesions, leading to small bowel obstruction.

T   Intravenous neostigmine may be beneficial at reducing time to resolution of acute colonic pseudo-obstruction. It is not currently recommended as first-line treatment, only when conservative management has failed. Continuous cardiac monitoring is required due to the risk of bradycardia, which usually responds well to atropine boluses.

T   Small bowel loops are dilated if >3cm wide. Large bowel loops are dilated if >6cm (or >9cm at the caecum) on plain abdominal X-rays.

1.   Waldmann C, Soni N, Rhodes A. *Oxford Desk Reference Critical Care.* Oxford, UK: Oxford University Press, 2008.

2.   Elsner JL, Smith JM, Ensor CR. Intravenous neostigmine for postoperative acute colonic pseudo-obstruction. *Ann Pharmacother* 2012; 46(3): 430-5.

Answer 21: Intra-abdominal sepsis: True a, c & d

T   Peritonitis may be subtle with acute or insidious onset. Signs include: malaise, pain, nausea, fever, anorexia and diarrhoea. Persistently raised inflammatory markers and abdominal pain may be the only sign of intra-abdominal sepsis and peritonism.

F   In peritonitis caused by ruptured viscus, acute appendicitis or diverticulitis, CT and ultrasound give limited yield and increase time to laparotomy, thereby delaying definitive management. Ultrasound may be helpful in primary bacterial peritonitis in liver disease to aid paracentesis and assess portal flow. CT imaging with contrast is useful in identifying bowel leaks and collections, which may be amenable to percutaneous drainage or re-laparotomy.

T   In acute peritonitis, laparoscopy or laparotomy are often required to investigate and treat.

T   Failure of sepsis resolution following laparotomy may be indicative of abscess or fistula formation, warranting re-laparotomy and washout.

F   Abdominal compartment syndrome may commonly present in the closed septic abdomen. Intra-abdominal pressures >25mmHg with organ dysfunction, particularly in patients who are sedated and ventilated, warrants urgent laparostomy/re-laparotomy.

1.   Waldmann C, Soni N, Rhodes A. *Oxford Desk Reference Critical Care*. Oxford, UK: Oxford University Press, 2008.

Answer 22: Variant Creutzfeldt-Jakob disease (vCJD): True a-d

T   Cellular prion protein (PrP^C) occurs naturally in humans and animals. The prion protein gene (PRNP) is located on chromosome 20 and encodes cellular prion protein. Accumulation of abnormal prion protein is associated with neurodegenerative diseases which can be transmitted, are progressive and are uniformly fatal.

T   The scrapic isoform of prion protein (PrP^Sc) is the abnormal form of prion protein. It can be acquired from external inoculation or ingestion or arise through inherited mutations. Once PrP^Sc is present it converts normal PrP^C into abnormal prion protein, which accumulates and is associated with loss of synapses and neuronal death.

T   vCJD is caused by the same prion strain that causes bovine spongiform encephalopathy (BSE) in cattle, concluding that human transmission is from dietary exposure.

T   A blood test has been recently developed by the NHS National Prion Clinic and can detect abnormal prion protein in blood with a sensitivity of 70%. Tonsillar biopsy has 100% sensitivity, but is not routinely recommended. The World Health Organisation has criteria for the diagnosis of vCJD: a progressive psychiatric disorder of clinical duration greater than 6 months, with no alternative diagnosis from routine investigations, is suggestive of vCJD.

F   Prion protein cannot be completely destroyed by autoclaving, so surgical instruments need to be quarantined or destroyed.

1.   Porter MC, Leemans M. Creutzfeldt-Jakob disease. *Contin Educ Anaesth Crit Care Pain* 2012; 13(4): 119-24.

Answer 23: Gastroparesis: True b-e

F   Gastroparesis is a symptomatic, chronic disorder characterised by delayed gastric emptying in the absence of mechanical obstruction.

T   Both hyponatraemia (due to excessive sodium loss in vomitus) and hypernatraemia (due to dehydration) can present. Loss of H^+ and Cl^- may result in a hypochloraemic alkalosis. Urinary potassium loss in exchange for H^+ may exacerbate hypokalaemia further.

T   Gastroparesis may be idiopathic. Patients are often female (around 80%).

T   Type I diabetes, abdominal surgery (vagotomy, fundoplication, bariatric surgery), hypothyroidism and rheumatological disorders (scleroderma, systemic lupus erythematosus and amyloidosis) are risk factors for secondary gastroparesis development.

T   Management of gastroparesis often fails. It includes dietary manipulation, optimising glycaemic control, antiemetics and prokinetics. Refractory gastroparesis may require enteral feeding and gastrostomy.

1.   Waldmann C, Soni N, Rhodes A. *Oxford Desk Reference Critical Care*. Oxford, UK: Oxford University Press, 2008.

Answer 24: The Child-Pugh score: True e

F   Consists of five clinical features (total bilirubin, serum albumin, prothrombin time [PT] or international normalised ratio [INR], ascites and hepatic encephalopathy) and is used to assess the prognosis of chronic liver disease and cirrhosis. Each factor is scored 1 to 3 depending on severity.

F   Albumin >35g/L is scored 1, 28-35g/L is scored 2, <28g/L is scored 3 points.

F   Class A (score 5-6) = 100% 1-year survival; Class B (score 7-9) = 80% 1-year survival; Class C (score 10-15) = 45% 1-year survival.

F   The Child-Pugh score is not as accurate at predicting prognosis in the critically ill patient with chronic liver disease. Intensive care unit-specific scoring systems such as the Acute Physiology and Chronic Health Evaluation II (APACHE II) and Sequential Organ Failure Assessment (SOFA) score are more accurate.

T   Class C (score 10-15) has a 45% predicted 1-year survival.

1.   http://www.2minutemedicine.com/the-child-pugh-score-prognosis-in-chronic-liver-disease-and-cirrhosis-classics-series.

2.   Flood S, Bodenham A, Jackson P. Mortality of patients with alcoholic liver disease admitted to critical care: a systemic review. *J Intensive Care Soc* 2012; 13(2): 130-5.

Answer 25: Industrial chemical poisoning: True a & c

T   Paraquat was withdrawn from sale in the EU after 2005 and withdrawn from medical supplies in 2008. Severe paraquat poisoning >20mg/kg, usually after ingestion, causes severe multi-organ failure. Pulmonary fibrosis is the major cause of respiratory failure and death. Supplemental oxygen during resuscitation may worsen lung injury.

F   Strychnine acts as an antagonist of glycine. It was banned in rodenticides in the United Kingdom from 2006. It remains permitted as a below-ground pesticide to control rodents in the United States. It has been found as a contaminant in herbal preparations and drugs of abuse (e.g. heroin). Strychnine is highly toxic with systemic features presenting 5 minutes after inhalation. Increased muscle tone, twitching and seizures are predominant features.

T   Chlorine is a pungent irritant gas which is denser than air so remains at ground level. It causes pneumonitis, stridor, laryngeal oedema, tachypnoea and acute pulmonary oedema.

F   Anhydrous ammonia (liquid or gas) reacts with tissue water to form the strongly alkaline solution, ammonium hydroxide. This reaction is exothermic causing thermal burns, with alkali causing liquefaction necrosis and deep tissue penetration.

F   Atropine and pralidoxime are used in the acute management of organophosphate poisoning. 'DUMBBBELS' is used as a mnemonic to describe the muscarinic features of cholinergic toxic syndrome: Diarrhoea, Urination, Miosis, Bronchorrhoea, Bronchoconstriction, Bradycardia (unreliable sign as tachycardia can occur), Emesis, Lacrimation and Salivation.

1.   www.toxbase.org.

2.   Geoghegan J, Tong JL. Chemical warfare agents. *Contin Educ Anaesth Crit Care Pain* 2006; 6(6): 230-4.

Answer 26: Causes of hyperlactaemia include: All True

T   Acute pancreatitis may be a cause of Type B hyperlactaemia. Type B lactic acidosis is defined classically by Cohen and Wood to occur when no clinical evidence of poor tissue perfusion or oxygenation exists. In reality, occult tissue hypoperfusion often coexists. Type B is divided into three subtypes: B1 occurs in association with systemic disease such as renal and hepatic failure, diabetes and malignancy; B2 is caused by drugs and toxins (e.g. alcohols, iron, isoniazid, zidovudine, biguanides and salicylates); and B3 is due to inborn errors of metabolism.

T   Short bowel syndrome (rise in D-lactate) causes a Type B hyperlactaemia.

T   Metformin can cause a drug-induced lactic acidosis.

T   Linezolid can cause lactic acidosis.

T   Thiamine deficiency and glucose-6-dehydrogenase deficiency can cause Type B hyperlactaemia. Regional infarction, ischaemia, hypotension, cardiac arrest and septic shock are causes of Type A hyperlactaemia. Type A lactic acidosis occurs in association with clinical evidence of poor tissue perfusion or oxygenation/hypoxia.

1.   Gunnerson KJ, Pinsky MR. Lactic acidosis. Medscape reference, 2013. http://emedicine.medscape.com/article/167027-overview.

2.   Waldmann C, Soni N, Rhodes A. *Oxford Desk Reference Critical Care*. Oxford, UK: Oxford University Press, 2008.

3.   http://www.evidence.nhs.uk/formulary/bnf/current/5-infections/51-antibacterial-drugs/517-some-other-antibacterials/linezolid/linezolid?q=LINEZOLID.

Answer 27: Baclofen toxicity: All False

F   Severe baclofen poisoning may result in long-lasting (days to weeks) coma which may mimic brain death with fixed dilated pupils. Generalised hypotonia, areflexia, drowsiness, hypotension and hypothermia may occur, which can progress to myoclonic jerks, grand mal convulsions, rhabdomyolysis, respiratory depression and respiratory/cardiac arrest.

F   Intubation and ventilation are often required in all but minor intrathecal overdoses. Intrathecal doses of 10mg and 30mg have been reported to cause profound coma.

F   If early airway intervention is undertaken, the prognosis is often excellent despite prolonged coma.

F   Baclofen toxicity often presents with hypotension and hypothermia. Baclofen withdrawal symptoms may occur following overdose and can present with hypertension, hyperthermia and hallucinations.

F   Haemodialysis should be considered for the management of acute baclofen toxicity.

1.   www.toxbase.org.

Answer 28: Risk factors for cerebral oedema in acute liver failure include: True a, c-e

T   The higher the grade of encephalopathy (Grade III/IV), the greater the risk of cerebral oedema development in acute liver failure.

F   Cerebral oedema development is rare in patients with an ammonia level <75µmol/L. A level of >100µmol/L increases the risk of encephalopathy, and a level of >200µmol/L is associated with raised intracranial pressure. Kumar *et al* looked at 295 patients with acute liver failure and found that those with levels >122µmol/L for 3 consecutive days since admission, had lower rates of survival and a higher incidence of cerebral oedema, infection and seizures compared with those whose ammonia levels decreased. Patients with persistent hyperammonaemia >85µmol/L for 3 days were also more likely to have complications or die.

T   In liver failure, the faster the onset of jaundice to encephalopathy, the greater the incidence of cerebral oedema development. Patients with hyper-acute liver failure have a greater risk of cerebral oedema development compared to those with acute liver failure.

T   The requirement for renal replacement therapy is associated with an increased risk of cerebral oedema in patients with acute liver failure.

T   Vasopressor support is associated with increased cerebral oedema development and is a reflection of disease severity.

1.   Wang DW, Yin YM, Yao YM. Advances in the management of acute liver failure. *World J Gastroenterol* 2013; 19(41): 7069-77.

2.   Kumar R, Harish Sharma S, Prakash S, *et al.* Persistent hyperammonemia is associated with complications and poor outcomes in patients with acute liver failure. *Clin Gasteroenterol Hepatol* 2012; 10(8): 925-31.

3. Maclure P, Salman B. Management of acute liver failure in critical care. Anaesthesia Tutorial of the Week 251, 2012. www.aagbi.org/education/educational-resources/tutorial-week.

Answer 29: Hyperthermia: All False

F   Hyperthermia is the elevation of body temperature due to loss of thermoregulatory control. Hyperpyrexia is where the set point for temperature is raised.

F   Antipyretics are not indicated in heat stroke (hyperthermic patient with neurological impairment such as altered consciousness or seizure), as abnormal body temperature control mechanisms are not a feature. Treatment involves basic resuscitation, cooling and removing from the source of heat.

F   Malignant hyperpyrexia (MH) occurs following exposure to a triggering agent (e.g. volatile anaesthetics and suxamethonium), which results in uncoupling of calcium metabolism with subsequent sustained muscle contraction and hypermetabolic state. MH presents with tachycardia, hypertension, hypercapnia, muscle rigidity and hyperthermia. It may progress to severe acidaemia, hyperkalaemia, renal failure, rhabdomyolysis, disseminated intravascular coagulation, myoglobinuria, arrhythmias and cardiac arrest. Resuscitation, removal of the triggering agent and dantrolene, as recommended by the Association of Anaesthetists of Great Britain and Ireland (AAGBI), is required. Dantrolene is given as an initial intravenous bolus of 2.5mg/kg followed by 1mg/kg as required up to a maximum of 10mg/kg. Dantrolene inhibits calcium ion release through inhibition of ryanodine receptors in the sarcoplasmic reticulum.

F   Ecstasy use is thought to cause central release of dopamine resulting in sympathetic over-activity. The drug's tendency to cause hyperthermia, and the environment in which it is taken, predisposes to hyperthermia development and deterioration.

F   Hyperthermia, rigidity and autonomic dysregulation are seen in neuroleptic malignant syndrome (NMS), which is caused by antagonism of dopamine (D2) receptors in the hypothalamus, nigrostriatal pathways and spinal cord by antipsychotic drugs. D2-receptor blockade results in an elevated temperature set point (hyperpyrexia) and impairment of heat-dissipating mechanisms (hyperthermia). Increased calcium release results in increased muscle contractility, hyperthermia, rigidity and muscle breakdown. Antipsychotics which may cause NMS include olanzapine, haloperidol, risperidone and quetiapine. Management involves removing the trigger and resuscitation. Bromocriptine (dopamine agonist) and dantrolene have been used in the management of NMS with varying success.

1.   Waldmann C, Soni N, Rhodes A. *Oxford Desk Reference Critical Care*. Oxford, UK: Oxford University Press, 2008.

2.   http://www.aagbi.org/sites/default/files/MH%20guideline%20for%20web%20v2.pdf.

3.   Tonkonogy J, Sholevar DP. Neuroleptic malignant syndrome. Medscape reference, 2013. http://emedicine.medscape.com/article/288482-overview#showall.

Answer 30: Status epilepticus (SE): True a-d

T   Classically, SE is defined as continuous seizure activity lasting greater than 30 minutes or intermittent seizures without regaining consciousness lasting for 30 minutes or longer. However, recently another definition of any seizure lasting more than 5 minutes should be considered as SE, with treatment undertaken to limit morbidity and mortality.

T   Within the first 5-10 minutes (early phase), the initial management of seizures follows the ABC resuscitation algorithm. 50ml of 50% dextrose should be given if hypoglycaemic seizures are suspected. Lorazepam (0.1mg/kg) is currently the gold standard for early seizure control. Lorazepam is more effective than phenytoin, phenobarbital and phenytoin with diazepam for SE management.

T   Parenteral phenobarbitone is highly alkaline with extravascular or intra-arterial injection causing pain, necrosis and potential gangrene. Second-line agents for established SE are: phenytoin (15-18mg/kg intravenously at a rate of 50mg/min) or fosphenytoin (15-20mg/kg intravenously at a rate of 50-100mg/min) and/or phenobarbital (bolus of 10-15mg/kg intravenously at a rate of 100mg/min). Extravasation of phenytoin can also result in extensive tissue necrosis and it must be given via a large-bore intravenous cannula or central vein.

T   Ketamine can be effective in cases of refractory SE unresponsive to other drugs.

F   The anti-epileptic mechanisms of action of levetiracetam (Keppra®) are still relatively unknown. However, studies have shown that it does not exhibit classic anti-epileptic mechanisms, with no effect on voltage-dependent Na^+ channels, GABA-ergic transmission or affinity for either GABA or glutamate receptors. Levetiracetam is thought to act on neurotransmitter release, synaptic vesicle protein 2 (SV2A) synaptic sites and influences Ca^{2+} signalling. It may be useful in refractory SE due to its minimal side effects and drug interaction profile.

1.   National Institute for Health and Care Excellence (NICE). The epilepsies: the diagnosis and management of the epilepsies in adults and children in primary and secondary care. NICE Clinical Guideline 137, 2013. London, UK: NICE, 2013. http://www.nice.org.uk/nicemedia/live/13635/57779/57779.pdf.

2.   Deshpande LS, DeLorenzo RJ. Mechanisms of levetiracetam in the control of status epilepticus and epilepsy. *Front Neurol* 2014; 5(11): 1-5.

3.   Perks A, Cheema S, Mohanraj R. Anaesthesia and epilepsy. *Br J Anaesth* 2012; 108(4): 562-71.

Answer 31: Regarding pathophysiological mechanisms of diarrhoea: True c & d

F   See explanation below.

F

T

T

F   Infection is a cause of diarrhoea, not a mechanism.

The four pathophysiological mechanisms of diarrhoea are:

1.   Osmotic: failure of the gut to absorb osmotically active solutes results in retention of water within the gut lumen, e.g. due to ingested compounds (certain laxatives, magnesium), inefficient gut mucosa (bile salt malabsorption due to bacterial overgrowth), or inadequate gut length (short gut syndrome).

2. Secretory: increased secretion or reduced absorption of salts and water across the gastrointestinal mucosa, e.g. due to bacterial endotoxins and certain laxatives.
3. Inflammatory: loss of mucosal integrity due to colitis. This often leads to bloody diarrhoea if the colorectum is involved.
4. Dysmotility: impaired gut motility causing fluid and electrolyte retention within the small bowel overwhelms the colon's ability to absorb, resulting in diarrhoea.

1. Waldmann C, Soni N, Rhodes A. *Oxford Desk Reference Critical Care*. Oxford, UK: Oxford University Press, 2008.

Answer 32: Acute adult encephalitis: True: a, d & e

T   Any concurrent or recent febrile illness with altered mental state, conscious level or behaviour, or new seizures or focal neurological signs should raise the possibility of encephalitis and be investigated accordingly.

F   In industrialised nations, *Herpes simplex* virus (HSV) is the most commonly diagnosed infectious cause of viral encephalitis. Most HSV is due to HSV-1 infection with 10% being caused by HSV-2 infection. HSV-2 infection is more common in the immunocompromised and neonates.

F   The pattern of neurological deficit can provide clues to the possible underlying aetiology: autonomic dysfunction, myoclonus and cranial neuropathies, may indicate brainstem encephalitis, which is seen with listeriosis, brucellosis, tuberculosis and some viral infections. Tremors or movement disorders occur with thalamic or basal ganglia involvement. They may be seen in some flavivirus infections (West Nile virus/Japanese encephalitis). Polio is associated with flaccid paralysis and encephalitis.

T   Aciclovir (10mg/kg intravenously tds) has been shown to improve outcomes in HSV encephalitis, reducing mortality from >70% to <20-30% with treatment. Aciclovir is usually continued for 14-21 days, with repeat lumbar puncture performed prior to cessation to confirm negative HSV polymerase chain reaction (PCR). In *Varicella zoster* virus (VZV) encephalitis, although the evidence is limited, aciclovir (10-15mg/kg intravenously tds) is recommended for up to 14 days, usually with a short course of steroids due to the propensity for inflammation. Aciclovir can cause a reversible nephropathy through crystalluria, resulting in an obstructive nephropathy after 4 days of intravenous therapy, affecting up to 20% of patients.

T   Less than 50% of patients with encephalitis have an identifiable infectious cause (direct central nervous system infection or systemic infection). Other causes include metabolic derangement, inherited metabolic encephalopathies, toxins, hypoxia, trauma and vasculitis. Autoimmune encephalitis may be responsible for up to 8% of encephalitis cases. Antibodies against the target voltage-gated potassium channel (VGKC) complex and the NMDA receptor have been identified and emerged as important causes of encephalitis. These encephalitides may be treatable with immunotherapy/immunosuppression with prompt diagnosis and treatment improving or even reversing symptoms. Untreated autoimmune encephalitis often progresses to irreversible cognitive deficits, ongoing seizures and death.

1.   Soloman T, Michael BD, Smith PE, *et al.* Management of suspected viral encephalitis in adults - Association of British Neurologists and British Infection Association National Guidelines. *J Infect* 2012; 64: 347-73.

2.   Irani SR, Schott JM. Autoimmune encephalitis. *Br Med J* 2011; 11: 342.

Answer 33: Delirium in the intensive care unit: True a & b

T   The diagnostic and statistical manual of mental disorders (DSM-IV) lists four domains of delirium: disturbance of consciousness, change in cognition, development over a short period and fluctuation. The National Institutes of Health defines delirium as a "sudden severe confusion and rapid changes in brain function that occur with physical or mental illness".

T   The presence of delirium is associated with increased mortality in adult critical care patients (estimated as a 10% increase in relative risk of death for each day of delirium).

F   The HOPE study found that regular haloperidol use (2.5mg intravenously tds) versus placebo, irrespective of coma or delirium state, did not modify the duration of delirium in critically ill patients. It was concluded that intravenous haloperidol is safe but should be reserved for short-term management of acute agitation only.

F   Studies have shown that minimising sedation, using sedatives with low delirium potential (α2-agonists), monitoring for delirium and treating when recognised, and using early mobility/exercise may help prevent delirium and associated adverse outcomes. The use of an 'ABCDE' care bundle and other such evidence-based interventions, may influence delirium development and improve overall outcomes.

F   There are two distinct types of delirium: hypoactive (inattention, disordered thinking, decreased consciousness without agitation) and hyperactive (purely agitated). Both forms can exist intermittently in an individual and is termed mixed delirium. Hyperactive delirium is the most clinically obvious and accounts for <2% of patients with delirium. The majority of patients with delirium suffer from hypoactive delirium, which may be subtle and more difficult to diagnose. Patients with hypoactive delirium are least likely to survive, but if they do, they may have better long-term function compared to hyperactive or mixed delirium.

1.   Reade MC, Finfer S. Sedation and delirium in the intensive care unit. *New Engl J Med* 2014; 370: 444-54.

2.   Page V, Ely W, Gates S, *et al.* Effect of intravenous haloperidol on the duration of delirium and coma in the critically ill patients (Hope-ICU): a randomised, double-blind, placebo controlled trial. *Lancet* 2013; 1(7): 515-23.

3.   Morandi A, Brummel NE, Ely EW. Sedation, delirium and mechanical ventilation: the 'ABCDE' approach. *Curr Opin Crit Care* 2011; 17: 43-9.

4.   Barr J, Puntillo K, Ely EW, *et al.* Clinical practice guidelines for the management of pain, agitation, and delirium in adult patients in the intensive care unit. *Crit Care Med* 2013; 41(1): 263-306.

Answer 34: Vaughan-Williams classification: True a & b

T   Lidocaine is a Class Ib Na^+ channel blocker. It shortens the refractory period of cardiac muscle. Other agents in this group are mexiletine and phenytoin.

T   Propranolol is a Class II β-adrenoceptor blocker. It also blocks peripheral conversion of T4 to T3.

F   Amiodarone was designed as a Class III anti-arrhythmic agent but also demonstrates Class I, II and IV activity. By blocking K^+ channels it slows the rate of ventricle repolarisation, increasing the action potential duration and refractory period.

F   Flecainide and propafenone are Class Ic Na^+ blockers. They have no effect on the refractory period of cardiac muscle.

F   Verapamil and diltiazem are Class IV Ca^{2+} channel blockers.

1.   Waldmann C, Soni N, Rhodes A. *Oxford Desk Reference Critical Care*. Oxford, UK: Oxford University Press, 2008.

Answer 35: Regarding sedatives used in critical care: True c-e

F   Midazolam is a GABA-A (gamma-aminobutyric acid) receptor agonist potentiating chloride channel opening. It has a half-life of 3 to 11 hours. Active metabolites accumulate with prolonged infusion. It is metabolised by hepatic oxidation with renal excretion. There is a higher risk of delirium with benzodiazepine use than with other sedatives.

F   Lorazepam has a slower onset of action compared to midazolam (5-20 minutes versus 2-5 minutes). The half-life of lorazepam is 8-15 hours and it is metabolised by hepatic glucuronidation with no active metabolites. It is the first-line treatment of seizures and may be useful in alcohol withdrawal.

T   Dexmedetomidine is a complete agonist at α2-adrenoceptors. Its use is becoming more popular in critical care due to favourable sedative properties. Dexmedetomidine can cause bradycardia and biphasic blood pressure response. There is relative preservation of airway patency and ventilation, no effect on intracranial or cerebral perfusion pressures, reduction in gastric transit, decreased shivering and no effect on adrenocortical function.

T   The AnaConDa® system is inserted between the endotracheal tube and Y-piece in the ventilator circuit. Dosing is facilitated by using an isoflurane syringe pump with the gas concentration controlled through a gas monitor. Use of the volatile isoflurane in this way allows easy use in critical care. It can be used for short-duration procedures allowing fast recovery.

T   Hypertriglyceridaemia may complicate propofol use, warranting an alternative sedative to be used.

1.   Reade MC, Finfer S. Sedation and delirium in the intensive care unit. *New Engl J Med* 2014; 370: 444-54.
2.   Roberts M, Stuart G. Dexmedetomidine in paediatric anaesthesia and intensive care. Anaesthesia Tutorial of the Week 293, 2013. www.aagbi.org/education/educational-resources/tutorial-week.
3.   http://www.sedanamedical.com/aboutanaconda_icu.php.
4.   Gommers D, Bakker J. Medications for analgesia and sedation in the intensive care unit: an overview. *Crit Care* 2008; 12(suppl 3): S4.
5.   Barr J, Puntillo K, Ely EW, *et al*. Clinical practice guidelines for the management of pain, agitation, and delirium in adult patients in the intensive care unit. *Crit Care Med* 2013; 41(1): 263-306.

Answer 36: Drugs which may cause drug-induced liver injury include: All True

The most common drug causing drug-induced liver injury is amoxicillin/clavulanate (co-amoxiclav) worldwide. Drug-induced liver injury can occur with antituberculosis drugs, antiepileptics, antibiotics, statins, non-steroidal anti-inflammatories and many other drugs. The list of non-paracetamol drugs which may cause acute liver failure is long. Examples include: propylthiouracil, isoniazid, simvastatin, halothane, phenytoin, valproate, nitrofurantoin, ibuprofen, diclofenac, cotrimoxazole and azathioprine. 3,4,-methylenedioxy-N-methylamphetamine or MDMA (ecstasy) can cause significant liver injury due to acute ischaemic hepatocellular damage.

1.   Leise MD, Poterucha JJ, Talwalkar JA. Drug-induced liver injury. *Mayo Clin Proc* 2014; 89(1): 95-106.
2.   Bernal W, Wendon J. Acute liver failure. *New Engl J Med* 2014; 369: 2525-34.
3.   Wang DW, Yin YM, Yao YM. Advances in the management of acute liver failure. *World J Gastroenterol* 2013; 19(41): 7069-77.
4.   Bernal W, Auzinger G, Dhawan A, Wendon J. Acute liver failure. *Lancet* 2010; 376: 196-201.

Answer 37: Drug pharmacokinetics: True a, d & e

T   Phase 1 reactions are almost entirely oxidative. Phase 2 reactions include glucuronidation, sulphation, acetylation, methylation and glycination.

F   This is first-order kinetics. Zero-order kinetics occurs when a constant amount of drug is eliminated per unit time, for example, ethanol and phenytoin.

F   Plasma concentration must be plotted <u>logarithmically</u> (log plasma concentration to time), to calculate these values.

T   The volume of distribution is the theoretical volume the drug would occupy if the concentration throughout the body was the same as the concentration in the plasma.

T   The pKa is the pH at which 50% of the drug is ionized. A base, for example, a local anaesthetic, will be more ionized at a pH less than the pKa, hence the reduced efficacy of local anaesthetic in infected tissue.

1.   Peck TE, Hill SA, Williams M. *Pharmacology for Anaesthesia and Intensive Care*, 3rd ed. Cambridge, UK: Cambridge University Press, 2008.

Answer 38: Donation after cardiac death (DCD): True b

F   Functional warm ischaemic time begins when the patient's systolic arterial pressure decreases below 50mmHg and/or the arterial oxygen saturation content decreases below 70%, ending with cold perfusion of organs. The maximum functional warm ischaemic times in the United Kingdom with regards to different organs are: kidney (120 minutes, plus a further 120 minutes in selected donors), liver (20-30 minutes), lung (60 minutes — time to re-inflation of the lungs rather than cold perfusion) and pancreas (30 minutes). The outcomes following DCD liver transplantation are acceptable but there is a greater postoperative morbidity, higher incidence of graft failure and biliary complications compared to livers donated after brain death (DBD).

T   The decision to withdraw cardiorespiratory support should always be independent and made before any consideration for organ donation.

F   Cardiopulmonary resuscitation (CPR) is an <u>unacceptable</u> intervention in a potential DCD donor if cardiac arrest occurs prior to the retrieval team being ready.

F   It is unacceptable for the donor coordinator to care for the potential donor whilst they are still alive. This is a conflict of interest.

F   Kidneys retrieved from DCD donors have a higher incidence of early graft dysfunction but have the same long-term outcomes as kidneys donated from DBD donors.

1.   Manara AR, Murphy PG, O'Callaghan G. Donation after circulatory death. *Br J Anaesth* 2012; 108 Suppl 1: i108-21.

2.   Dunne K, Doherty P. Donation after circulatory death. *Contin Educ Anaesth Crit Care Pain* 2011; 11(3): 82-6.

Answer 39: Do not attempt resuscitation (DNAR) orders: True b, c & e

F   There are three options for managing a DNAR order peri-operatively: 1) The DNAR decision is discontinued. Surgery and anaesthesia are to proceed with cardiopulmonary resuscitation (CPR) being used in the event of an arrest; 2) The DNAR decision is to be modified to permit the use of drugs and techniques commensurate with the provision of anaesthesia; 3) No changes to be made to the DNAR decision. Under most circumstances this option is not compatible with the provision of general anaesthesia for any type of surgical intervention.

T   The DNAR decision should be reinstated when the patient returns to the ward unless in exceptional circumstances.

T   Referrals to the critical care outreach team that result in an end-of-life decision being made with no admission to critical care are estimated to comprise about one third of all referrals.

F   The General Medical Council (GMC) UK recommends that if a patient is admitted to hospital acutely unwell, or becomes clinically unstable, and they are at foreseeable risk of cardiac or respiratory arrest, a judgement about the likely benefits, burdens and risks of CPR should be made as early as possible.

T   GMC guidance states that "Emergencies can arise when there is no time to make a proper assessment of the patient's condition and the likely outcome of CPR; when no previous DNAR decision is in place; and when it is not possible to find out the patient's views. In these circumstances, CPR should be attempted, unless you are certain you have sufficient information about the patient to judge that it will not be successful".

1. Pattison N, O'Gara G. Making appropriate decisions about admission to critical care: the role of critical care outreach and medical emergency teams. *British Association of Critical Care Nurses* 2014; 19(1): 4-6.

2. The Association of Anaesthetists of Great Britain and Ireland. Do not attempt resuscitation (DNAR) decisions in the perioperative period, 2009. www.aagbi.org.

3. http://www.gmc-uk.org/guidance/ethical_guidance/end_of_life_DNACPR_decision. asp.

Answer 40: Caustic ingestion: True b, c & e

F   Acids cause coagulative necrosis, which results in a self-limiting burn pattern. Alkalis induce liquefactive necrosis with saponification of fats and solubilization of proteins. Alkalis are hygroscopic and absorb water from tissues, resulting in deeper tissue penetration and extensive burns. Cleaning and dishwasher products, paint strippers and alkalis contained in hair straighteners and relaxers are most commonly implicated.

T   Due to increased tissue adherence, alkali ingestion causes more damage to the oesophagus, whereas acid tends to result in more severe gastric injury. Ingestion of a large alkali volume will damage the stomach and small bowel.

T   Full personal protective equipment should be worn by medical staff as it is likely that the chemical will be toxic to skin and eyes. Early intubation is advisable due to the ongoing evolving nature of the caustic injury. Injuries may involve the airway and face, and may include oesophageal and gastrointestinal burns, splash injuries and ocular injuries.

F   Repeated endoscopies are often required to monitor changes and for therapeutic purposes. Oesophageal strictures and pyloric stenosis may develop within 2 months. Tracheo-oesophageal fistula may develop, and early tracheostomy may be required due to permanent tracheal damage.

T   Following caustic injury there is an increased risk of oesophageal cancer (up to 1000x higher than the general population).

1. Weigert A, Black A. Caustic ingestion in children. *Contin Educ Anaesth Crit Care Pain* 2006; 5(1): 5-8.

Answer 41: Paediatric trauma: True b-e

F   Cervical spine injury is uncommon in paediatric trauma (<2%), but traumatic brain injury is high (75%).

T   See below for explanation.

T

T

T

Over 80% of paediatric injuries are caused by blunt trauma. Orotracheal intubation with manual in-line immobilisation and rapid sequence induction should be used to secure the airway in blunt trauma with an uncleared C-spine. Ketamine (1-2mg/kg intravenously), thiopental (2-5mg/kg intravenously), etomidate (0.3mg/kg intravenously) and fentanyl (0.5-1µg/kg intravenously) with suxamethonium (1-2mg/kg intravenously) are appropriate agents for rapid sequence induction. Isotonic crystalloid (20ml/kg intravenous bolus) should be given as initial fluid resuscitation in hypovolaemic shock. Non-accidental injury is the most common cause of head injury in the first year of life.

1.   Cullen PM. Paediatric trauma. *Contin Educ Anaesth Crit Care Pain* 2012; 12(3): 157-61.

Answer 42: Regarding *Plasmodium falciparum* malaria: True a & d

T   Most malarial deaths are caused by *Plasmodium falciparum*. The other species responsible are *Plasmodium vivax*, *Plasmodium malariae*, *Plasmodium ovale* and *Plasmodium knowlesi*.

F   *P. falciparum* malaria initially develops in the liver, after which red cells are invaded by parasites.

F   Generally, the incubation period is normally 9-14 days, but may be longer.

T   Thick and thin blood films remain the gold standard for diagnosis and can be used to monitor the efficacy of treatment.

F   The World Health Organisation (WHO) recommends combination drug therapy for the treatment of *P. falciparum* malaria, to reduce the threat of resistance and improve treatment outcomes — artemisinin-based combination therapy is recommended for uncomplicated *P. falciparum* malaria.

1.   Bersten AD, Soni N. *Oh's Intensive Care Manual*, 6th ed. Butterworth Heinemann Elsevier, 2009.

Answer 43: Tuberculosis (TB): True b & e

F   TB causes close to 3 million deaths annually.

T   The majority of primary TB infections are asymptomatic. Secondary TB occurs following reactivation, also known as reactivation disease and is responsible for 90% of TB cases in patients not infected with HIV.

F   Computed tomography is more sensitive than chest radiography — it can demonstrate infiltrates, cavitations and lymphadenopathy.

F   Thick and thin blood films are used in the diagnosis of malaria. Acid-fast staining and culture of all potential sites should be performed for TB.

T   Lumbar puncture findings in TB meningitis include: a raised protein, lymphocytosis and low glucose.

1.   Bersten AD, Soni N. *Oh's Intensive Care Manual*, 6th ed. Butterworth Heinemann Elsevier, 2009.

Answer 44: Botulism and tetanus: True a & e

T   Botulism causes an acute descending motor paralysis. It affects mainly cranial, respiratory and autonomic nerves.

F   In botulism, a toxin blocks <u>acetylcholine</u> release from the presynaptic junction.

F   Botulin exotoxin can be identified by a number of techniques including: enzyme-linked immunosorbent assay (ELISA), electrochemiluminescent (ECL) tests, mouse inoculation and tissue cultures.

F   Tetanus is a toxin-mediated disease caused by the bacteria *Clostridium tetani*. It results in skeletal muscle rigidity and spasm with autonomic instability, due to inhibition of presynaptic GABA-ergic inhibitory interneurons.

T   Management of tetanus involves: supportive treatment, human immunoglobulin, antibiotics to kill tetanus spores (e.g. metronidazole intravenously), sedation and endotracheal intubation/ventilation with neuromuscular blockade and benzodiazepines, clonidine and morphine to manage associated autonomic dysfunction.

1.   Waldmann C, Soni N, Rhodes A. *Oxford Desk Reference Critical Care.* Oxford, UK: Oxford University Press, 2008.

2.   Bersten AD, Soni N. *Oh's Intensive Care Manual,* 6th ed. Butterworth Heinemann Elsevier, 2009.

Answer 45: *Clostridium difficile*: True c & e

F   *Clostridium difficile* is a spore-forming, Gram-positive <u>anaerobic</u> bacillus.

F   The organism was originally given its descriptive name 'difficile', because it grew slowly in culture and was difficult to isolate.

T   Duodenal infusion with donor faeces via a nasogastric/nasoduodenal tube is significantly more effective for the treatment of recurrent *Clostridium difficile* infection than vancomycin use.

F   *Clostridium difficile* toxins (enterotoxin A and cytotoxin B) do not affect intracellular levels of cyclic adenosine monophosphate (cAMP) or cyclic guanosine monophosphate (cGMP). It is thought that Rho proteins are the target within colonic eukaryotic cells leading to diarrhoea.

T   Chemotherapy for cancer may predispose to *Clostridium difficile* infection due to disruption of colonic microflora.

1.   Kelly CP, LaMont T. *Clostridium difficile* infection. *Ann Rev Med* 1998; 49: 375-90.

2.   van Nood E, Vriez A, Nieuwdorp M, *et al.* Duodenal infusion of donor feces for recurrent *Clostridium difficile*. *New Engl J Med* 2013; 368(10): 407-15.

Answer 46: Multi-drug-resistant (MDR) bacteria: True b, c & e

F   In the past 15 years, a large number of new antibiotic agents have been produced with activity against Gram-positive cocci. However, relatively few agents have been developed against Gram-negative rods. Tackling multi-drug-resistant Gram-negative rods in the future is likely to be a major problem, due to lack of effective antibiotics.

T   Vancomycin-resistant enterococci (VRE) have evolved mutated penicillin binding proteins (PBP), conferring resistance to β-lactam antibiotics (penicillins, cephalosporins, carbapenems and monobactams). Methicillin-resistant *Staphylococcus aureus* (MRSA) and penicillin-resistant *Streptococcus pneumoniae* also contain mutated PBP.

T   The genes for extended spectrum β-lactamase (ESBL) enzymes are transferrable between bacteria via chromosomes or plasmids. The most common bacteria carrying ESBLs are *Klebsiella* species and *Escherichia coli*, and less commonly *Enterobacter*, *Serratia*, *Morganella*, *Proteus* and *Pseudomonas*. ESBL bacteria are often resistant to aminoglycosides and quinolones.

F   *Pseudomonas aeruginosa* and *Acinetobacter* species are Gram-negative bacteria. They have minimal nutritional requirements, can be difficult to eradicate and pose a great risk to critically ill patients. Colistin, carbapenems and tigecycline have some success against MDR *Pseudomonas* and *Acinetobacter*.

T   Currently, there is a lack of evidence and wide variation in strategies to prevent infection and spread of MDR organisms.

1.   Parsons PE, Wiener-Kronish JP. *Critical Care Secrets*, 5th ed. Missouri, USA: Elsevier Mosby, 2013.

2.   Brusselaers N, Vogelaers D, Blot S. The rising problem of antimicrobial therapy resistance in the intensive care unit. *Ann Intensive Care* 2011; 1: 47.

Answer 47: Electrical safety: True a & d

T   During synchronised cardioversion, the shock is timed to the R-wave of the electrocardiogram. The risk of precipitating ventricular fibrillation (VF) is greatest if the current passes through the heart during repolarization.

F   Class II equipment is either double-insulated or has a single layer of reinforced insulation. An earth wire is not required.

F   Type CF equipment contains electrodes which may contact the heart directly. The leakage current through its intracardiac connection must be under 50μA.

T   Type B equipment should have a leakage current under 500μA.

F   Dry skin has a resistance in excess of 100,000Ω. This may be reduced to approximately 1000Ω if the skin is wet, increasing electrical conductivity and electrocution risk.

1.   Davis PD, Kenny GC. *Basic Physics and Measurement in Anaesthesia*, 5th ed. Edinburgh: Butterworth Heinemann, 2007.

2.   Bersten AD, Soni N. *Oh's Intensive Care Manual*, 6th ed. Butterworth Heinemann Elsevier, 2009.

Answer 48: Venous thromboembolism in pregnancy: True b & d

F   Plasma concentrations of fibrinogen and the majority of clotting factors increase, apart from Factors XI and XIII, which fall.

T   Platelet function remains normal. However, the platelet count falls despite increased platelet production, due to haemodilution and increased activity and consumption in normal pregnancy.

F   There is a 10x increased risk of venous thromboembolism during pregnancy and a 25x increased risk in the postpartum period.

T   Obesity is the most important risk factor for thromboembolism in pregnancy.

F   There are no data to support an increased rate of foetal or maternal morbidity/mortality with thrombolysis. Recombinant tissue plasminogen activator does not cross the placenta and can be used in the management of massive acute pulmonary embolism.

1.   Centre for Maternal and Child Enquiries (CMACE). Saving mothers' lives: reviewing maternal deaths to make motherhood safer: 2006-08. The Eighth Report of the Confidential Enquiries into Maternal Deaths in the United Kingdom. *Br J Obstet Gynaecol* 2011; 118(Suppl. 1): 1-203.

2.   Bersten AD, Soni N. *Oh's Intensive Care Manual*, 6th ed. Butterworth Heinemann Elsevier, 2009.

3.   Heidemann BH, McClure JH. Changes in maternal physiology during pregnancy. *Contin Educ Anaesth Crit Care Pain* 2003; 3(3): 65-8.

Answer 49: Intubation of the pregnant patient: True a & e

T   This is due to capillary engorgement of nasal and pharyngeal mucosa.

F   Reduced colloid oncotic pressure contributes to airway oedema.

F   Pregnant women have a reduced gastro-oesophageal sphincter pressure and increased intragastric pressure. This reduces the barrier pressure, increasing the risk of pulmonary aspiration.

F   Mendelson's syndrome is aspiration pneumonitis, an inflammatory reaction of lung parenchyma following aspiration of gastric contents. Particulate antacids may be associated with pneumonitis if aspirated.

T   This is due to increased blood volume and reduced oncotic pressure.

1.   Rucklidge M, Hinton C. Difficult and failed intubation in obstetrics. *Contin Educ Anaesth Crit Care Pain* 2012; 12(2): 86-91.

2.   Bersten AD, Soni N. *Oh's Intensive Care Manual*, 6th ed. Butterworth Heinemann Elsevier, 2009.

3.   Yentis SM, Hirsch NP, Smith GB. *Anaesthesia and Intensive Care A-Z. An Encyclopaedia of Principles and Practice*, 3rd ed. Edinburgh, UK: Elsevier Butterworth Heinemann, 2004.

Answer 50: Sepsis in pregnancy: True b-d

F   The death rate from sepsis in pregnancy is rising. Infection is largely due to community-acquired group A streptococcal infection.

T   There are limited data on the risk of foetal malformations associated with the use of quinolones in pregnancy; therefore, it is recommended to avoid their use unless no other option exists.

T   The most common sources of infection are chorioamnionitis, postpartum endometritis, urinary tract infections, pyelonephritis and septic abortions.

T   Management of septic shock in the pregnant patient follows normal Surviving Sepsis guidelines.

F   The Surviving Sepsis guidelines recommend that empiric combination therapy should not be used for more than 3-5 days. De-escalation to appropriate single therapy should be performed as soon as the susceptibility profile of the causative organism is known.

1. Centre for Maternal and Child Enquiries (CMACE). Saving mothers' lives: reviewing maternal deaths to make motherhood safer: 2006-08. The Eighth Report of the Confidential Enquiries into Maternal Deaths in the United Kingdom. *Br J Obstet Gynaecol* 2011; 118 (Suppl. 1): 1-203.
2. Bersten AD, Soni N. *Oh's Intensive Care Manual*, 6th ed. Butterworth Heinemann Elsevier, 2009.
3. Dellinger RP, Levy MM, Rhodes A, *et al*. Surviving Sepsis Campaign: international guidelines for management of severe sepsis and septic shock: 2012. *Crit Care Med* 2013; 41: 580-637.

Answer 51: Pulse oximetry and oxygen measurement: True c-e

Γ   These are the isobestic points (590nm and 805nm), at which absorption of a certain wavelength of light by two substances is equal. The wavelengths of red light and infrared light are 660nm and 940nm, respectively.

F   This is Lambert's law. Beer's law states that the absorption of radiation by a given thickness of solution, of a given concentration, is the same as that of twice the thickness of a solution of half the concentration.

T   Methaemoglobin is counted as deoxygenated haemoglobin, with a pulse oximetry SpO_2 value approaching 85%.

T   The Clark electrode contains a platinum cathode and silver/silver chloride anode and is used to measure oxygen concentration. The fuel cell contains a gold cathode and lead anode, and is an alternative device for measuring oxygen concentration.

T   Oxygen is a paramagnetic gas. The concentration of oxygen in gases can therefore be measured with a paramagnetic analyser.

1. Davis PD, Kenny GNC. *Basic Physics and Measurement in Anaesthesia*, 5th ed. Edinburgh, UK; Butterworth Heinemann, 2003.

Answer 52: Endocrine physiology: True a & d

T   The anterior lobe of the pituitary gland secretes growth hormone, prolactin, adrenocorticotropic hormone, thyrotrophin, luteinising and follicle-stimulating hormones. The posterior lobe secretes vasopressin and oxytocin.

F Catecholamine metabolites, for example, metanephrine, can be measured in urine to aid in the diagnosis of phaeochromocytoma. Plasma catecholamines are not measured.

F Glucocorticoids are secreted by the zona fasciculata of the adrenal cortex. The outer zona glomerulosa secretes aldosterone and the inner zona reticularis secretes androgen sex hormones. The adrenal medulla secretes catecholamines.

T Glucagon is produced by α-cells of the islets of Langerhans, and acts to oppose insulin via the second messenger, cyclic adenosine monophosphate (cAMP).

F Iodine initially reacts with tyrosine to form monoiodotyrosine, a reaction catalysed by thyroid peroxidase. Further iodination leads to the formation of diiodotyrosine (DIT).

1. Smith T, Pinnock C, Lin T. *Fundamentals of Anaesthesia*, 3rd ed. Cambridge, UK: Cambridge University Press, 2009.

Answer 53: During resuscitation of a full-term neonate: True b & c

F Evaluation consists of assessment of colour, tone, respiratory and heart rate.

T A compression: ventilation ratio of 3:1 is appropriate.

T A size 3.5mm endotracheal tube is appropriate for a full-term neonate.

F There is one umbilical vein available for vascular access, and two umbilical arteries.

F Adequate ventilation and reversal of hypoxia is usually sufficient to resuscitate and stabilise a neonate post-delivery. Circulatory support, including chest compressions, is rarely required.

1. Resuscitation Council (UK). European paediatric life support (EPLS) for use in the UK, 3rd ed. London, UK: Resuscitation Council (UK), 2011. www.resus.org.uk.

Answer 54: Indications for synchronised DC cardioversion include: True b & c

F   Sinus tachycardia with syncope is not an indication for cardioversion.

T   Atrial fibrillation with a systolic blood pressure of 75mmHg is a sign of compromise. Cardioversion is indicated as per the Advanced Life Support adult tachycardia algorithm.

T   Ischaemic chest pain with atrial flutter is a sign of compromise and an indication for DC cardioversion.

F   Cardiopulmonary resuscitation should be commenced and defibrillation performed in patients with pulseless ventricular tachycardia.

F   Mobitz Type II atrioventricular block should be managed with pharmacological therapy (e.g. atropine and isoprenaline), or transcutaneous pacing.

1.   Resuscitation Council (UK). Advanced life support, 6th ed. London, UK: Resuscitation Council (UK), 2011. www.resus.org.uk.

Answer 55: Following liver transplantation: True b & c

F   There are many causes of graft dysfunction including: primary non-function (a form of reperfusion injury), rejection, preservation injury, vascular and biliary complications, drug-induced dysfunction, infection and recurrence of chronic disease.

T   A typical regime of methylprednisolone would be 1g daily for 3 days, followed by tapering of the dose.

T   In the absence of antiviral prophylaxis, 23-85% of patients will develop *Cytomegalovirus* (CMV) infection after orthotopic liver transplantation. Ganciclovir remains the treatment of choice for CMV disease.

F   Following liver transplantation, calcineurin inhibitors (ciclosporin and tacrolimus) AND a steroid form the classical mainstay of immunosuppressive treatment, particularly in the early stages. With time after transplantation, drugs such as azathioprine or mycophenolate mofetil (MMF) may be added to allow dose reduction in calcineurin inhibitors and steroids. Other agents, such as antilymphocyte antibodies (ALA), monoclonal antibodies (basiliximab) and/or sirolimus, may be used as part of the immunosuppressive regimen post-liver transplant.

F   Approximately 20% of liver transplant recipients require readmission to intensive care. Readmission correlates with reduced patient survival and graft function. Predictors of readmission to critical care include: an abnormal pre-discharge chest X-ray, high central venous pressure, tachypnoea, increasing patient age, abnormal pre-transplant synthetic function, abnormal bilirubin, large intra-operative blood product requirement and renal dysfunction. The commonest cause for readmission is cardiorespiratory failure due to fluid overload and infection. Graft dysfunction, severe sepsis, bleeding, biliary anastomotic leaks and other surgical complications are other important causes of readmission.

1.   Bersten AD, Soni N. *Oh's Intensive Care Manual*, 6th ed. Butterworth Heinemann Elsevier, 2009.

Answer 56: A 70kg male presents to the emergency department having fallen into a running bath. He has sustained scalds to his head, torso and both arms: All False

F   If we use the Wallace Rule of Nines he has sustained approximately 63% BSA burns.

F   He should receive about 18L of crystalloid, as per the Parkland formula (4ml x kg x BSA), over the 24-hour period from the <u>time of sustaining the burn</u> and not the time from presentation to the emergency department. Half the fluid volume (9L) should be ideally given within the first 8 hours of the burn, with the remaining 9L being given over the next 16 hours.

F   There is no evidence to support prophylactic antibiotics. Routine bacteriological surveillance is essential in burns patients to target antibiotics accordingly.

F   The main cause of mortality in burns injuries is infection.

F   'Burn-specific criteria' for the diagnosis of sepsis was developed in 2007 by the American Burn Association (ABA). Severe burn injury is accompanied by a systemic inflammatory response, making traditional indicators of sepsis insensitive and non-specific. The

American Burn Association criteria include: temperature (>39°C or <36°C), progressive tachycardia (>110 beats per minute), progressive tachypnoea (>25 breaths per minute not ventilated or minute ventilation >12L/min ventilated), thrombocytopenia (<100,000/μl; not applied until 3 days after initial resuscitation), hyperglycaemia (untreated plasma glucose >200mg/dL, >7 units of insulin/hr intravenous drip, or >25% increase in insulin requirements over 24 hours), and feed intolerance >24 hours (abdominal distension, residuals 2x the feeding rate, or diarrhoea >2500ml/day). Meeting >3 of these criteria should trigger concern for infection. A recent retrospective review by Hogan *et al* found that the ABA trigger for sepsis did not correlate strongly with bacteraemia (receiver operating curve for meeting >3 ABA sepsis criteria is 0.638). Further evaluation of the ABA sepsis criteria is required.

1.   Bishop S, Maguire S. Anaesthesia and intensive care for major burns. *Contin Educ Anaesth Crit Care Pain* 2012; 12(3): 118-22.

2.   Bersten AD, Soni N. *Oh's Intensive Care Manual*, 6th ed. Butterworth Heinemann Elsevier, 2009.

3.   Greenhalgh DG, Saffle JR, Holmes JH, *et al*. American Burn Association Consensus Conference on Burn Sepsis and Infection Group. American Burn Association consensus conference to define sepsis and infection in burns. *J Burn Care Res* 2007; 28(6): 776-90.

4.   Hogan BK, Wolf SE, Hospenthal DR, *et al*. Correlation of American Burn Association sepsis criteria with the presence of bacteraemia in burned patients admitted to the intensive care unit. *J Burn Care Res* 2012; 33(3): 371-8.

Answer 57: Spinal and neurogenic shock: True a & b

T   Cord injury above T1 will remove intercostal function. Breathing will be entirely diaphragmatic.

T   The anterior spinal artery is formed from vertebral artery branches. It runs along the anterior aspect of the spinal cord. The two posterior spinal arteries arise from the vertebral arteries, adjacent to the medulla oblongata.

F   Approximately 14% of vertebral column fractures result in damage to the spinal cord.

F   Spinal injury causing interruption of autonomic pathways within the spinal cord may result in hypotension and/or bradycardia and is termed <u>neurogenic</u> shock. Neurogenic shock is a distributive type of shock. Hypotension occurs due to loss of vascular sympathetic tone causing a low systemic vascular resistance. Bradycardia occurs due to unopposed vagal activity. Spinal shock is the loss of sensation and muscle paralysis, with initial loss but gradual recovery of reflexes below the level of spinal injury. Spinal shock does not refer to circulatory collapse and should not be confused with neurogenic shock.

F   90% of SCI patients will develop deep vein thrombosis. 10% will develop pulmonary embolism.

1.   Bonner S, Smith C. Initial management of acute spinal cord injury. *Contin Educ Anaesth Crit Care Pain* 2013; 13(6): 224-31.

Answer 58: Postoperative care of the cardiac transplant patient: True a & d

T   Milrinone may be useful in managing low cardiac output post-transplantation, particularly where β-receptor downregulation has occurred due to chronic overstimulation.

F   The use of an intra-aortic balloon pump peri-operatively can improve left ventricular function where other measures have failed.

F   There is uncertain gut absorption with ciclosporin and bioavailability is poor.

T   Cardiac biopsies are performed via the right internal jugular vein and are classified using the Billingham classification.

F   In patients with cardiac tamponade, a raised central venous pressure (jugular venous distension) is more likely due to impaired venous return. Other signs include: hypotension due to decreased stroke volume, muffled heart sounds, pulsus paradoxus, tachycardia and dyspnoea. Low-voltage QRS complexes and ST segment changes may also occur.

1.   Bersten AD, Soni N. *Oh's Intensive Care Manual*, 6th ed. Butterworth Heinemann Elsevier, 2009.

2.   Morgan-Hughes NJ, Hood G. Anaesthesia for a patient with a cardiac transplant. *Br J Anaesth CEPD Rev* 2002; (3): 74-8.

Answer 59: In the adult trauma patient: True c & e

F   Loss of 15-30% blood volume would be Class II haemorrhagic shock. Class III haemorrhagic shock occurs when 30-40% blood volume is lost.

F   Pulse pressure is initially normal in Class I haemorrhage, and decreases with Classes II, III and IV haemorrhage.

T   Appropriate sites of intraosseous (IO) access do include the sternum, proximal and distal tibia, and proximal humerus.

F   Bone fracture at a potential site for IO access is a contraindication to this technique, due to the risk of extravasation. An alternate site must be chosen for IO placement.

T   All resuscitation drugs can be given via the IO route.

1.   Geeraerts T, Chhor V, Cheisson G, et al. Clinical review: initial management of blunt pelvic trauma patients with haemodynamic instability. Crit Care 2007; 11(1): 204.

Answer 60: The following are recognised causes of a raised anion gap acidosis: True: a, d & e

T   The anion gap is calculated using the formula $[Na^+ + K^+] - [Cl^- + HCO_3^-]$ and is in the range 8-12mEq/L in health. Ethylene glycol poisoning is a cause.

F   Raised anion gap acidosis occurs due to an increase in the plasma concentration of organic acids or toxins including: methanol and ethylene glycol, ketones, lactate, salicylates, paraldehyde and urea. It is not typically raised in renal tubular acidosis.

F   Normal anion gap acidosis occurs due to disorders of sodium and chloride regulation, and is seen with excess chloride administration, severe diarrhoea and excess gastrointestinal losses, renal tubular acidosis and administration of certain drugs, such as carbonic anhydrase inhibitors.

T

T

1.   Waldmann C, Soni N, Rhodes A. Oxford Desk Reference Critical Care. Oxford, UK: Oxford University Press, 2008.

Answer 61: Consent and confidentiality: True b & e

F   In the situation where a patient is unable to give consent, treatment that is lifesaving or in their best interests can be provided without consent.

T   Any adult judged to be competent can refuse treatment against the advice of their doctor.

F   Enduring powers of attorney can make decisions regarding the financial affairs of a patient but not with regards to treatment.

F   For anonymised data analysis for internal quality control procedures, individual patient consent is not necessary.

T   If information regarding a patient is to be shared with a third party, this should only occur following consent from the patient to do so.

1.   British Medical Association. Consent. Report of the working party 2001. London, UK: British Medical Association, 2001.

2.   British Medical Association. Advanced statements about medical treatment. Report of the working party 1995. London, UK: British Medical Association, 1995.

3.   British Medical Association. Confidentiality and disclosure of health information. Report of the working party 1999. London, UK: British Medical Association, 1999.

Answer 62: The following are recognised tests for analysis of non-parametric data: True b, d & e

F   Parametric data are data derived from a continuum or distribution (such as a normal distribution).

T   Non-parametric data look at a rank order of values.

F   Unpaired t-tests and Pearson's tests are both utilised in the analysis of parametric data.

T   Mann-Whitney U tests, Wilcoxon matched pairs tests and Spearman's rank coefficient tests may all be utilised to analyse non-parametric data.

T   See above.

1.   Greenhalgh T. How to Read a Paper - the Basics of Evidence-based Medicine. Oxford, UK: Wiley-Blackwell, 2014.

⬤ Answer 63: Complications of extracorporeal membrane oxygenation (ECMO): True a, c & e

T   About one third of patients on ECMO suffer an acute stroke event (usually haemorrhagic).

F   Clots in the circuit are an emergency but can be managed successfully.

T   Bleeding is the most common complication of ECMO.

F   Although there should always be a second back-up pump on the circuit, pump failure is an acute emergency and requires a well-practised protocol to be in place, to ensure pump change is undertaken quickly to avoid patient harm or death.

T   Sudden cannula migration and dislodgement quickly results in massive haemorrhage, air embolism and death. Personnel need to be trained for this event. For example: clamping the arterial end then venous end of the circuit, applying pressure to the dislodged cannulae site, starting cardiopulmonary resuscitation, gaining immediate surgical support and undertaking of procedures to quickly resite the cannulae and get the patient back onto ECMO. The bedside ventilator and inotropes/vasopressors should be started, if there is any delay in getting the patient back onto ECMO.

1.   Martinez G, Vuylsteke A. Extracorporeal membrane oxygenation in adults. *Contin Educ Anaesth Crit Care Pain* 2011; 12(2): 57-61.

2.   Waldmann C, Soni N, Rhodes A. *Oxford Desk Reference Critical Care.* Oxford, UK: Oxford University Press, 2008.

⬤ Answer 64: The following are included in Well's criteria for the risk of pulmonary embolism (PE): True a, c & e

T   Well's criteria is a scoring system that stratifies the risk of PE being present according to the presence of the following clinical factors: clinical symptoms of deep vein thrombosis, other diagnosis less likely than PE (3 points); heart rate >100/minute, recent immobilisation or surgery, previous DVT or PE (1.5 points); haemoptysis, malignancy (1 point). A score of 6 points or more indicates a high probability of PE (87.4%). A score of less than 2 points indicates a low risk of PE (3.4%). Pleuritic chest pain and ECG changes are not included in the scoring system.

F

T

F

T

1. Ouellette DR, Harrington A, Kamangar N, *et al*. Pulmonary embolism clinical scoring systems. Medscape reference, 2011. http://emedicine.medscape.com/article/1918940-overview.

Answer 65: Tracheostomy: True a, c & d

T High-volume low-pressure cuffs provide a wider surface area for cuff pressure to be dissipated, reducing the incidence of cuff-related mucosal damage.

F Cuff pressure should not exceed >25cmH$_2$O (18mmHg) to reduce the risk of impaired mucosal perfusion, tissue necrosis and tracheal stenosis.

T In dual-lumen tracheostomies, the inner cannula should be removed for cleaning every 7-14 days or earlier if secretions are problematic.

T Tracheostomy decannulation should be considered when the patient has a satisfactory respiratory drive and effective cough.

F Tracheal stenosis is a rare but significant complication following tracheostomy, causing stridor and potential voice changes if the larynx is involved.

1. Bhandary R, Niranjan N. Tracheostomy. Anaesthesia Tutorial of the Week 241, 2011. www.aagbi.org/education/educational-resources/tutorial-week.

Answer 66: Physiotherapy: True a & e

T There is an association with reduced rates of ventilator-associated pneumonia (VAP) in patients treated with physiotherapy.

F A pressure of 40cmH$_2$O is the recommended upper limit for hyperinflation techniques.

F Sedation, an artificial airway and inadequate humidification alter mucociliary clearance.

F   Patients with <u>expiratory muscle</u> weakness or fatigue, for example, in neuromuscular disease, may benefit from cough assist techniques.

T   Intrapulmonary percussive ventilation is a technique that has no effect on sputum weight or mucociliary transport.

1.   Waldmann C, Soni N, Rhodes A. *Oxford Desk Reference Critical Care*. Oxford, UK: Oxford University Press, 2008.

Answer 67: When assessing a pleural effusion, it is deemed exudative if: True a-d

T   Classically, an exudative pleural effusion is defined as having a protein level >30g/L, with transudate <30g/L. Unfortunately, the protein level often lies very close to the 30g/L cut-off requiring the use of further criteria to differentiate, such as Light's criteria. Light's criteria: pleural fluid is an exudate when one or more of the following are present: pleural fluid protein/serum protein ratio >0.5, pleural fluid lactate dehydrogenase (LDH)/serum LDH ratio >0.6 and when pleural fluid LDH is more than two thirds the upper limit of normal serum LDH. False positives can occur in patients with left ventricular failure and/or diuretic use.

T   Pleural fluid LDH/serum LDH ratio >0.6.

T   Pleural fluid LDH more than two thirds the upper limit of normal serum LDH.

T   When the pleural fluid protein is >30g/L it is termed an exudate.

F   Low pH is more likely to indicate a pleural effusion that is an exudate, but not always. A pleural fluid pH <7.2 is associated with infection and is an indication for drainage. It may also be low in malignancy and inflammatory conditions.

1.   Maskell NA, Butland RJA. BTS guidelines for the investigation of a unilateral pleural effusion in adults. *Thorax* 2003; 58 (suppl II): ii8-17.

Answer 68: Regarding irregularities in serum potassium: True a-d

T   Thiazide and loop diuretics promote delivery of sodium to the collecting ducts where sodium is reabsorbed by the amiloride-sensitive Na⁺ channel. A favourable gradient is thus created for potassium channel secretion of potassium and resultant hypokalaemia.

T   In Bartter's syndrome, there is an inherited defect in the thick ascending limb of the loop of Henle, with normotensive patients displaying renal potassium loss and increased aldosterone secretion due to activation of the renin-angiotensin system. The high serum bicarbonate in this context is seen in Bartter's syndrome (or Gitelman's syndrome); a low serum bicarbonate may indicate a renal tubular acidosis.

T   A concentration in excess of this is strongly associated with peripheral vein damage. An infusion pump or other rate-limiting device must always be used.

T   Severe hyperkalaemia (potassium >7.0mmol/L) may cause the following ECG changes: peaked T-waves, flattening and widening of the P-wave, PR prolongation, loss of P-waves, prolonged QRS complex with abnormal morphology, high-grade AV block with slow junctional and ventricular escape rhythms, conduction block, sinus bradycardia, atrial fibrillation, and sine-wave pre-terminal rhythm.

F   In severe hyperkalaemia, membrane stabilisation is achieved by calcium. Insulin-dextrose therapy shifts potassium into the intracellular compartment.

1.   Rastergar A, Soleimani M. Hypokalemia and hyperkalemia. *Postgrad Med J* 2001; 77: 759-64.

Answer 69: Pulmonary function tests: True d & e

F   The Fowler method is used to measure anatomical dead space. Helium dilution or nitrogen washout is used to measure functional residual capacity (FRC).

F   Vital capacity (VC) measurement is useful in predicting the need for intubation in Guillain-Barré syndrome (VC <15ml/kg), but is less useful in other conditions.

F   The ratio of respiratory frequency to tidal volume (f/VT) or Rapid Shallow Breathing Index (RSBI) is a reliable predictor of weaning and extubation outcome. A value <80 suggests a high likelihood of successful weaning. Values >105 suggest that weaning may be difficult at this time.

T   If the expiratory time is too short or expiratory resistance is increased, intrinsic PEEP (PEEPi) may develop during mechanical ventilation.

T   Respiratory drive can be assessed by measuring airway pressure 0.1 sec after occluding the airway against inspiratory effort.

1.   Waldmann C, Soni N, Rhodes A. *Oxford Desk Reference Critical Care.* Oxford, UK: Oxford University Press, 2008.

Answer 70: End-tidal carbon dioxide (CO_2) monitoring: True a, d & e

T   Capnography is an AAGBI standard of monitoring.

F   Raman spectroscopy can be used to measure CO_2, but infra-red (IR) spectroscopy is used at the bedside.

F CO_2 selectively absorbs infra-red light at a wavelength of 4.3μm. Absorption of this wavelength of light is proportional to CO_2 concentration and can be used to calculate end-tidal CO_2 in kPa or mmHg.

T   Capnography is the gold standard for confirming endotracheal tube placement.

T   The difference between $PaCO_2$ and end-tidal $PetCO_2$ is 0.2-0.6kPa (2-5mmHg).

1.   Waldmann C, Soni N, Rhodes A. *Oxford Desk Reference Critical Care.* Oxford, UK: Oxford University Press, 2008.

Answer 71: Calcium: True c & e

F   Greater than 98% of total body calcium is found within the bones.

F   Although widened T-waves may be seen, the QT interval tends to be shortened.

T   Patients with secondary hyperparathyroidism are often normocalcaemic, but can be hypercalcaemic or hypocalcaemic. Tertiary hyperparathyroidism occurs when parathyroid hyperplasia becomes so severe that removal of the underlying cause does not eliminate the stimulus for parathyroid hormone (PTH) secretion and hypertrophic chief cells become autonomous.

F   Thiazide diuretics are associated with hypercalcaemia.

T   These agents are all recognised treatments in the management of hypercalcaemia. Mithramycin and glucocorticoids are used in malignancy-related hypercalcaemia.

1.   Manoj PM, Webb ST. Cations: potassium, calcium, and magnesium. *Contin Educ Anaesth Crit Care Pain* 2012; 12 (4): 195-8.

Answer 72: Propofol infusion syndrome (PRIS): True b-e

F   Prospective studies have suggested an incidence of PRIS of 1.1% in adult intensive care patients.

T   New-onset metabolic acidosis is the commonest presenting feature of PRIS and tends to be due to a combination of renal failure and lactic acidosis.

T   Brugada syndrome-like ECG changes may be seen in PRIS along with atrial tachyarrhythmias, bradycardias, bundle branch block and eventually asystole.

T   Severe head injury, sepsis, high exogenous or endogenous catecholamine and glucocorticoid levels, low carbohydrate to high lipid intake and inborn errors of fatty acid oxidation are all risk factors for the development of PRIS.

T   Serial monitoring of serum CK, triglycerides and lactate are appropriate in patients who are on high-dose propofol infusions and in those who are at higher risk of developing PRIS. Risk factors for developing PRIS include: traumatic brain injuries, sepsis, high catecholamine and glucocorticoid levels, low carbohydrate to high lipid intake and inborn errors of fatty acid oxidation.

1.   Loh NHW, Nair P. Propofol infusion syndrome. *Contin Educ Anaesth Crit Care Pain* 2013; 13(6): 200-2.

Answer 73: Magnesium: True b, c & e

F   Two grams of magnesium sulphate is equivalent to 8mmol of magnesium ions.

T   Diuretics, ACE inhibitors, aminoglycosides, amphotericin, cyclosporin and cisplatin are all associated with hypomagnesaemia.

T   These are indications to consider immediate cessation of intravenous magnesium therapy.

F   These are characteristic electrocardiogram (ECG) findings in hypermagnesaemia.

T   Increased magnesium levels inhibit acetylcholine release.

1.   Parikh M, Webb ST. Cations: potassium, calcium, and magnesium. *Contin Educ Anaesth Crit Care Pain* 2012; 12(4): 195-8.

Answer 74: Infection control and critical care: True b

F   Patients on the intensive care unit (ICU) are approximately five to ten times more likely to develop a nosocomial infection than patients receiving ward care.

T   Distance between bed spaces and utilisation of cubicles are important factors in the design of intensive care units, for preventing transmission of infection.

F   Transducer sets should be changed at least every 48 hours.

F   Recent trials and meta-analyses have failed to demonstrate any mortality benefit using biomarkers such as pro-calcitonin (PCT) in infection control.

F   The Ostrosky-Zeichner rule has a high <u>negative</u> predictive value and is useful in identifying low-risk patients who are not likely to develop invasive candidiasis.

1.   Afshari A, Pagani L, Harbarth S. Year in review 2011: Critical care - infection. *Crit Care* 2012; 16(6): 242.

2.   Jensen JU, Hein L, Lundgren B, *et al*. Procalcitonin and Survival Study (PASS) Group: procalcitonin-guided interventions against infections to increase early appropriate antibiotics and improve survival in the intensive care unit: a randomized trial. *Crit Care Med* 2011; 39: 2048-58.

⬤ Answer 75: Renal replacement therapy (RRT) is indicated in overdose of the following drugs: True a & d

T
F
F
T
F

A guiding principle is that drugs are generally cleared by RRT if they are water-soluble and not highly protein bound. Common toxins that may require RRT include: vancomycin, gentamicin, lithium, aspirin, theophylline, carbamazepine, valproic acid, metformin, methotrexate, ethylene glycol and methanol. RRT is less useful if the poison is a large or charged (polar) molecule, has a large volume of distribution or is extensively protein bound (e.g. digoxin, phencyclidine, warfarin, amitriptyline).

1. Goodman JW, Goldfarb DS. The role of continuous renal replacement therapy in the treatment of poisoning. *Semin Dial* 2006; 19(5): 402-7.

2. http://www.merckmanuals.com/professional/injuries_poisoning/poisoning/_general _principles_of_poisoning.html.

⬤ Answer 76: Colitis: True b, c & e

F   Systemic symptoms such as fever, anorexia and weight loss are more associated with inflammatory bowel disease (ulcerative colitis and Crohn's disease).

T   Bloody diarrhoea is a common presenting complaint of colitis.

T   Ischaemic colitis and bowel infarction is a complication, which can present following abdominal aortic aneurysm repair. The duration and difficulty of surgery, cross-clamp placement (supra- versus infra-renal), duration of cross-clamp placement and whether the blood supply to the bowel was compromised (superior and inferior mesenteric artery) influences the risk of colitis development.

F   Antidiarrhoeal drugs (loperamide/codeine), anticholinergics and non-steroidal anti-inflammatory drugs (NSAIDs) increase the risk of perforation in severe acute colitis. Perforation may be indicated by the presence of severe pain.

T High-dose steroids and immunosuppressive therapy (cyclosporin/ azathioprine) may be beneficial and prevent the need for colectomy.

1. Waldmann C, Soni N, Rhodes A. *Oxford Desk Reference Critical Care.* Oxford, UK: Oxford University Press, 2008.

Answer 77: Kidney structure and function: True a, b & e

T The kidney contains approximately 1 million nephrons.

T Cortical nephrons have shorter loops of Henle. Approximately 20% of loops of Henle are long enough to enter the inner medulla. These are found in the deep juxtamedullary nephrons.

F Renal blood flow equates to 20-25% of the cardiac output. The high renal blood flow maintains a high glomerular filtration rate and hence a very low arteriovenous O_2 difference.

F The GFR (total volume of fluid filtered by the glomerulus per unit time) is approximately 180L/day.

T 99% of the glomerular filtrate returns to the extracellular compartment. Approximately 1% of glomerular filtrate is the mean fractional excretion of water, which equates to about 1-2L/day.

1. Despopoulos A, Silbernagl S. *Colour Atlas of Physiology*, 6th ed. Thieme publishing, 2008.

Answer 78: 5mg of prednisolone is equivalent to: True c

F Prednisolone has a relative potency of four in relation to hydrocortisone and has an intermediate duration of action versus short-acting hydrocortisone. 5mg of prednisolone is equivalent to 20mg of hydrocortisone.

F Prednisone 5mg is equivalent to 5mg prednisolone.

T Methylprednisolone 4mg is equivalent to 5mg prednisolone.

F Dexamethasone 0.75mg is equivalent to 5mg of prednisolone.

F Betamethasone 0.75mg is equivalent to 5mg of prednisolone.

Note that these values do not take mineralocorticoid effects into account.

1. British National Formulary 6.3.2 and 13.4. http://www.bnf.org.
2. http://www.accessdata.fda.gov/drugsatfda_docs/label/2011/011856s103s104lbl. pdf.

⬤ **Answer 79: In relation to patients with HIV and critical care: True c**

F   25-50% of acute respiratory failure in patients admitted to critical care with HIV is caused by infection with *Pneumocystis jiroveci*.

F   Anti-retroviral therapy should be stopped or staggered during critical illness or toxicity to minimise the risk of resistance. Specialist advice from clinicians and pharmacists with expertise in managing HIV infection on critical care should be sought.

T   Of HIV-positive patients admitted to critical care, studies suggest that between 3 and 23% were admitted due to sepsis. Sepsis in HIV patients is associated with a high mortality.

F   Up to 70% of lower GI bleeding in HIV-positive patients is related directly to HIV infection. Such infections include: associated opportunistic infection (*Cytomegalovirus* [CMV] colitis, *Mycobacterium avium*) or associated malignant processes (Kaposi sarcoma, AIDS-associated lymphoma). HIV infection is also associated with idiopathic colonic ulcers.

F   *Cryptococcus neoformans* infection is the most common cause of meningitis in HIV-patients admitted to critical care.

1. Crothers K, Huang L. Critical care of patients with HIV. HIV Insite, 2006. UCSF. http://hivinsite.ucsf.edu/InSite?page=kb.
2. Hare CB. Clincal overview of HIV disease. HIV Insite, 2006. UCSF. http://hivinsite.ucsf.edu/InSite?page=kb.

⬤ **Answer 80: Concerning the confirmation of brainstem death in the UK: All False**

F   Brainstem death should only be confirmed at least 6 hours after the onset of apnoeic coma.

F   Testing must be confirmed by two medical practitioners with at least 5 years of registration with the General Medical Council (GMC), and experience in conducting brainstem death tests. However, there is no statutory time interval that must pass between performing the two sets of tests.

F   Death is confirmed after performing the second set of tests, but the official time of death is the time at which the first set of tests were completed. This is in relation to UK criteria.

F   Prior to testing for brainstem death, it is necessary to correct reversible causes of brainstem depression, such as the presence of alcohol or sedative drugs or hypothermia <34°C. The Academy of Medical Royal Colleges state that changes in sodium may occur as a result of brainstem death, rather than a cause and do not preclude brainstem death testing. However, unresponsiveness may occur in patients with severe hyponatraemia (<115mmol/L) and hypernatraemia (>160mmol/L), with caution being advised if considering brainstem death testing. Therefore, it would be prudent to correct extremes of sodium prior to these tests.

F   Neither doctor performing the brainstem death tests should have any connection to the transplant team.

1.   Academy of Medical Royal Colleges. A code of practice for the diagnosis and confirmation of death, 2010. http://www.aomrc.org.uk/publications/statements/doc_details/42-a-code-of-practice-for-the-diagnosis-and-confirmation-of-death.html.

Answer 81: Critical care and haematological malignancies: True d & e

F   Neutrophils play an important role in the pathogenesis of ARDS, thus in patients with low levels of functioning neutrophils, the risk of ARDS is effectively reduced.

F   Neutropenic sepsis can be diagnosed in patients who are receiving anticancer treatment and have a neutrophil count less than 0.5 x 10^9 per litre and either a temperature greater than 38°C or signs and/or symptoms consistent with clinical sepsis.

F   Patients can be successfully treated with antibiotics infused through the catheter, particularly if the infection is caused by coagulase-negative *Staphylococci*. However, removal of the catheter should always be considered.

T   This is appropriate for low-grade disease. Treatment for more severe disease includes ciclosporin, tacrolimus, methotrexate and thalidomide.

T   Allopurinol blocks the conversion of hypoxanthine and xanthine to uric acid by xanthine oxidase enzyme and prevents new uric acid formation.

1.   Bersten AD, Soni N. *Oh's Intensive Care Manual*, 6th ed. Butterworth Heinemann Elsevier, 2009.

2.   National Institute for Health and Care Excellence. Neutropenic sepsis: prevention and management of neutropenic sepsis in cancer patients. NICE Clinical Guideline, CG151. London, UK: NICE, 2012. http://www.nice.org.uk.

Answer 82: Anti-neutrophil cytoplasmic antibody (ANCA): True: b, c & e

F   Two forms of ANCA exist: cytoplasmic (c-ANCA) and perinuclear (p-ANCA).

T   If ANCA is positive, two target antigens should be checked (myeloperoxidase [MPO] and serine proteinase-3 [PR3]). This may aid further differentiation and diagnosis of connective tissue disease/vasculitis. The simultaneous presence of PR3 ANCA and cANCA has a specificity for granulomatosis with polyangiitis (GPA) of >99%.

T   A positive p-ANCA may be associated with cystic fibrosis. It is often MPO negative.

F   Microscopic polyarteritis may present with positive ANCA (either c-ANCA or p-ANCA). It is often myeloperoxidase (MPO) and serine proteinase-3 (PR3) positive also.

T   Drug-induced ANCA vasculitis may occur with minocycline, hydralazine and propylthiouracil.

1.   Parsons PE, Wiener-Kronish JP. *Critical Care Secrets*, 5th ed. Missouri, USA: Elsevier Mosby, 2013.

Answer 83: In relation to pregnancy and critical care the following are true: True a-c & e

T

T   See Table 4.1.

Table 4.1. Physiological changes in pregnancy.	
System	**Physiology**
Respiratory	Increased alveolar ventilation (70%), relative hypocarbia ($PaCO_2$ of 25-32mmHg), reduced functional residual capacity (20%), increased O_2 consumption and reduced venous oxygen saturation (SvO_2)
Cardiovascular	Increased cardiac output (40%), increased stroke volume (25%), increased heart rate (25%), reduced total peripheral resistance, normal CVP in superior vena cava distribution, elevated CVP in inferior vena cava distribution, aorto-caval compression, increased circulating volume, increased plasma volume (40-50%), increased red cell mass (20%) and physiologic anaemia
Gastrointestinal	Reduced lower oesophageal sphincter tone, elevated risk of gastro-pulmonary aspiration, increased metabolism of carbohydrate +++, protein ++ and fat +, and hyperglycaemia (due to insulin resistance)
Haematopoietic	Reduced haemoglobin concentration (functional anaemia despite elevated red cell mass), slightly elevated leucocyte count, slightly reduced platelet count, increased clotting tendency
Renal	Increased renal blood and plasma flow (50-60%), increased glomerular filtration (50-60%), reduced serum urea and creatinine, glycosuria and mild proteinuria

T   Major obstetric haemorrhage is the leading cause of maternal mortality worldwide and is the most frequent indication for pregnancy-related critical care admission.

F   HELLP syndrome is a constellation of findings that include haemolysis with a microangiopathic haemolytic anaemia, elevated liver function tests and thrombocytopenia (low platelets).

T   In addition to very high mortality rates (up to 85% in some series), the majority of survivors unfortunately have chronic neurological deficits.

1.   Neligan PJ, Laffey JG. Clinical review: special populations - critical illness and pregnancy. *Crit Care* 2011; 15: 227.

Answer 84: Considering propofol: True a, b & e

T   Propofol is 2,6-diisopropylphenol, a phenol derivative, commonly used for induction of anaesthesia and sedation on critical care.

T   The vasodilation that is frequently seen following administration of propofol occurs secondary to several mechanisms, including the increased production and release of nitric oxide from vascular endothelium.

F   It has a calorific value of 1 calorie per ml mainly due to the lipid component of the emulsion. It is important to consider the calorific and lipid content of propofol as part of any sedated patient's daily nutritional intake to protect against overfeeding.

F   Propofol may provoke involuntary movements but these are not accompanied by seizure activity on the EEG.

T   Propofol is rapidly metabolised in the liver to inactive glucuronide and sulphate and glucuronide conjugates of the hydroxylated metabolite. However, despite being metabolised by the liver, metabolism of propofol does not appear to be impaired by hepatic disease.

1.   Peck TE, Hill SA, Williams M. *Pharmacology for Anaesthesia and Intensive Care*, 3rd ed. Cambridge, UK: Cambridge University Press, 2008.

Answer 85: Inotropes and vasopressors: True a

T   Dopamine administration in adult patients with septic shock is associated with greater mortality and a higher incidence of arrhythmic events compared to noradrenaline.

F   Vasopressin (up to 0.03 units/min) may be used in septic shock as an adjunct to noradrenaline or to help reduce overall noradrenaline dose. The VASST study found no mortality benefit using low-dose vasopressin as the single initial vasopressor in septic shock compared to noradrenaline.

F   Dobutamine doses in excess of 20µg/kg/min usually provide little additional benefit in septic shock.

F   Dopamine has predominantly β-adrenergic effects at lower doses and α-adrenergic effects at higher doses; therefore, the use of dopamine at low doses may cause hepatosplanchnic and renal circulation dilatation. Controlled trials have shown no protective effect of dopamine on renal function and its routine use for this purpose is no longer recommended.

F   Adrenaline has predominantly β-adrenergic effects at low doses and α-adrenergic effects at higher doses. In septic shock, its use is recommended by the Surviving Sepsis Campaign group as a second-line agent, to add to or potentially substitute noradrenaline, when an additional agent is needed to maintain adequate blood pressure. Adrenaline use has been shown to be no better than noradrenaline in septic shock. It is arrhythmogenic, reduces splanchnic blood flow and can increase blood lactate levels.

1.   Vincent JL, De Backer D. Circulatory shock. *New Engl J Med* 2013; 369: 1726-34.

2.   De Backer D, Cesar A, Hassane N, Vincent JL. Dopamine versus norepinephrine in the treatment of septic shock: a meta-analysis. *Crit Care Med* 2012; 40(3): 725-30.

3.   Kinnear J. Adrenaline (epinephrine). Anaesthesia Tutorial of the Week 226, 2011. www.aagbi.org/education/educational-resources/tutorial-week.

4.   Russell JA, Walley KR, Singer J, et al. Vasopressin versus norepinephrine infusion in patients with septic shock. *New Engl J Med* 2008; 358(9): 877-87.

5.   Sharman A, Low J. Vasopressin and its role in critical care. *Contin Educ Anaesth Crit Care Pain* 2008; 8(1): 134-7.

6.   Dellinger RP, Levy MM, Rhodes A, et al. Surviving Sepsis Campaign: international guidelines for management of severe sepsis and septic shock: 2012. *Crit Care Med* 2012; 41(2): 580-637.

Answer 86: Ultrasound in critical care: True a, c-e

T   In patients who are mechanically ventilated, the absence of inferior vena cava (IVC) diameter variation during the ventilatory cycle on focused echocardiography is suggestive that the patient is well filled and would not benefit from further fluid boluses. An increase in the IVC diameter of 12% or more during lung inflation is suggestive that the patient is likely to be a fluid-responder.

F   In 2010, the Advanced Life Support (ALS) resuscitation guidelines recognised that echocardiography during pulseless electrical activity (PEA)/asystolic cardiac arrest may aid the detection of potentially reversible causes of cardiac arrest. No studies have yet shown that the use of echocardiography in this way improves outcome.

T   Diagnosis of pneumothorax is made on ultrasound, when normal lung artefacts are absent and normal lung movement of the visceral pleura with respiration is lost. In pneumothorax, normal lung sliding and comet tail artefacts are lost due to air preventing propagation of ultrasound waves.

T   Echocardiography findings in acute massive pulmonary embolism include right ventricular dilatation and impairment of free wall contraction, paradoxical septal wall motion and/or dilatation of right pulmonary artery. Depending on the clinical context, this could indicate the need for urgent thrombolysis.

T   The National Institute for Health and Care Excellence (NICE) recommends that all central venous catheters should be inserted using ultrasound guidance.

1.   Wilson S, MacKay A. Ultrasound in critical care. *Contin Educ Anaesth Crit Care Pain* 2012; 12(4): 190-4.

2.   Noble VE, Nelson BP. *Manual of Emergency and Critical Care Ultrasound*, 2nd ed. Cambridge, UK: Cambridge University Press, 2011.

Answer 87: Indications for intubation and ventilation after traumatic brain injury prior to transfer include: All True

T   GCS ≤8 in traumatic brain injury is a formal indication for intubation and ventilation. The Association of Anaesthetists of Great Britain and Ireland (AAGBI) in their 2006 document state that: "Tracheal intubation during transfer is difficult and dangerous. All patients with a GCS of 8 or less require intubation prior to transfer. In addition, whatever the baseline GCS, intubation should be considered if the GCS has fallen by 2 or more points. Intubation is essential if there is a fall of 2 or more points in the motor score. Intubation requires adequate sedation and muscle relaxation to avoid an increase in [ICP], and measures to prevent aspiration of gastric contents. This will normally involve rapid sequence induction with in-line stabilisation of the cervical spine". If the GCS has fallen from a baseline of 15 to 12, this is an indication for intubation, particularly if transfer is being considered.

T A decrease in motor response score of >2 points indicates a deteriorating conscious level and a likely need for intubation prior to transfer.

T Bilateral mandibular fractures pose a bleeding risk to the airway and potential difficult airway.

T If spontaneous hyperventilation reduces $PaCO_2$ to less than 4.0kPa, the subsequent vasoconstriction may worsen cerebral perfusion. This warrants intubation and ventilation for neuroprotection.

T Seizures are an indication for intubation and ventilation.

1. Dinsmore J. Traumatic brain injury: an evidence-based review of management. *Contin Educ Anaesth Crit Care Pain* 2013; 13(6): 189-95.

2. The Association of Anaesthetists of Great Britain and Ireland (AAGBI). Recommendations for the safe transfer of patients with brain injury, 2006. http://www.aagbi.org/sites/default/files/braininjury.pdf.

Answer 88: Anaphylaxis: True b, d & e

F IgE is the immunoglobulin often responsible in anaphylaxis. In some cases IgG anaphylaxis may be responsible.

T An intramuscular dose of 0.5-1mg or intravenous dose of 50-100μg (by those familiar with the use of IV adrenaline) is recommended.

F Adrenaline/epinephrine increases levels of cyclic adenosine monophosphate (cAMP) in leukocytes and mast cells, inhibiting histamine release, and improves cardiac contractility, peripheral vascular and bronchial smooth muscle tone and mast cell stabilisation.

T   Risk factors for latex anaphylaxis include being a healthcare worker, a history of spina bifida and an allergy to kiwi fruit.

T   Suxamethonium carries the highest risk.

1.   Yentis SM, Hirsch NP, Smith GB. *Anaesthesia and Intensive Care A-Z. An Encyclopaedia of Principles and Practice*, 3rd ed. Edinburgh, UK: Elsevier Butterworth Heinemann, 2004.

2.   Bersten AD, Soni N. *Oh's Intensive Care Manual*, 6th ed. Butterworth Heinemann Elsevier, 2009.

3.   Mills ATD, Sice PJA, Ford SM. Anaesthesia-related anaphylaxis: investigation and follow-up. *Contin Educ Anaesth Crit Care Pain* 2014; 14(2): 57-62.

Answer 89: Diagnostic criteria for sepsis, severe sepsis and septic shock include: True b-e

F   Raised plasma procalcitonin levels (> two standard deviations above the upper limit of normal) are associated with sepsis.

T   White cell count >12,000/mm^3 or <4000/mm^3 is suggestive of sepsis. Also, a normal white cell count with >10% immature forms, may be seen as part of the inflammatory variables associated with sepsis.

T   Elevated mixed venous oxygen saturations >70% is a haemodynamic variable suggestive of sepsis.

T   Severe sepsis is sepsis plus organ dysfunction.

T   Septic shock is sepsis plus either hypotension refractory to fluid therapy or hyperlactaemia.

1.   Angus DC, van der Poll T. Severe sepsis and septic shock. *New Engl J Med* 2013; 369: 840-51.

Answer 90: Drowning: True b, d & e

F   Submersion in icy water may lead to protective hypothermia, but this is not common.

T   The diving reflex is thought to occur due to cold water stimulation of the ophthalmic division of the trigeminal nerve and is characterised by apnoea, vasoconstriction and bradycardia.

F   Attempts should be made to raise the body temperature of hypothermic patients during resuscitation, as severe hypothermia may impede successful resuscitation. If return of spontaneous circulation (ROSC) is achieved, it is then recommended that rewarming targets following out-of-hospital cardiac arrest be undertaken according to local policy (e.g. therapeutic hypothermia or normothermia).

T   Five rescue breaths should be delivered when commencing CPR.

T   An immersion time greater than 10 minutes indicates prolonged asphyxia.

1.   Carter E, Sinclair R. Drowning. *Contin Educ Anaesth Crit Care Pain* 2011; 11(6): 210-3.

2.   Resuscitation Council (UK). Advanced life support, 6th ed. London, UK: Resuscitation Council (UK), 2011. www.resus.org.uk.

5 MCQ Paper 5: Questions

Question 1: Inadvertent intra-arterial thiopental injection:

a   When suspected, the indwelling catheter should be removed.

b   A slow infusion of 0.9% saline should be started via the catheter.

c   Anticoagulation with heparin may be beneficial.

d   Opioids and non-steroidal analgesia may provide symptomatic relief.

e   Damage is caused solely by crystal formation in distal vessels.

Question 2: Cardiopulmonary exercise testing (CPET):

a   A standard seven-panel plot is used to display physiological results graphically.

b   Peak VO_2 (oxygen consumption) is independent of patient motivation.

c   The anaerobic threshold (AT) is the point at which the rate of oxygen consumption (VO_2) increase exceeds the rate of carbon dioxide output.

d   An AT <14ml/kg/min is associated with worse outcomes following major surgery.

e   Multivariate analysis can be applied to CPET data to predict 5-year survival after major surgery.

Question 3: Transurethral resection of prostate (TURP) syndrome:

a   Irrigation fluid can cause haemolysis.
b   Is caused by absorption of pure water used in irrigation fluid intra-operatively.
c   Presents acutely with pulmonary oedema and hypernatraemia.
d   Hypertonic saline may be required if associated with neurological signs.
e   Central pontine myelinolysis may occur with management.

Question 4: Regarding myocardial blood supply:

a   The right coronary artery (RCA) arises from the posterior aortic sinus.
b   The left coronary artery (LCA) arises from the anterior aortic sinus.
c   The anterior cardiac veins drain into the right atrium via the coronary sinus.
d   The posterior descending artery (PDA) and anterior interventricular artery is normally a branch of the left coronary artery.
e   Coronary artery dominance is determined by the marginal branch.

Question 5: In relation to central venous cannulation (CVC) insertion:

a   The internal jugular vein (IJV) runs from the jugular foramen to its termination behind the lateral border of the sternoclavicular joint.
b   Ultrasound-guided cannulation improves first-pass success and reduces complications.
c   The internal jugular vein site is associated with a reduced incidence of CVC infection compared with the subclavian vein site.
d   The subclavian vein runs from the apex of the axilla behind the border of the clavicle and underneath the first rib to join the internal jugular vein.
e   Ultrasound can be used for subclavian vein puncture.

Question 6: Hypoxia:

a   Anatomical shunt due to a ventricular septal defect (VSD) is a cause of hypoxaemic hypoxia.

b   Stagnant hypoxia occurs due to impaired cellular metabolism.

c   Cyanide poisoning can present with normal circulatory and ventilatory indices.

d   Carbon monoxide poisoning is a cause of anaemic hypoxia.

e   Methaemoglobinaemia is a cause of histotoxic hypoxia.

Question 7: A porphyric crisis may present with:

a   Severe abdominal pain which is poorly localised.

b   Proximal weakness greater than distal weakness.

c   Psychosis.

d   Hyponatraemia.

e   Tachycardia.

Question 8: In heparin-induced thrombocytopenia (HIT):

a   Heparin irreversibly binds to anti-thrombin III.

b   HIT may result from the interaction of heparin with platelet factor 4 (PF4).

c   HIT is caused by an IgM antibody.

d   HIT can be ruled out if the platelet count falls within 48 hours of commencing heparin.

e   The Warkentin criteria may be used to determine the patient's pretest probability of HIT.

Question 9: Considering the management of patients with haematological malignancies:

a   Patients with Hodgkin's lymphoma require irradiated blood products for life.

b   *Cytomegalovirus* (CMV)-negative blood products should be requested for all potential recipients of allogenic stem cell and bone marrow transplants.

c   Cisplatin is an alkylating agent.

d   Tumour lysis syndrome may result in hyperkalaemia and hypercalcaemia.

e   Patients who have received bleomycin are at lifelong risk of pulmonary toxicity provoked by high inspired fractions of oxygen.

Question 10: Focused assessment with sonography in trauma (FAST):

a   Is performed using three views.
b   A linear 5.0-10.0MHz probe is most commonly used.
c   On extended FAST (eFAST) exam, normal lung sliding and the presence of comet tail artifact rule out pneumothorax with 100% negative predictive value.
d   A negative scan excludes intra-abdominal injury.
e   Diagnostic peritoneal lavage (DPL) is more sensitive for detecting small volumes of intraperitoneal blood.

Question 11: Regarding haemoglobinopathies and coagulation disorders:

a   Idiopathic thrombobocytopenic purpura (ITP) occurs due to IgG autoantibody activity against platelets.
b   ITP can be managed with long-term steroid therapy.
c   Thrombotic thrombocytopenic purpura (TTP) results in a macroangiopathic haemolytic anaemia.
d   Therapeutic plasma exchange in a 70kg male would involve the removal and replacement of 2-3L of plasma in a single exchange.
e   TTP is associated with *Cytomegalovirus* (CMV) and HIV infection.

Question 12: Local anaesthetic toxicity:

a   May present with altered mental state.
b   The maximum safe dose of levobupivacaine is 3.5mg/kg.
c   Usually occurs immediately after local anaesthetic injection.
d   15ml/kg of Intralipid® 2% should be given immediately.
e   Propofol may be used as a substitute for Intralipid®.

Question 13: Regarding cardiac troponins I and T (cTnI and cTnT):

a   Troponin I or T is the gold standard biomarker for acute coronary syndrome diagnosis.

b   A troponin rise is seen within 2-4 hours of the onset of cardiac ischaemic damage.

c   Troponins may remain elevated for up to 2 weeks after myocardial injury.

d   Yield a negative predictive value of 95% as a single test on admission.

e   Elevated troponins are associated with increased mortality and morbidity in non-cardiac critically ill patients.

Question 14: Non-ST elevation acute coronary syndrome (NTE-ACS):

a   Has a lower long-term mortality compared to STEMI.

b   Revascularisation should be performed within 24 hours of NTE-ACS for very high-risk patients.

c   A normal electrocardiogram (ECG) excludes the diagnosis.

d   The GRACE score has 6 variables and may be used to assess risk of death following myocardial infarction.

e   Ticagrelor is indicated in all patients suffering NTE-ACS.

Question 15: Considering atrial fibrillation (AF) and the risk of stroke:

a   The CHA2DS2-VASc score has a maximum score of 6.

b   Low-dose aspirin is associated with a 22% relative risk reduction in stroke events.

c   Warfarin reduces the relative risk of stroke in AF by about 60%.

d   Intracranial haemorrhage risk is approximately 3% per year in those on warfarin for AF.

e   Antithrombotic therapy is not recommended in patients with lone AF (e.g. no other pathology) and age <65.

Question 16: Long QT syndrome (LQTS):

a A corrected QT interval (QTc) of over 0.30 seconds is considered prolonged.

b Patients with LQTS are at risk of developing polymorphic ventricular tachycardia (VT).

c Jervell-Lange-Nielsen syndrome is an autosomal dominant condition that causes LQTS.

d Romano-Ward syndrome is an autosomal recessive condition that causes LQTS.

e Magnesium sulphate may be effective in preventing recurrent torsade de pointes.

Question 17: Drugs associated with the development of torsade de pointes include:

a Droperidol.

b Clarithromycin.

c Haloperidol.

d Fluoxetine.

e Fluconazole.

Question 18: Considering the management of advanced cardiac failure:

a Dobutamine stimulates D1 and β1 receptors.

b Levosimendan opens smooth muscle K^+ channels.

c A serum N-terminal pro-B-type natriuretic peptide (NTproBNP) level >2000pg/ml carries a poor prognosis in chronic heart failure.

d Administration of β-blockers in patients with acute myocardial infarction and cardiogenic shock is associated with an increased 30-day mortality.

e Pre-operative natriuretic peptides are not useful for predicting postoperative cardiac complications.

Question 19: Management of ascites in chronic liver disease:

a   Persistent ascitic leak at the site of ascitic tap puncture may occur following paracentesis.

b   A serum-ascites albumin gradient (SAAG) >1.1g/dL suggests ascites is caused by portal hypertension.

c   A paracentesis drain should be removed after 12 hours.

d   Patients who have more than 2L removed by paracentesis should receive 8g of albumin per litre of ascites removed.

e   A low sodium diet and diuretics effectively control ascites in the majority of patients.

Question 20: Cardiopulmonary bypass:

a   Bubble oxygenators are associated with less blood component damage than membrane oxygenators.

b   pH stat management will result in a higher cerebral blood flow.

c   The incidence of postoperative cognitive deficits following cardiopulmonary bypass is approximately 40%.

d   Ten milligrams (10mg) of protamine is required to neutralise 100 units of heparin.

e   The use of aprotinin to reduce blood loss in patients receiving cardiac bypass is not recommended.

Question 21: In relation to the management of pre-eclampsia:

a   Mild pre-eclampsia should be managed with antihypertensive medications.

b   Magnesium sulphate should be used as the antihypertensive of choice in severe pre-eclampsia.

c   Once commenced, magnesium sulphate should be continued until the time of delivery.

d   Knee jerk reflexes can be used to monitor magnesium therapy instead of testing serum levels.

e   Thromboprophylaxis should be withheld in order to allow for regional anaesthesia.

Question 22: Considering splanchnic ischaemia:

a   Blood flow to the brain and heart is maintained at the expense of the mesenteric circulation in shock.

b   The rectum is supplied by the superior mesenteric artery (SMA).

c   Worsening lactic acidosis is an early sign.

d   Noradrenaline has been shown to reduce splanchnic perfusion.

e   Gut reperfusion may cause deleterious effects.

Question 23: With regards to the acute surgical abdomen in the intensive care unit:

a   Mortality as predicted by the Acute Physiology And Chronic Health Evaluation II (APACHE II) score is increased in ICU patients with an acute surgical abdomen.

b   Unexplained or rising lactate may be indicative of an anastomotic leak following primary bowel anastomosis.

c   Analysis of abdominal drain content is a reliable indicator of bleeding or anastomotic leak.

d   Following intestinal perforation, serial laparotomy and surgical toilet every 2-3 days is warranted.

e   Intra-abdominal haematoma is a focus for infection and best drained radiologically.

Question 24: The following may be associated with high levels of serum natriuretic peptide:

a   Suspected heart failure.

b   Liver cirrhosis.

c   Obesity.

d   A glomerular filtration rate (GFR) <60ml/min.

e   Age >70.

Question 25: According to the modified King's College criteria, indications for liver transplantation following paracetamol-induced acute liver failure include:

a   Arterial lactate >3.5mmol/L after early fluid resuscitation.

b   Arterial pH of <7.3 after fluid resuscitation.

c   The presence of Grade III encephalopathy, an international normalised ratio (INR) >6.5 and creatinine >300μmol/L occurring within a 24-hour period.

d   Age <10 years or >40 years, with an INR >3.5 and serum bilirubin >300μmol/L.

e   An INR <6.5 and the presence of encephalopathy.

Question 26: Complications of acute aneurysmal subarachnoid haemorrhage (SAH) on critical care include:

a   Rebleeding.

b   Hydrocephalus.

c   Seizures.

d   Vasospasm.

e   Delayed cerebral ischaemia (DCI) in the absence of vasospasm.

Question 27: Hepatitis A virus (HAV) infection:

a   Is enterically transmitted.

b   Infection does not confer life-long immunity.

c   Is a double-stranded RNA virus.

d   Has a high mortality rate.

e   Vaccination has poor efficacy for HAV prevention.

Question 28: Categories of shock:

a   Hypovolaemic shock is characterised by a profound reduction in cardiac output and vascular tone.

b   Tachycardia, hypotension, cool peripheries, low mixed venous oxygen saturation (SvO_2) and elevated central venous pressure are consistent with cardiogenic shock.

c   Hypotension, skin vasoconstriction, dilated jugular veins and pulsus paradoxus are associated with distributive shock.

d   Anaphylaxis is associated with decreased vascular tone and tachycardia.

e   Spinal shock is associated with bradycardia and hypotension.

Question 29: Mixed venous oxygen saturation (SvO_2):

a   Is low (<65%) if O_2 delivery is reduced or O_2 consumption increases.

b   Is high (>75%) if O_2 extraction is decreased.

c   Central venous oxygen saturation ($ScvO_2$) is often less than SvO_2 in the critically ill.

d   In the first 6 hours of septic shock, targeting an SvO_2 of at least 70% was found to be associated with decreased mortality.

e   Normal SvO_2 (65-75%) rules out persistent tissue hypoxia.

Question 30: Withdrawal phenomena on the intensive care unit:

a   Signs of acute alcohol withdrawal typically include abdominal pain, piloerection, mydriasis, irritability, fever and hypertension.

b   Flumazenil may induce symptoms of anxiety, hyperactive delirium and seizures following long-term exposure to benzodiazepines.

c   Dexmedetomidine does not cause withdrawal symptoms.

d   Opioid and sedative withdrawal is overlooked and often attributed mistakenly to alcohol in critical care patients.

e   Nicotine replacement therapy in critical care is completely safe.

Question 31: Necrotising fasciitis:

a   Type I infections are caused by group A *Streptococci*.

b   Clindamycin is an appropriate antibiotic.

c   Blistering and bulla formation are early features of necrotising fasciitis.

d   Patients who are immunocompromised are at greater risk of development.

e   Surgery to remove necrotic and damaged tissue should be delayed until the patient is stabilised.

Question 32: Considering inhalational poisoning:

a   Carbon monoxide (CO) poisoning may initially present with headache, myalgia and/or neurological impairment.

b   A cherry red skin discolouration appearance is rarely seen with CO toxicity.

c   The elimination half-life of CO in room air is over 4 hours.

d   Hyperbaric O_2 therapy (3 atmospheres) for CO poisoning should be considered in patients with carboxyhaemoglobin (HbCO) levels above 40%.

e   Elevated lactate and a raised anion gap may be suggestive of cyanide poisoning.

Question 33: In patients with decompensated chronic liver disease:

a   Hyperglycaemia is common.

b   Oesophageal varices are a contraindication to fine-bore nasogastric tube (NG) insertion.

c   Sodium restriction should be undertaken in the presence of ascites.

d   Hypoaldosteronism often results in chronic liver disease.

e   Up to 50% of patients develop renal dysfunction due to hepatorenal syndrome (HRS).

Question 34: Regarding lumbar puncture (LP) in suspected meningoencephalitis:

a   CT scanning should always be undertaken prior to performing an LP in suspected meningoencephalitis.

b   Opening pressure is often very high in fungal infections.

c   Following a 'traumatic tap', peripheral red blood cells in cerebrospinal fluid (CSF) may artificially increase the white cell count and confound diagnosis.

d   A CSF lactate less than 2mmol/L is said to rule out bacterial disease.

e   If the first CSF is normal in patients with *Herpes simplex* virus (HSV) encephalitis, a second LP is unlikely to be helpful.

Question 35: Regarding microscopic examination of cerebrospinal fluid (CSF):

a   A cell count of 36,000/mm^3 is associated with tuberculous infection.

b   Viral infection is associated with a neutrophilic pleocytosis.

c   A 'gin' clear colour is seen in fungal infection.

d   Typically, with bacterial meningitis a CSF to plasma glucose ratio of 0.50 to 0.66 is found.

c   A protein count of <1.0g/L is normal.

Question 36: Controversies in the management of septic shock (2012-2014):

a   Targeting a mean arterial blood pressure of 80-85mmHg compared with 65-70mmHg during resuscitation of patients in septic shock does not improve mortality.

b   Albumin replacement in septic shock, in addition to crystalloids, improves overall mortality.

c   High-volume haemofiltration improves haemodynamic profile and mortality in patients with septic shock.

d   Drotrecogin alfa (activated) reduced mortality at 28 days in septic shock.

e   Protocol-based early goal-directed therapy (EGDT) with crystalloids in early septic shock results in less fluid being given.

Question 37: Considering mechanisms of antibiotic action:

a   Penicillins inhibit the enzyme transpeptidase which forms the lattice cross-links of bacterial cell walls.

b   Co-trimoxazole induces the enzyme dihydrofolate reductase.

c   Metronidazole damages bacterial RNA function.

d   Vancomycin inhibits cell wall production.

e   Rifampicin prevents RNA transcription.

Question 38: Regarding intravenous anaesthetic agents:

a   Thiopental can be safely used in patients with porphyria.

b   Ketamine (4-10mg/kg) may be given intramuscularly for anaesthetic induction.

c   Propofol should be avoided in patients with a known egg allergy.

d   Etomidate suppresses 11 β-hydroxylase and 17 α-hydroxylase following a single dose.

e   Thiopentone is predominantly excreted unchanged via the kidneys.

Question 39: Propofol:

a   A dose of 1-2mg/kg IV is often used for induction of anaesthesia.

b   Metabolic alkalosis and cardiac instability are the most common presenting features of propofol infusion syndrome (PRIS).

c   Has a small volume of distribution.

d   Intra-arterial injection may cause tissue necrosis.

e   Increasing levels of creatine kinase (CK) after 24-48 hours of propofol infusion should raise a suspicion of PRIS.

Question 40: Regarding the principles of pharmacokinetics:

a   Bioavailability is defined as the concentration of a drug reaching the systemic circulation following a single oral dose.

b   Drugs absorbed from the buccal mucosa are subject to first-pass metabolism.

c   The intrinsic activity of a drug is represented by the position of the dose-response curve on the x-axis.

d   Competitive and non-competitive antagonists shift the dose response curve to the right.

e   The therapeutic index is the ratio given by the median effective dose (ED50) divided by the median lethal dose (LD50).

Question 41: Regarding drugs used on the intensive care unit:

a   Laudanosine is cleared primarily by the liver.

b   Clonidine is an agonist at α2-receptors.

c   Rifampicin inhibits cytochrome p450.

d   Procainamide is a Class Ia antiarrhythmic.

e   Midazolam possesses an imidazole ring which opens at a pH greater than 4.

Question 42: Suggested physiological goals for the active management of a heart-beating donor include:

a   Heart rate of 80-100 beats per minute and systolic blood pressure >100mmHg.

b   Arterial pH 7.35-7.45, $PaCO_2$ 4.7-6kPa and PaO_2 greater than or equal to 10.7kPa.

c   Serum sodium between 130-160mmol/L.

d   Serum glucose of 4-8mmol/L.

e   A cardiac index of 2.4L/min/m².

Question 43: Organ donation and consent:

a   The modified Maastricht classification is used to classify donation after brain-death patients (DBD).

b   In the UK, the consent rate for organ donation is >75%.

c   An advance statement, the organ donor register and exploring any previously held views may help determine consent for donation in a patient who lacks capacity.

d   The Mental Capacity Act provides a statutory framework for actions which may be required to allow donation.

e   When approaching those close to the patient, one should be open and apologetic.

Question 44: Absolute contraindications to trans-oesophageal echo (TOE) include:

a   Atlantoaxial joint disease.

b   Hiatus hernia.

c   Prior chest irradiation.

d   Oesophageal stricture.

e   Active upper GI bleeding.

Question 45: Congenital disorders associated with difficult airways in children include:

a   Pierre-Robin syndrome.

b   Treacher-Collins syndrome.

c   Apert syndrome.
d   Down's syndrome.
e   Osteopetrosis.

Question 46: Intubation of the critically ill child:

a   Haemodynamic compromise which has failed to respond to fluid resuscitation is an indication for intubation.
b   Up to 40% of a child's cardiac output may be required to support the work of breathing.
c   The child should always be moved to a place of safety and familiarity (e.g. theatres) prior to intubation.
d   In extremis, intramuscular ketamine (5-10mg/kg) and suxamethonium (3-4mg/kg) may be used for rapid sequence induction.
e   Endotracheal internal diameter size can be estimated with the formula: [age+4]/4.

Question 47: Regarding disseminated fungal infections:

a   *Candida* species are the most common causative fungal pathogens.
b   The use of total parenteral nutrition on the ICU is a risk factor.
c   A single positive fungal blood culture is likely to be a contaminant.
d   Asymptomatic candiduria should be always treated.
e   Antifungal therapy should be delayed in suspected cases, until blood cultures are positive to reduce the development of resistant organisms.

Question 48: Antifungal drugs:

a   Amphotericin B binds irreversibly to cholesterol causing fungal cell death.
b   Fluconazole inhibits C-14 α-demethylase.
c   Caspofungin inhibits ergosterol.
d   Fluconazole is nephrotoxic.
e   Fluconazole is active against *Aspergillus* species.

Question 49: Considering connective tissue disorders and critical care:

a   A prolonged Russell viper venom time and false-positive test for syphilis (VDRL) are often seen with Goodpasture's disease.

b   Scleroderma may present with diffuse alveolar haemorrhage (DAH).

c   Scleroderma renal crisis is a medical emergency and classically presents with an abrupt onset of hypotension and acute renal failure.

d   A presentation of a malar/discoid rash with renal involvement is seen with systemic sclerosis.

e   Anti-RNP (ribonuclear protein) is associated with polymyositis.

Question 50: The intra-aortic balloon pump (IABP) and clinical practice:

a   Use of an IABP is contraindicated in patients with severe aortic regurgitation.

b   The balloon should be positioned to lie proximal to the subclavian artery.

c   IABP use reduces mortality in patients with cardiogenic shock complicating acute myocardial infarction, for whom an early revascularisation strategy is planned.

d   The IABP should be discontinued during attempted defibrillation.

e   Patients should be positioned no greater than 30°C head up with an IABP in place.

Question 51: In relation to the human immunodeficiency virus (HIV):

a   HIV-1 is a single-stranded DNA virus.

b   Acute respiratory failure accounts for >60% of critical care admissions in patients with HIV.

c   Binding of viral surface envelope protein (Env) to CD4 receptors on the cell initiates infection.

d   Therapies aim to inhibit viral replication, reverse transcription and/or protein cleavage.

e   CD4 counts <650 cells/µl indicate significant impairment of immune function.

Question 52: Mechanisms of blast injury:

a   Secondary injury is caused by displacement of the victim.
b   Solid organs are more vulnerable to a blast wave than air-containing organs.
c   Surgical intervention is not required for bowel contusion sustained by blast injury.
d   The presence of a primary blast injury strongly suggests that secondary and tertiary injuries will be present.
e   Benzylpenicillin is an appropriate prophylactic and therapeutic antibiotic in the management of gunshot wounds sustained in the field.

Question 53: In a patient with carbon monoxide poisoning:

a   Carbon monoxide is directly toxic to the lungs.
b   The oxyhaemoglobin dissociation curve will be shifted to the left.
c   The arterial PO_2 will drop, stimulating the aortic and carotid bodies.
d   The normal elimination half-life of carbon monoxide in air is 2 hours.
e   Hyperbaric oxygen therapy is contraindicated in pregnant women with carbon monoxide poisoning.

Question 54: The following physiological changes are seen in pregnancy:

a   Plasma albumin decreases by approximately 10g/L.
b   Systolic arterial pressure decreases to a greater extent than diastolic arterial pressure.
c   Respiratory acidosis is considered normal in pregnancy.
d   Oxygen consumption is increased by approximately 20%.
e   The uterine vascular bed is responsive to vasoconstrictors.

Question 55: The Confidential Enquiry into Maternal Deaths in the UK 2006-2008 (Centre for Maternal and Child Enquiries: CEMACE):

a   Demonstrated a decline in the overall maternal mortality rate in the UK.

b   Substandard care was implicated in approximately a third of direct and indirect maternal deaths.

c   Thrombosis and thromboembolism was the leading cause of direct death identified in this report.

d   Cardiac disease was identified as the leading cause of indirect maternal death.

e   Deaths due to anaesthesia all involved difficulties with the airway.

Question 56: Obstetric haemorrhage:

a   Is no longer a major cause of maternal death globally.

b   Women who have had two or more Caesarean sections and placenta praevia are deemed to be at high risk of placenta accreta.

c   Patient safety guidelines recommend that a level 2 critical care bed should be available for women at high risk of placenta accreta undergoing Caesarean section.

d   Primary postpartum haemorrhage (PPH) is defined as the loss of 1000ml or more of blood from the genital tract within 24 hours of the birth of a baby.

e   Recombinant Factor VIIa is an appropriate adjuvant treatment in the management of major PPH.

Question 57: Electrocardiography findings in electrolyte disorders include:

a   Prolonged PR interval in hyperkalaemia.

b   Shortened QT interval in hyperkalaemia.

c   J-waves in hypokalaemia.

d   Prolonged QT interval in hypocalcaemia.

e   Tachycardia in hypermagnesaemia.

Question 58: Regarding fluids used for resuscitation:

a   The transvascular exchange of fluid is determined by hydrostatic and oncotic pressures across capillaries and the interstitial space.

b   The structure and function of the endothelial glycocalyx layer is a key determinant of membrane permeability in pathophysiological states.

c   Fluid resuscitation with boluses of albumin or saline, in febrile children with poor perfusion, is associated with improved outcomes.

d   The use of hydroxyethyl starch (HES) may be beneficial in early sepsis.

e   Albumin use is associated with increased mortality among patients with traumatic brain injury.

Question 59: Following liver transplantation:

a   Patients who undergo transplant for acute liver failure and encephalopathy are no longer at risk of intracranial hypertension following successful transplantation.

b   Mortality in those who require renal replacement therapy (RRT) is approximately 40%.

c   Aspartate aminotransferase (AST) levels should fall by 50% each day.

d   Primary non-function presents approximately 24 hours post-transplant.

e   Ultrasound should be undertaken if there is a suspicion of hepatic artery thrombosis.

Question 60: Regarding heart-lung transplantation:

a   Eisenmenger's syndrome is an indication for heart-lung transplantation.

b   Postoperatively there will be an abnormal cough.

c   Rejection is more likely to manifest in the heart first rather than the lungs.

d   Rejection is the leading cause of mortality in the 6 months following transplantation.

e   In the first 24 hours postoperatively, the presence of infiltrates on chest X-ray suggests rejection.

Question 61: Following severe crush injuries:

a   Rhabdomyolysis may occur resulting in hyperkalaemia, hypercalcaemia and hyperphosphataemia.

b   Creatinine levels are the most sensitive indicators of muscle damage.

c   The addition of mannitol and bicarbonate have no impact on the development of acute kidney injury, need for dialysis or mortality in patients with a creatine kinase level >5000U/L.

d   Compartment pressures exceeding 30mmHg are an indication for fasciotomy.

e   Fat embolism syndrome cannot be detected on a chest X-ray.

Question 62: Regarding the Injury Severity Score (ISS):

a   The maximum score is 90.

b   The six body regions included are as follows: head, face, chest, abdomen, extremity and external.

c   In patients with multiple injuries, the worst Abbreviated Injury Scale (AIS) score from each region of the body is added together.

d   A patient with an AIS of 6, in any body region, is given an ISS of 75.

e   The Injury Severity Score is linear.

Question 63: The following may cause a raised urinary sodium and plasma hyponatraemia:

a   Post-transurethral resection of prostate (TURP) syndrome.

b   Hypothyroidism.

c   Syndrome of inappropriate anti-diuretic hormone (SIADH).

d   Psychogenic polydipsia.

e   Cerebral salt wasting.

Question 64: Regarding pelvic trauma:

a   Most pelvic fractures result from falls.

b   The superior and inferior gluteal arteries arise from the external iliac artery.

c   There are generally three different types of mechanism of pelvic injury in trauma.

d   The superior gluteal artery is the artery most frequently damaged in association with pelvic fracture.

e   An 'open book' fracture can quadruple the volume of the retroperitoneal space.

Question 65: Withdrawal of treatment:

a   Should consider the potential futility of continuing treatment.

b   Should consider the equity in the use of ICU resources.

c   Discussions should involve the patient if at all possible.

d   In some cases a court of law may be needed to rule on withdrawal of treatment.

e   Anxiolytic and analgesic drugs should not be used if they are likely to hasten the death of the patient following withdrawal of care.

Question 66: The following are acceptable methods of randomisation of patients for a randomised controlled trial (RCT):

a   Use of the last digit of the patient's date of birth with odd and even numbers being assigned to different groups.

b   Toss of coin with heads and tails being used to assign to different groups.

c   Date that the patient is consented to the trial with odd and even numbers being assigned to different groups.

d   Sequentially numbered sealed envelopes containing a computer-generated number that is used to assign to different groups.

e   Sequential allocation of patients to groups as they are recruited to the study.

Question 67: The following may introduce inaccuracy in the recording of oxygen saturations via pulse oximetry:

a   Oxygen saturations below 70%.

b   Hypothermia.

c   Atrial fibrillation.

d   Hyperbilirubinaemia.

e   Methaemoglobinaemia.

Question 68: Acute severe asthma:

a   Worsening gas trapping with hypoinflation is responsible for the pathophysiology of life-threatening asthma.

b   Large negative pressures generated by inspiratory effort can impede left atrial filling and cardiac output.

c   Magnesium 1.2-2g intravenously over 20 minutes is recommended in addition to oxygen and medical therapy.

d   Initial ventilatory settings should adopt relatively low rates (12-14 breaths/min), little or no positive end-expiratory pressure (PEEP) (<5cmH$_2$O) and relatively long expiratory times (I:E 1:4).

e   Extracorporeal CO$_2$ removal (ECCO$_2$R) devices may be considered in cases of refractory hypercarbia.

Question 69: The following have been demonstrated to reduce the incidence of ventilator-associated pneumonia (VAP):

a   Prophylactic antibiotics in ventilated patients.

b   Head-up patient positioning.

c   Daily sedation holds.

d   Subglottic irrigation devices.

e   Low tidal volume ventilation.

Question 70: Regarding the Berlin definition for acute respiratory distress syndrome (ARDS):

a   The timing of ARDS must occur within 5 days of a known clinical insult and new or worsening respiratory symptoms.

b   Bilateral opacities are evident on chest imaging, which are not attributable to effusions, lobar collapse or pulmonary nodules.

c   The respiratory failure seen cannot be fully explained by cardiac failure or fluid overload.

d   ARDS is classified into mild and severe according to the PaO$_2$/FiO$_2$ ratio.

e   Severe ARDS is defined by a PaO$_2$/FiO$_2$ ratio of <150mmHg with a positive end-expiratory pressure (PEEP) >5cmH$_2$O.

Question 71: Predictors of successful extubation:

a   A 2-hour spontaneous breathing trial (SBT) is a more sensitive predictor of successful extubation than a 30-minute SBT.

b   A rapid shallow breathing index of >105 during SBT predicts successful extubation.

c   Increased age increases the risk of failed extubation.

d   Failed extubation is more likely in patients with upper airway abnormalities.

e   Negative fluid balance prior to extubation increases the likelihood of successful extubation.

Question 72: Relating to the control of solutes and water in the kidney:

a   Approximately 75% of the filtered sodium load is reabsorbed daily.

b   The highest proportion of sodium reabsorption occurs in the distal convoluted tubule.

c   Both the thick and thin ascending limbs of the loop of Henle are mostly impermeable to water.

d   Filtered glucose is reabsorbed in the proximal convoluted tubule.

e   The collecting ducts have a high natural permeability to water allowing for final adjustment of urine volume in combination with anti-diuretic hormone (ADH).

Question 73: The following are true in the management of diabetic ketoacidosis (DKA):

a   Cerebral oedema is the commonest cause of UK mortality associated with DKA.

b   Measurement of capillary blood ketones at the bedside, using a ketone meter, is the method of choice for monitoring response to treatment.

c   Insulin infusions form the cornerstone of management and often may need to run in excess of 15 units of insulin per hour.

d   Introduction of 10% dextrose infusions are not recommended until the blood glucose has fallen to less than 10mmol/L.

e   In patients in whom the arterial pH has fallen to <7.10, an infusion of bicarbonate is likely to be beneficial.

Question 74: In relation to hyperosmolar hyperglycaemic state (HHS) in adults with diabetes, the following statements are correct:

a HHS has a higher mortality than diabetic ketoacidosis (DKA).

b Characteristic features of HHS include: hypovolaemia, marked hyperglycaemia (>30mmol/L) without significant hyperketonaemia (<3mmol/L) and serum osmolality <320mOsm/kg.

c Fluid losses in HHS are estimated to be between 50-100ml/kg.

d The rate of fall of plasma sodium should not exceed 10mmol/L in 24 hours.

e The fall in blood glucose should be no more than 10mmol/L/hr.

Question 75: The following conditions are currently (2013-14) recommended indications for the institution of therapeutic hypothermia (TH):

a Out-of-hospital cardiac arrest with ventricular fibrillation or pulseless ventricular tachycardia as the presenting rhythm.

b Acute ischaemic stroke (AIS).

c Subarachnoid haemorrhage.

d Perinatal asphyxia.

e Sepsis syndrome.

Question 76: In relation to hyponatraemia, the following statements are true:

a Acute 'profound' hyponatraemia can be defined as the biochemical finding of a serum sodium concentration of <125mmol/L, which is documented to exist for <72 hours.

b When correcting serum sodium concentration for the presence of hyperglycaemia, the serum sodium concentration will rise.

c In a patient with hypotonic hyponatraemia with a urine osmolality ≤100mOsm/kg, beer potomania is a possible diagnosis.

d   In a patient with hypotonic hyponatraemia with a urine osmolality ≥100mOsm/kg, the finding of a urine sodium concentration >30mmol/L would be consistent with both the syndrome of inappropriate anti-diuretic hormone (SIADH) and cerebral salt wasting.

e   The initial management of hyponatraemia with severe symptoms should include the use of 3% hypertonic saline (or equivalent) regardless of whether the hyponatraemia is acute or chronic.

Question 77: Concerning patient safety initiatives:

a   Historic data suggest that less than 20% of bloodstream infections are likely to be central line-related.

b   As part of care bundles to prevent ventilator-associated pneumonia (VAP), the head of the bed should be elevated to between 15-30°.

c   As part of care bundles to prevent VAP, sedation should be interrupted at least every 2 days to assess readiness for extubation.

d   As part of care bundles to prevent central line infection, 0.5% chlorhexidine should be used for skin antisepsis.

e   Total parenteral nutrition (TPN) should only be administered via a separate line not a multi-lumen central line.

Question 78: Transpulmonary pressure (TPP) and ventilator-associated lung injury:

a   At end-inspiration, the TPP is the principal force maintaining inflation.

b   TPP is calculated from the alveolar pressure minus the pleural pressure.

c   The use of oesophageal TPP monitoring to set positive end-expiratory pressure (PEEP), to achieve an end-expiratory TPP of 0-10cmH$_2$O, may be associated with improved outcomes in acute respiratory distress syndrome (ARDS).

d   During non-invasive ventilation (NIV), TPPs may be dangerously high, despite low delivered airway pressures.

e   Barotrauma is directly due to high airway pressures.

Question 79: The following statements are true in relation to renal replacement therapy (RRT) and vascular access:

a   In a patient with Goodpasture's syndrome presenting to critical care for RRT, the subclavian vein should be the first choice for catheter access.

b   Femoral vein catheters of adequate length are likely to provide good flow rates.

c   Femoral vein catheters are significantly more likely to cause catheter-related blood stream infections (CRBSI) than other central line sites.

d   Arteriovenous fistulae should not be used for intermittent RRT on critical care.

e   High-access pressure alarms may indicate a problem with the vascular access catheter or inadequate blood pump flow rates.

Question 80: When prescribing continuous renal replacement therapy (CRRT), the following statements are correct:

a   High-volume haemofiltration (HVHF) at 70ml/kg/hr is likely to be beneficial with regard to mortality in septic shock patients.

b   High-volume haemofiltration (HVHF) at 70ml/kg/hr is likely to be beneficial with regard to mortality in non-septic shock patients.

c   Too high a filtration ratio is associated with clotting in the haemofilter.

d   Increasing pre-dilution may prolong filter life and increase solute clearance.

e   Bicarbonate-based replacement solutions can be prepared well in advance for patients on CRRT.

Question 81: Regarding anticoagulation and continuous renal replacement therapy (CRRT):

a   A pre-filter infusion of unfractionated heparin remains the most common method of anticoagulation for CRRT worldwide.

b   In patients with heparin-induced thrombocytopenia (HIT), direct thrombin inhibitors (e.g. argatroban) or Factor Xa inhibitors (e.g. danaparoid or fondaparinux) should be used rather than no anticoagulation in CRRT.

c   Citrate provides anticoagulation by chelation of ionised calcium.
d   Citrate anticoagulation requires an exogenous infusion of calcium to replace that lost in the effluent.
e   Severe liver impairment is a contraindication for citrate anticoagulation.

Question 82: Hypernatraemia:

a   Hypernatraemia is most often due to unreplaced water loss from the gastrointestinal tract, sweat or urine.
b   Over-rapid correction of hypernatraemia especially if chronic in onset (>48 hours) can result in brain oedema.
c   Hypovolaemic patients with hypernatraemia should initially be managed with hypotonic solutions.
d   Central diabetes insipidus is caused by the kidney failing to respond correctly to anti-diuretic hormone (ADH).
e   In patients with nephrogenic diabetes insipidus, desmopressin is the treatment of choice.

Question 83: Regarding temporary cardiac pacing:

a   Transcutaneous pacing always requires a general anaesthetic.
b   The pacemaker code 'VVD' is for ventricular pacing only.
c   'Capture' describes the ability of the electrical impulse to initiate myocardial depolarisation.
d   Pacing output should be set at the capture threshold.
e   Increasing the sensitivity dial increases pacemaker sensitivity.

Question 84: Anaesthesia and MRI:

a   Involves X-ray radiation.
b   In a T1-weighted image, fat appears dark and water bright.
c   Standard pulse oximeters may cause burns.
d   Standard infusion pumps work in the MRI environment.
e   Switching of gradient fields may cause hearing loss.

Question 85: Concerning intracranial pressure (ICP) monitoring:

a   ICP monitoring should be instituted in all salvageable patients with severe traumatic brain injury and an abnormal CT scan.

b   ICP monitoring should be instituted in salvageable patients with severe traumatic brain injury and a normal CT scan.

c   There is level I evidence to support decision making on whether to insert an ICP bolt or not.

d   The Brain Trauma Foundation (BTF) guidelines recommend the ventricular catheter as the most accurate and reliable method of measuring ICP, as compared to intraparenchymal devices.

e   Treatment should be initiated above an ICP threshold of 30mmHg.

Question 86: Regarding acid-base balance:

a   The use of 0.9% sodium chloride for resuscitation may result in an increased plasma strong ion difference.

b   In renal tubular acidosis, urinary strong ion difference is high whilst plasma strong ion difference is low.

c   In Type 2 renal tubular acidosis, there is increased proximal tubular chloride resorption.

d   Acetazolamide increases urinary strong ion difference.

e   Metabolic alkalosis is a cause of cerebral vasospasm.

Question 87: In relation to thyroid function tests, which of the following statements are true?:

a   In overt hyperthyroidism, free T4 and free T3 levels are always high.

b   Increased thyroid-stimulating hormone (TSH) in the presence of normal or low free T4 suggests primary hypothyroidism.

c   In the euthyroid sick syndrome, reverse T3 levels tend to be high.

d   T4 levels may be decreased in the euthyroid sick syndrome.

e   Euthyroid hyperthyroxinaemia is characterised by increased T4 with variable T3 and TSH, with increased peripheral conversion of T4 to T3.

Question 88: Non-invasive ventilation (NIV):

a   Decreases the work of breathing and may aid weaning from mechanical ventilation.
b   Can reduce the need for intubation and hospital morbidity.
c   Failure is associated with a higher mortality in respiratory failure.
d   Greatest benefit is seen in acute hypercapnic chronic obstructive pulmonary disease (COPD) exacerbation or cardiogenic pulmonary oedema.
e   Severe acidosis is a contraindication.

Question 89: Rotational thromboelastometry (ROTEM®):

a   Uses two disposable cups.
b   EXTEM uses contact activator.
c   INTEM assesses the extrinsic clotting pathway.
d   FIBTEM contains the platelet inhibitor cytochalasin D and calcium.
e   The normal range for clotting time (CT) is: INTEM 40-100s and EXTEM 46-148s.

Question 90: Biological weapon poisoning:

a   Ricin inhibits protein synthesis causing cell death and multi-organ failure.
b   Following inhalational exposure to anthrax, person-to-person transmission can occur.
c   VX phosphorylates the serine hydroxyl group in the active site of acetylcholinesterase (AChE).
d   *Yersinia pestis* can be rapidly detected to confirm a pneumonic plague aerosolized attack.
e   An erythematous macular rash which progresses to papules, then pustules in a centrifugal pattern, may indicate *Variola major* exposure.

Answer overview: Paper 5

Question:	a	b	c	d	e		Question:	a	b	c	d	e
1	F	T	T	T	F		46	T	T	F	T	F
2	F	F	F	F	T		47	T	T	F	F	F
3	F	F	F	T	T		48	F	T	F	F	F
4	F	F	F	F	F		49	F	T	F	F	F
5	F	T	F	F	T		50	T	F	F	F	T
6	T	F	T	T	F		51	F	F	T	T	F
7	T	T	T	T	T		52	F	F	F	T	T
8	F	T	F	F	T		53	F	T	F	F	F
9	T	F	T	F	T		54	F	F	F	T	T
10	F	F	T	F	T		55	T	F	F	T	F
11	T	F	F	T	T		56	F	F	T	F	T
12	T	F	F	F	F		57	T	T	F	T	F
13	T	T	T	T	T		58	F	T	F	F	T
14	F	F	F	F	T		59	F	T	T	F	F
15	F	T	T	F	T		60	T	T	F	F	F
16	F	T	F	F	T		61	F	F	T	T	F
17	T	T	T	T	T		62	F	T	F	T	F
18	F	T	T	T	F		63	F	T	T	F	T
19	T	T	F	F	F		64	F	F	T	T	T
20	F	T	T	F	F		65	T	T	T	T	F
21	F	F	F	T	F		66	F	F	F	T	F
22	T	F	F	F	T		67	T	T	T	F	T
23	T	T	F	F	F		68	F	F	T	T	T
24	T	T	F	T	T		69	F	T	T	T	F
25	T	T	T	F	F		70	F	T	T	F	F
26	T	T	T	T	T		71	F	F	T	T	T
27	T	F	F	F	F		72	F	F	T	T	F
28	F	T	F	T	F		73	T	T	F	F	F
29	T	T	F	T	F		74	T	F	F	T	F
30	F	T	F	T	F		75	T	F	F	T	F
31	F	T	F	T	F		76	F	T	T	T	T
32	T	T	T	T	T		77	F	F	F	F	F
33	F	F	T	F	F		78	T	T	T	T	F
34	F	T	T	T	F		79	F	T	F	F	T
35	F	F	F	F	F		80	F	F	T	F	F
36	T	F	F	F	F		81	T	T	T	T	T
37	T	F	F	T	T		82	T	T	F	F	F
38	F	T	F	T	F		83	F	T	T	F	F
39	T	F	F	F	T		84	F	F	T	F	T
40	F	F	F	F	F		85	T	T	F	T	F
41	T	T	F	T	F		86	F	T	T	T	T
42	F	T	F	T	T		87	F	T	T	T	T
43	F	F	T	T	F		88	T	T	T	T	F
44	F	F	F	T	T		89	F	F	F	T	F
45	T	T	T	T	T		90	T	F	T	F	T

5 MCQ Paper 5: Answers

Answer 1: Inadvertent intra-arterial thiopental injection: True b-d

F   The catheter should be left in place for diagnostic and treatment strategies. Common clinical signs of thiopental intra-arterial injection are pain on injection, anaesthesia or muscle weakness distal to injection in awake patients and skin pallor or cyanosis, distal to the injection site.

T   An isotonic solution such as 0.9% saline should be used to maintain catheter patency for access to surgical tissues and vasculature.

T   No formal guideline for management of intra-arterial injection exists but heparinisation is recommended as it may reduce vasospasm and clot formation.

T   Analgesia with paracetamol, NSAIDs and opiates may provide symptom relief; regional nerve plexus blockade may also be utilised to relieve symptoms of intra-arterial injection.

F   The underlying pathophysiology of arterial damage is unclear. It may be related to a combination of endothelial inflammation, crystal formation, thrombus, high osmolarity, lipid solubility, direct cytotoxic effect and vasospasm.

1.   Sen S, Chini EN, Brown MJ. Complications after unintentional intra-arterial injection of drugs: risks, outcomes, and management strategies. *Mayo Clin Proc* 2005; 80(6): 783-95.

Answer 2: Cardiopulmonary exercise testing (CPET): True

e

F A standard nine-panel plot is used to graphically present CPET results. Panels 2, 3 and 5 relate to the cardiovascular system; panels 1, 4 and 7 examine ventilation and panels 6, 8 and 9 examine ventilation perfusion relationships.

F The anaerobic threshold (AT) is independent from patient motivation and provides a reliable measure of dynamic functional capacity specific to that patient. Peak VO_2 represents the maximum VO_2 that is measured, usually at the point where exercise is terminated, and therefore may be influenced by patient motivation to continue exercising. Peak VO_2 correlates with postoperative cardiopulmonary complications after oesophagectomy and abdominal aneurysm surgery.

F The anaerobic threshold (AT) is the point at which the rate of increase of carbon dioxide output exceeds the rate of increase in oxygen consumption (VO_2). It is the point where aerobic metabolism alone is no longer adequate and is supplemented by anaerobic production of adenosine triphosphate (ATP).

F Patients with a peak VO_2 less than 14ml/kg/min have a worse overall prognosis than those with a peak VO_2 above 14ml/kg/min in patients with heart failure. Patients with an anaerobic threshold (AT) <11ml/min/kg are considered high risk, as there is a higher associated morbidity and mortality following major abdominal surgery. Patients with a pre-operative AT <11ml/kg/min should be admitted to critical care following major surgery.

T Multivariate analysis and model generation techniques can be applied to CPET data to predict 5-year survival after major surgery.

1.   Agnew N. Preoperative cardiopulmonary exercise testing. *Contin Educ Anaesth Crit Care Pain* 2010; 10(2): 33-7.

2.   Drury N, Carlisle J. Cardiopulmonary exercise testing. Anaesthesia Tutorial of the Week 217, 2011. www.aagbi.org/education/educational-resources/tutorial-week.

3.   Older P, Hall A, Hader R. Cardiopulmonary exercise testing as a screening test for perioperative management of major surgery in the elderly. *Chest* 1999; 116: 355-62.

4.   Colson M, Baglin J, Bolsin S, Grocott MPW. Cardiopulmonary exercise testing predicts 5-year survival after major surgery. *Br J Anaesth* 2012; 109(5): 735-41.

Answer 3: Transurethral resection of prostate (TURP) syndrome: True d & e

F   Irrigation fluid (usually glycine 1.5%, mannitol 5% or sorbitol 3.5%) is both non-conductive (so diathermy current is concentrated at the cutting point) and non-haemolytic (if fluid enters the circulation).

F   Pure water is not suitable for irrigation as it is conductive and of poor optical density. TURP syndrome is caused by the excessive absorption of irrigation fluid such as glycine 1.5%.

F   Presents acutely with pulmonary oedema, cerebral oedema, seizures and hyponatraemia (acute fall in Na^+ sometimes <120mmol/L). It tends to be detected earlier in awake patients. If unrecognised and untreated, mortality can be high. Intubation and ventilation, seizure management and furosemide may be warranted for the acute management of TURP syndrome.

T   Hypertonic saline (1.8-3%) may be required acutely to correct hyponatraemia in patients who have a Na^+ <120mmol/L and neurological signs. Resuscitation with consideration of endotracheal intubation and cautious correction of Na^+ to 125mmol/L are the initial treatment aims. Aim for a rise in Na^+ of 1-2mmol/hr and no more than a maximum of 10mmol/L in 24 hours.

T   Central pontine myelinolysis (permanent neurological damage) can occur when severe acute hyponatraemia and chronic hyponatraemia are corrected too rapidly.

1.   O'Donnell AM, Foo ITH. Anaesthesia for transurethral resection of the prostate. *Contin Educ Anaesth Crit Care Pain* 2009; 9(3): 92-6.
2.   Allman KG, Wilson IH, O'Donnell A. *Oxford Handbook of Anaesthesia*, 3rd ed. Oxford, UK: Oxford University Press, 2011.

Answer 4: Regarding myocardial blood supply: All False

F   The right coronary artery (RCA) arises from the anterior aortic sinus or right coronary sinus and provides blood supply to the inferior and posterior areas of the myocardium.

F   The left coronary artery (LCA) arises from the posterior aortic sinus or left coronary sinus. It divides into the left anterior descending and circumflex arteries, and provides blood supply to the antero-apical, lateral and septal areas of the myocardium.

F   The majority of cardiac veins that accompany the coronary arteries ultimately drain into the right atrium via the coronary sinus (tributaries: great cardiac vein, middle cardiac vein, small cardiac vein and the oblique vein). The anterior cardiac veins drain directly into the right atrium.

F   The posterior descending artery (PDA) is a branch of the RCA. The anterior interventricular artery is normally a branch of the LCA.

F   Coronary artery dominance is determined by the PDA. Right dominance (80% incidence) occurs when the PDA branches off the RCA. Left dominant circulation (20%) is when the PDA is a branch of the left circumflex artery.

1.   Moore KL, Dailey AF. *Clinically Orientated Anatomy*, 4th ed. Lippincott Williams & Wilkins, 1999.

2.   http://www.cardiologysite.com/ppchtml/lca_dom.html.

Answer 5: In relation to central venous cannulation (CVC) insertion: True b & e

F   The posterior border of the sternoclavicular joint is where the IJV combines with the subclavian vein to become the brachiocephalic vein.

T   Ultrasound-guided cannulation of the IJV has been demonstrated to reduce time to successful cannulation, increase the rate of first-pass success and reduce complications associated with CVC insertion.

F   The subclavian vein for CVC access is associated with a lower rate of CVC infection than the IJV site. However, subclavian access has a higher rate of procedure-related complications and may not be as easily visualised by ultrasound.

F   The subclavian vein runs above the first rib to join the IJV.

T   Ultrasound may be used to puncture the subclavian vein with a more lateral approach, than that used with the landmark technique.

1.   Waldmann C, Soni N, Rhodes A. *Oxford Desk Reference Critical Care*. Oxford, UK: Oxford University Press, 2008.

Answer 6: Hypoxia: True a, c & d

T   Anatomical shunt due to a ventricular septal defect (VSD) is a cause of hypoxaemic hypoxia.

F   Stagnant hypoxia occurs when there is failure to transport sufficient oxygen due to impaired blood flow, and may result from left ventricular failure, pulmonary embolism and hypovolaemia.

T   Histotoxic hypoxia is when impaired tissue and cellular metabolism of oxygen occurs, despite normal oxygen delivery, resulting in acidosis and lactataemia. Cyanide toxicity is an example of histotoxic hypoxia.

T   Carbon monoxide poisoning impairs circulating haemoglobin functionally, causing anaemic hypoxia.

F   Methaemoglobinaemia is also a cause of anaemic hypoxia.

1.   Cosgrove JF, Fordy K, Hunter I, Nesbitt ID. Thomas the Tank Engine and Friends improve the understanding of oxygen delivery and the pathophysiology of hypoxaemia. *Anaesthesia* 2006; 61: 1069-74.

2.   McLellan SA, Walsh TS. Oxygen delivery and haemoglobin. *Contin Educ Anaesth Crit Care Pain* 2004; 4(4): 123-6.

3.   Waldmann C, Soni N, Rhodes A. *Oxford Desk Reference Critical Care*. Oxford, UK: Oxford University Press, 2008.

Answer 7: A porphyric crisis may present with: All True

T   Porphria may present with an acute crisis. Signs and symptoms include: recurrent, severe, poorly localised abdominal pain (see below).

T   Proximal weakness is more marked than distal weakness with the upper limbs affected more than the lower. Up to 20% of patients will develop respiratory failure and bulbar paresis.

T   Mood disturbance, psychosis and confusion may all be seen during a porphyric crisis.

T   Low sodium and magnesium are biochemical features of a porphyric crisis.

T   Tachycardia, tachyarrhythmias and hypertension may be observed during a crisis.

1.   Findley H, Philips A, Cole D, Nair A. Prophyrias: implications for anaesthesia, critical care, and pain medicine. *Contin Educ Anaesth Crit Care Pain* 2012; 12(3): 128-33.

Answer 8: In heparin-induced thrombocytopenia (HIT): True b & e

F   Heparin binds reversibly to antithrombin III.

T   It results from an immune response triggered by the interaction of heparin and platelet factor 4 (PF4).

F   It is caused by an IgG antibody which recognises the complex of heparin and PF4 on the platelet surface.

F   HIT typically presents 5-10 days after starting heparin; however, if the patient has been recently exposed to heparin (within 3 months), the platelet count may drop earlier.

T   The Warkentin criteria assigns points to the degree of thrombocytopenia, timing of platelet drop, development of thrombosis or other sequelae and the likelihood of other causes for thrombocytopenia. The pretest probability score is then classed as high, intermediate or low.

1.   Parsons PE, Wiener-Kronish JP. *Critical Care Secrets*, 5th ed. Missouri, USA: Elsevier Mosby, 2013.

Answer 9: Considering the management of patients with haematological malignancies: True a, c & e

T   Patients with Hodgkin's lymphoma require irradiated blood products for life as they have an increased risk of transfusion-related graft versus host disease (GVHD) with non-irradiated products.

F   CMV-negative blood products are only required for patients who are CMV-negative prior to transplant.

T   Cisplatin is an alkylating agent used in chemotherapy regimens for several haematological malignancies. It exerts its cytotoxic effects via generation of DNA cross-links and prevention of cell replication.

F   Rapid turnover of tumour cells following administration of cytotoxic agents may result in massive release of intracellular contents. Many metabolic derangements may occur including: hyperkalaemia, hyperuricaemia, hyperphosphataemia, hypermagnesaemia and initially hypocalacaemia due to calcium phosphate precipitation in myocytes.

T Patients who have received bleomycin are at risk of oxygen toxicity and should have an alert card and an alert sticker in their medical notes.

1. Bersten AD, Soni N. *Oh's Intensive Care Manual*, 6th ed. Butterworth Heinemann Elsevier, 2009.
2. Allan N, Siller C, Breen A. Anaesthetic implications of chemotherapy. *Contin Educ Anaesth Crit Care Pain* 2012; 12(2): 52-6.
3. Tiu RV, Mountantonakis SE, Dunbar AJ, Schreiber MJ. Tumour lysis syndrome. *Sem Thromb Hemostasis* 2007; 33(4): 397-407.

Answer 10: Focused assessment with sonography in trauma (FAST): True c & e

F FAST scanning is performed using four views: hepatorenal recess or Morison's pouch (RUQ), splenorenal or perisplenic view (LUQ), pelvic view and pericardial or subcostal/subxiphoid view.

F A phased array or curvilinear 2.5-5.0MHz probe is most commonly used for FAST scanning.

T FAST scanning is performed using four views as explained above. In the extended FAST (eFAST) exam, in addition to the standard four views, the probe is used to assess the left and right costophrenic angles, to assess for blood in the thorax pooling in the costophrenic space and for normal sliding of the lung pleura with respiration to rule out pneumothorax.

F A negative scan does not exclude intra-abdominal injury. One study found that 22% of abdominal injuries were not associated with free fluid.

T Diagnostic peritoneal lavage (DPL) is more sensitive for detecting small volumes of intraperitoneal blood than FAST scanning.

1. Noble VE, Nelson BP. *Manual of Emergency and Critical Care Ultrasound*, 2nd ed. Cambridge, UK: Cambridge University Press, 2011.
2. Wilson S, MacKay A. Ultrasound in critical care. *Contin Educ Anaesth Crit Care Pain* 2012; 12(4): 190-4.

Answer 11: Regarding haemoglobinopathies and coagulation disorders: True a, d & e

T   In idiopathic thrombocytopenic purpura (ITP), platelets are targeted by an IgG autoantibody. The platelets are subsequently destroyed by the monocyte-macrophage system resulting in thrombocytopenia.

F   Steroids are generally used in ITP for short-term therapy, with initial high doses followed by gradual weaning. In emergency situations where bleeding is present with ITP, immunoglobulin therapy may be considered, to rapidly increase platelet levels. For longer-term management, immunosuppressant therapy with rituximab or splenectomy may be required.

F   Thrombotic thrombocytopenic purpura (TTP) is characterised by platelet microthrombi in small vessels, resulting in a microangiopathic haemolytic anaemia and raised bilirubin. Evidence of mechanical red cell fragmentation is often seen on blood film. TTP is either primary (idiopathic) or secondary in origin.

T   Typically, 30-40ml/kg of plasma is removed and replaced during each exchange. Normally the plasma is replaced with albumin or albumin and normal saline. In TTP, the plasma is replaced with solvent-detergent fresh frozen plasma (SDFFP).

T   Secondary TTP, which is seen in approximately 40% of cases, is associated with several conditions including pregnancy, bone marrow transplantation, infection with CMV and HIV, and several drugs including immunosuppressants, hormone treatments and antiplatelet agents.

1.   Bersten AD, Soni N. *Oh's Intensive Care Manual*, 6th ed. Butterworth Heinemann Elsevier, 2009.

2.   UK Blood Transfusion and Tissue Transplantation Services. Transfusion Handbook. *Therapeutic Plasma Exchange*. Available at: http://www.transfusionguidelines.org/?Publication=HTM&Section=9&pageid=1137.

Answer 12: Local anaesthetic toxicity: True a

T   May present with tingling tongue/lips, dizziness, tinnitus, muscle twitching, altered mental state, agitation, loss of consciousness, seizures and cardiovascular collapse (VF arrest).

F   2mg/kg is the estimated safe dose for levobupivacaine. The safe dose is dependent on site of injection. Injection into a highly vascular site will result in toxicity at much lower doses of local anaesthetic.

F   Local anaesthetic toxicity often occurs some time after initial local anaesthetic injection and not immediately.

F   An initial bolus of 1.5ml/kg Intralipid® 20% should be given followed by an infusion of Intralipid® 20% at 15ml/kg/hr.

F   Propofol is not a suitable substitute for Intralipid®.

1.   http://www.aagbi.org/sites/default/files/la_toxicity_2010_0.pdf.

2.   Smith T, Pinnock C, Lin T. *Fundamentals of Anaesthesia*, 3rd ed. Cambridge, UK: Cambridge University Press, 2009.

Answer 13: Regarding cardiac troponins I and T (cTnI and cTnT): All True

T   Serum levels of troponin I and T are both elevated following myocardial damage. Due to their specificity for cardiac muscle damage, troponins are now considered the gold standard biomarker for diagnosis of acute coronary syndrome.

T   Troponins start to rise within 2-4 hours of myocardial damage and peak at 12-24 hours post-injury.

T   Minor elevations usually resolve within 2-3 days but with larger areas of necrosis, troponins may remain elevated for up to 2 weeks post-injury.

T   High sensitivity assays yield a negative predictive value of 95% as a single test on admission and nearly 100% by repeat sample after 3 hours.

T   A raised troponin in non-cardiac critically ill patients is associated with worse outcomes and longer hospital stay. Quenot *et al* demonstrated that in the absence of an acute coronary syndrome or cardiac dysfunction, myocardial injury was identified in 32% of critically ill patients. Those with a raised troponin (cTnI) had a 51% mortality rate compared with only 16% without.

1.   http://www.escardio.org/guidelines-surveys/esc-guidelines/GuidelinesDocuments/Essential%20Messages%20NSTE.pdf.

2.   Quenot JP, Le Teuff G, Quantin C, *et al.* Myocardial injury in critically ill patients. Relation to increased cardiac troponin I and hospital mortality. *Chest* 2005; 128: 2758-64.

3.   Wolfe Barry JA, Barth JH, Howell SJ. Cardiac troponins: their use and relevance in anaesthesia and critical care medicine. *Contin Educ Anaesth Crit Care Pain* 2008; 8(2): 62-6.

Answer 14: Non-ST elevation-acute coronary syndrome (NTE-ACS): True e

F   Initial mortality of NTE-ACS is lower compared to ST-elevation myocardial infarction (STEMI). However, NTE-ACS mortality at 6 months is equal to that of STEMI with long-term mortality being higher than STEMI.

F   Revascularisation (angioplasty/percutaneous coronary intervention [PCI]) timing is customised by risk in NTE-ACS. Within 72 hours, all patients at risk should be considered for revascularisation, but within 2 hours for 'very high-risk' patients with life-threatening symptoms and within 24 hours for 'high-risk' (Grace score >140, troponin release, ST-T changes) patients. Low-risk patients should be non-invasively evaluated.

F   A normal ECG does not exclude the diagnosis of NTE-ACS, and further investigation with serum biomarkers and coronary angiography may be required in some cases of ischaemia (e.g. hidden ischaemia in the circumflex artery and right ventricular involvement).

F   The GRACE score has 8 variables: age, heart rate, systolic BP, creatinine, congestive heart failure Killip class, cardiac arrest at admission, ST segment deviation and elevated cardiac enzymes or markers. The GRACE score gives an acute coronary syndrome (ACS) risk score for risk of in-hospital death and 6-month mortality, and is used to guide urgency of revascularisation in NTE-ACS.

T   Drug management of NTE-ACS includes: anti-ischaemic therapy (nitrates oral or IV); β-blockade in patients with tachycardia, hypertension or LV dysfunction; consideration of calcium channel blockade in those without heart failure; and antiplatelet therapy. Antiplatelet therapy should consist of lifelong aspirin and a P2Y12 inhibitor for 12 months. Anticoagulation and the use of a glycoprotein IIb/IIIa inhibitor in high-risk PCI patients should also be considered.

1.   http://www.escardio.org/guidelines-surveys/esc-guidelines/GuidelinesDocuments/ Essential%20Messages%20NSTE.pdf.

Answer 15: Considering atrial fibrillation (AF) and the risk of stroke: True b, c & e

F   The CHADS2 score has a maximum score of 6. However, the refined CHA2DS2-VASc score has a maximum of 9 and is used to estimate stroke risk per year in patients with non-valvular AF. A score >2 indicates the need for anticoagulation with warfarin due to an estimated 2.2% per year adjusted stroke rate.

T   There is an associated 22% relative risk reduction in stroke events with aspirin use in AF.

T   Anticoagulation with warfarin reduces the incidence of cardio-embolic events in patients with AF, and may reduce the relative risk of stroke by up to 60%.

F   The risk of intracranial haemorrhage in those on warfarin for AF is 0.3% per year.

T   Antithrombotic therapy is not recommended in patients with AF (irrespective of gender) who are aged <65 and have lone AF (e.g. no other associated pathology), as they have very low absolute stroke event rates.

1.   Olsen JB, Lip GYH, Hansen ML, *et al*. Validation of risk stratification schemes for predicting stroke and thromboembolism in patients with atrial fibrillation: nationwide cohort study. *Br Med J* 2011; 342: d124.

2.   Bersten AD, Soni N. *Oh's Intensive Care Manual*, 6th ed. Butterworth Heinemann Elsevier, 2009.

3.   Camm AJ, Lip GYH, De Caterina R, *et al*. Focused update of the ESC guidelines for the management of atrial fibrillation. An update of the 2010 ESC guidelines for the management of atrial fibrillation. *Eur Heart J* 2012; 33: 2719-47.

Answer 16: Long QT syndrome (LQTS): True b & e

F   A normal QTc is 0.30-0.44 seconds; greater than 0.44 seconds is considered prolonged.

T   Patients with LQTS are vulnerable to polymorphic ventricular tachycardia (VT) — also known as torsade de pointes — the development of which may result in sudden death.

F   Jervell-Lange-Nielsen syndrome is a congenital LQTS and is inherited as an autosomal recessive condition.

F   Romano-Ward syndrome is an inherited autosomal dominant cause of LQTS.

T   Many episodes of torsade de pointes are of short duration and self-terminating. However, immediate DC cardioversion should be performed in patients with torsade de pointes and haemodynamic instability. Magnesium sulphate 2g intravenously over 2-3 minutes may be effective in preventing recurrent torsade de pointes, even when serum magnesium concentration is normal.

1.   Hunter JD, Sharma P, Rathi S. Long QT syndrome. *Contin Educ Anaesth Crit Care Pain* 2008; 8(2): 67-70.

Answer 17: Drugs associated with the development of torsade de pointes include: All True

There are many drugs associated with a prolonged QT and subsequent torsade de pointes development including: droperidol, amiodarone, erythromycin, quinidine, clarithromycin, haloperidol, fluconazole, cisapride, methadone and fluoxetine.

1.   Hunter JD, Sharma P, Rathi S. Long QT syndrome. *Contin Educ Anaesth Crit Care Pain* 2008; 8(2): 67-70.

Answer 18: Considering the management of advanced cardiac failure: True b-d

F   Dobutamine stimulates $\beta1$ and $\beta2$ receptors in a 3:1 ratio. There is also some minor effect on $\alpha1$ receptors. It is a positive inotrope and chronotrope. It may decrease sympathetic tone overall, reducing peripheral vascular resistance and may induce mild vasodilatation at low doses.

T   Levosimendan improves Ca^{2+} sensitization of contractile proteins (positive inotrope effect) and opens smooth muscle K^+ channels (peripheral vasodilatation). Levosimendan may also have a phosphodiesterase inhibitor effect, increase stroke volume and cardiac output, reduce pulmonary wedge pressure, and decrease systemic vascular resistance and pulmonary vascular resistance.

T   High levels of serum natriuretic peptides (B-type natriuretic peptide, [BNP] or N-terminal pro-B-type natriuretic peptide [NTproBNP]) are associated with a poor prognosis in patients with suspected heart failure. Patients with a BNP level above 400pg/ml or an NTproBNP level above 2000pg/ml warrant urgent referral for echocardiography and cardiology assessment within 2 weeks.

T   van Diepen *et al* found that the administration of β-blockers prior to cardiogenic shock resolution was independently associated with higher 30-day mortality in patients with myocardial infarction and cardiogenic shock.

F   Natriuretic peptides are released by cardiac myocytes in response to ventricular wall stretch or myocardial ischaemia. Raised pre-operative natriuretic peptides are associated with postoperative cardiac complications. They may become a useful pre-operative screening tool for tailoring individual postoperative management in the future.

1.   Valchanov K, Parameshwar J. Inpatient management of advanced heart failure. *Contin Educ Anaesth Crit Care Pain* 2008; 8(5): 167-71.

2.   National Institute for Health and Clinical Excellence (NICE). Chronic heart failure: management of chronic heart failure in adults in primary and secondary care. NICE Clinical Guideline 108, 2010. London, UK: NICE, 2010. http://www.nice.org.uk/guidance/CG108.

3.   van Diepen S, Reynolds HR, Stebbins A, *et al.* Incidence and outcomes associated with early heart failure pharmacotherapy in patients with ongoing cardiogenic shock. *Crit Care Med* 2014; 42(2): 281-8.

4.   Minto G, Biccard B. Assessment of the high-risk perioperative patient. *Contin Educ Anaesth Crit Care Pain* 2014; 14(1): 12-7.

Answer 19: Management of ascites in chronic liver disease: True a & b

T   Paracentesis may result in persisting ascitic leak at the site of needle puncture and/or infection with skin organisms.

T   A serum-ascites albumin gradient (SAAG) >1.1g/dL suggests ascites is caused by portal hypertension. SAAG is calculated from the serum albumin minus the albumin concentration of ascitic fluid. Under normal circumstances the SAAG is <1.1 due to serum oncotic pressure counter-balancing serum hydrostatic pressure. A very high SAAG >2.5 can occur in heart failure and Budd-Chiari syndrome.

F   Paracentesis drains should be removed after 6-8 hours to reduce the risk of bacterial peritonitis.

F   Paracentesis up to 5L does not require albumin replacement but should be followed with fluid expansion. Paracentesis greater than 5L requires albumin replacement with 8g albumin per litre of ascites removed or 100ml 20% albumin per 3L of ascites removed.

F   A low sodium diet and diuretics are only effective at ascites control in about 10% of patients.

1.   Zetterman RK. Management of ascites. Medscape reference, 2011. http://www.medscape.com/viewarticle/739859_print.

2.   EASL. EASL clinical practice guidelines on the management of ascites, spontaneous bacterial peritonitis, and hepatorenal syndrome in cirrhosis. *J Hepatol* 2010; 53: 397-417.

3.   Waldmann C, Soni N, Rhodes A. *Oxford Desk Reference Critical Care*. Oxford, UK: Oxford University Press, 2008.

4.   Jackson P, Gleeson D. Alcoholic liver disease. *Contin Educ Anaesth Crit Care Pain* 2010; 10(3): 66-71.

5.   Lee J, Kwang-Hyub H, Sang H. Ascites and spontaneous bacterial peritonitis: an Asian perspective. *J Gasteroenterol Hepatol* 2009; 24(9): 1494-503.

Answer 20: Cardiopulmonary bypass: True b & c

F   Bubble oxygenators are thought to increase the risk of microscopic air emboli, blood component damage and consumption of coagulation factors.

T   pH stat management corrects arterial blood gases to patient temperature. This requires the addition of CO_2 to the oxygenator to counteract the increased gas solubility which naturally occurs at lower temperatures, resulting in cerebral vasodilation and increased cerebral blood flow.

T   Postoperative cognitive decline following cardiopulmonary bypass is common and may affect up to 40% of patients. This may be due to cerebral emboli, global hypoperfusion and inflammation. It may also be triggered by a pre-operative decline of cognitive function.

F   1mg of protamine will neutralise 100 units of heparin. The side effects include bradycardia, hypotension, increased pulmonary artery pressure and anaphylactoid reactions.

F   Marketing authorisations for aprotinin-containing medicines were suspended following the BART study, which appeared to show an increased death rate at 30 days in patients who had received aprotinin. However, the European Medicines Agency has subsequently recommended that aprotinin may still be used in patients undergoing cardiopulmonary bypass who are at high risk of major blood loss and recommends lifting the suspension.

1.   Yentis SM, Hirsch NP, Smith GB. *Anaesthesia and Intensive Care A-Z. An Encyclopaedia of Principles and Practice*, 3rd ed. Edinburgh, UK: Elsevier Butterworth Heinemann, 2004.

2.   Muzic DS, Chaney MA. What's new with alpha-stat vs. pH-stat? Society of Cardiovascular Anesthesiologists. Drug and Innovation Review, 2006. Available at: http://ether.stanford.edu/library/cardiac_anesthesia/Cardiac%20Surgery%20and%20CPB/Alpha-stat%20and%20ph-stat.pdf.

3.   Fudickar A, Peters S, Stapelfeldt C, *et al.* Postoperative cognitive deficit after cardiopulmonary bypass with preserved cerebral oxygenation: a prospective observational pilot study. *BMC Anesthesiology* 2011; 11(7). http://www.biomedcentral.com/1471-2253/11/7.

4.   Sasada M, Smith S. *Drugs in Anaesthesia and Intensive Care*, 3rd ed. Oxford, UK: Oxford Universiy Press, 2003.

5.   http://www.ema.europa.eu/ema/index.jsp?curl=pages/news_and_events/news/2012/02/news_detail_001447.jsp&mid=WC0b01ac058004d5c1.

Answer 21: In relation to the management of pre-eclampsia: True d

F   Treatment of mild pre-eclampsia is primarily supportive with frequent foetal monitoring and may include complete or partial bed rest.

F   Magnesium sulphate should be used as seizure prophylaxis or in the management of an acute eclamptic fit. Medications commonly used for blood pressure control in pre-eclampsia include hydralazine, labetalol and nifedipine.

F   Magnesium sulphate should be continued for at least 24 hours postpartum, due to the continued risk of eclampsia.

T   Signs of magnesium toxicity include loss of deep tendon reflexes, respiratory muscle weakness, dysrhythmias and cardiac arrest. Loss of the patellar reflex occurs at a plasma magnesium concentration of approximately 3.5-5mmol/L, respiratory muscle weakness at 5-6.5mmol/L, cardiac conduction defects at >7.5mmol/L and cardiac arrest at >12.5mmol/L.

F   Pregnancy and pre-eclampsia result in a hypercoagulable state. Thromboprophylaxis should be given, with appropriate timing borne in mind with regard to regional anaesthesia techniques. It should not be withheld unless there is associated significant bleeding/coagulation dysfunction and/or low platelets.

1.   Turner JA. Diagnosis and management of pre eclampsia - an update. *Int J Women's Health* 2010; 2: 327-37.

2.   Lu JF, Nightingale CH. Magnesium sulfate in eclampsia and pre-eclampsia: pharmacokinetic principles. *Clin Pharmacokinet* 2000; 38(4): 305-14.

Answer 22: Considering splanchnic ischaemia: True a & e

T   In shocked states, blood flow to the brain and heart is maintained at the expense of the mesenteric circulation, reducing bowel perfusion, exacerbating ischaemia and increasing the risk of infarction.

F   The superior mesenteric artery (SMA) supplies the jejunum, ileum and midgut up to the left colic flexure. The inferior mesenteric artery (IMA) supplies the hind gut, descending and sigmoid colon, dividing into the left colic, sigmoid and rectal arteries.

F	Worsening lactic acidosis is often a late sign of splanchnic ischaemia/infarction and therefore should not be used to exclude the diagnosis if normal. Significant bowel infarction may occur in the presence of a normal lactate, particularly if the blood supply to the damaged bowel is completely compromised.

F	There is no evidence that noradrenaline has a negative effect on gut perfusion. Vasoactive drugs such as noradrenaline may be necessary to ensure adequate gut perfusion. Adrenaline and dopamine have been shown to reduce splanchnic perfusion.

T	Reperfusion of the gut following an ischaemic insult can cause significant deleterious effects and cardiovascular instability, due to the release of toxic mediators and anaerobic metabolites.

1.	Waldmann C, Soni N, Rhodes A. *Oxford Desk Reference Critical Care*. Oxford, UK: Oxford University Press, 2008.

2.	http://sketchymedicine.com/2012/04/blood-supply-of-the-gi-tract.

Answer 23: With regards to the acute surgical abdomen in the intensive care unit: True a & b

T	Acute intra-abdominal surgical problems increase the probability of death as predicted by the APACHE II score in critical care patients.

T	An unexplained or rising lactate level following primary bowel anastomosis may be indicative of anastomotic leak or ischaemia, although a rise in lactate is often a late sign and such pathology may exist in the presence of a normal serum lactate.

F	Abdominal drains have a poor predictive value for anastomotic leak or intra-abdominal bleeding. Clinical findings, blood results and contrast-enhanced CT scanning of the abdomen will provide a more reliable indication.

F	Serial laparotomy and surgical toilet every 2-3 days is not advised following intestinal perforation and peritonitis. A selective approach instead should be taken for re-laparotomy and wash out depending on collection development and clinical progress.

F	Intra-abdominal haematoma formation following intra-abdominal bleeding may be a focus of infection and lead to abscess formation. Large haematomas warrant early surgical evacuation. Radiological drains are often ineffective for haematoma drainage as clots block even the largest of drains; therefore, a laparotomy may be required for large haematoma removal.

1.   Waldmann C, Soni N, Rhodes A. *Oxford Desk Reference Critical Care*. Oxford, UK: Oxford University Press, 2008.

Answer 24: The following may be associated with high levels of serum natriuretic peptide: True a, b, d & e

T   High levels of serum natriuretic peptides (B-type natriuretic peptide [BNP] or N-terminal pro-B-type natriuretic peptides [NTproBNP]) can occur in suspected heart failure. BNP <100pg/ml and NTproBNP <400pg/ml in an untreated patient makes heart failure unlikely.

T   BNP and NTproBNP do not differentiate between heart failure due to left ventricular systolic dysfunction and heart failure with preserved ejection fraction. High levels can be seen in left ventricular hypertrophy, ischaemia, tachycardia, right ventricular overload, hypoxaemia, pulmonary embolism, glomerular filtration rate (GFR) <60ml/min, sepsis, chronic obstructive pulmonary disease (COPD), diabetes, age greater than 70 and liver cirrhosis.

F   Obesity can reduce levels of serum natriuretic peptides. ACE inhibitors, β-blockers, angiotensin-receptor blockers and aldosterone antagonists can also reduce levels.

T   Natriuretic peptides and their metabolites are excreted in part via the renal system and thus serum levels are frequently elevated in patients with a GFR of less than 60ml/min.

T   BNP may be up to 3.5 times elevated in elderly patients without overt heart failure. This is thought to be due to the increased incidence of associated comorbidities that may also elevate serum BNP levels, such as renal impairment, ventricular hypertrophy and diastolic dysfunction.

1.   National Institute for Health and Care Excellence (NICE). Chronic heart failure: management of chronic heart failure in adults in primary and secondary care. NICE Clinical Guideline 108, 2010. London, UK: NICE, 2010. http://www.nice.org.uk/guidance/CG108.

Answer 25: According to the modified King's College criteria, indications for liver transplantation following paracetamol-induced acute liver failure include: True a-c

T   Patients with an arterial lactate >3.5mmol/L after early fluid resuscitation following paracetamol (acetaminophen)-induced acute liver failure should be strongly considered for transplantation.

T   Patients with an arterial pH of <7.3 after adequate fluid resuscitation should be considered for transplantation following paracetamol-induced acute liver failure.

T   If there is Grade III or IV encephalopathy, an INR >6.5 and creatinine >300µmol/L occurring within 24 hours, this is an indication for transplant listing following paracetamol-induced acute liver failure.

F   In patients with non-paracetamol-induced acute liver failure, the presence of any of the three following features warrants transplant listing: age <10 years or >40 years; INR >3.5; serum bilirubin >300µmol/L; interval from jaundice to encephalopathy >7 days; unfavourable aetiology, e.g. seronegative hepatitis, idiosyncratic drug reactions or Wilson's disease.

F   An INR of <6.5 and encephalopathy irrespective of grade is an indication for transplantation listing in patients with non-paracetamol-induced acute liver failure.

1.   Wang DW, Yin YM, Yao YM. Advances in the management of acute liver failure. *World J Gastroenterol* 2013; 19(41): 7069-77.

Answer 26: Complications of acute aneurysmal subarachnoid haemorrhage (SAH) on critical care include: All True

T   The risk of rebleeding following SAH is greatest immediately after the initial event with a rate of 5-10% within the first 72 hours.

T   20-30% of patients develop acute hydrocephalus within the first 3 days. Delayed hydrocephalus can also occur. Acute hydrocephalus requires immediate transfer to a neurosurgical centre for extra-ventricular drain (EVD) insertion.

T   Clinical seizures are an uncommon but well-recognised complication of SAH and affect up to 7% of patients. Seizures may be a sign of rebleeding in unprotected aneurysms.

T   Up to 70% of patients with SAH develop vasospasm on angiography, with 30% exhibiting symptoms (decreased conscious level, new focal neurology). The risk of vasospasm continues for up to 21 days post initial bleed but is highest between days 4 and 10. Severe vasospasm or rebleeding following an initial SAH is responsible for significant delayed neurological morbidity and mortality.

T   Delayed cerebral ischaemia (DCI) occurs in more than 60% of patients with acute SAH. The risk is greatest between days 4 and 10 post initial bleed and can occur in the absence of vasospasm.

1.   Luoma A, Reddy U. Acute management of aneurysmal subarachnoid haemorrhage. *Contin Educ Anaesth Crit Care Pain* 2013; 13(2): 52-8.

Answer 27: Hepatitis A virus (HAV) infection: True a

T   HAV is enterically transmitted, typically by faecal-oral route or via consumption of contaminated foodstuffs.

F   A single episode of HAV infection confers life-long immunity against reinfection.

F   HAV is a single-stranded RNA virus.

F   HAV has a low mortality rate, thought to be less than 0.1%. There is a higher risk of death seen in young children and older adults with chronic liver disease.

F   Vaccination is highly effective at preventing HAV infection with efficacy ranging between 80-100%.

1.   Yong HT, Son R. Hepatitis A virus - a general overview. *Int Food Res J* 2009; 16: 455-67.

2.   Gilroy RK, Wu GY, Talavera F, *et al.* Hepatitis A treatment and management. Medscape reference. http://emedicine.medscape.com/article/177484-treatment.

Answer 28: Categories of shock: True b & d

F   Hypovolaemic shock is characterised by a profound reduction in blood volume, associated with an initial decrease in preload compensated for by an increase in endogenous catecholamines, cardiac output and profound vasoconstriction. Eventually, if compensatory mechanisms are not sufficient, blood pressure and cardiac output will decrease.

T   Cardiogenic shock is characterised by tachycardia, hypotension, low cardiac output state, low mixed venous O_2 saturation, high cardiac filling pressures and increased systemic vascular resistance (SVR).

F   Obstructive shock is due to obstruction of the cardiovascular system, with pulmonary embolus or cardiac tamponade being the most common causes. Typical presentation is with hypotension, cold peripheries/vasoconstriction and dilated jugular veins. Pulsus paradoxus is common.

T   Anaphylactic shock is a form of distributive shock associated with decreased vascular tone, deranged blood flow distribution, hypovolaemia and often a high cardiac output state. Distributive shock is seen with anaphylaxis, sepsis and neurogenic shock.

F   Spinal shock is a loss of sensation and motor function following a spinal cord injury with gradual recovery of lost reflexes. Spinal shock is not associated with circulatory shock and should not be confused with neurogenic shock. Neurogenic shock is a form of distributive shock with hypotension due to loss of sympathetic autonomic pathways following spinal cord injury. This results in reduced SVR and bradycardia.

1.   Waldmann C, Soni N, Rhodes A. *Oxford Desk Reference Critical Care*. Oxford, UK: Oxford University Press, 2008.

2.   Mack EH. Neurogenic shock. *Open Paediatr Med J* 2013; 7 (suppl 1: M4): 16-8.

3.   Vincent JL, De Backer D. Circulatory shock. *New Engl J Med* 2013; 369: 1726-34.

Answer 29: Mixed venous oxygen saturation (SvO_2): True a, b & d

T SvO_2 is typically decreased in the presence of low O_2 delivery states (anaemia, haemorrhage, hypoxia, hypovolaemia, heart failure) due to increased O_2 extraction or in the presence of normal delivery but increased O_2 consumption (agitation, pain, fever, shivering, respiratory failure, increased metabolic demands).

T SvO_2 is increased in patients in states of decreased O_2 extraction (shunting, sepsis, cell death). It is also increased with increased O_2 delivery (O_2 therapy, blood transfusion, IV fluids, inotropes, increased cardiac output) and in states with decreased O_2 consumption (sedation, analgesia, hypothermia, mechanical ventilation.

F   The $ScvO_2$ reflects the O_2 saturation measured in the superior vena cava. Under normal circumstances the $ScvO_2$ is less than the SvO_2. However, in the critically ill, the $ScvO_2$ is often greater. Normal SvO_2 is 65-75%.

T   Rivers *et al* found that targeting an SvO_2 of at least 70% in the first 6 hours of septic shock was associated with a reduction in mortality. These findings are being evaluated in a number of ongoing clinical trials.

F   A normal SvO_2 does not rule out persistent tissue hypoxia.

1.   van Beest P, Wietasch G, Scheeren T, *et al*. Clinical review: use of venous oxygen saturations as a goal - a yet unfinished puzzle. *Crit* Care 2011; 15: 232.

2.   Vincent JL, De Backer D. Circulatory shock. *New Engl J Med* 2013; 369: 1726-34.

3.   Rivers E, Nguyen B, Havstad S, *et al*. Early goal-directed therapy in the treatment of severe sepsis and septic shock. *New Engl J Med* 2001; 345: 1368-77.

Answer 30: Withdrawal phenomena on the intensive care unit: True b & d

F   Opiate withdrawal typically presents with sweating, piloerection, mydriasis, lacrimation, rhinorrhoea, vomiting, diarrhoea, abdominal cramping, tachycardia, hypertension, fever, tachypnoea, yawning, restlessness, irritability, myalgias, hyperalgesia and anxiety. Acute severe alcohol withdrawal can present with degrees of neurologic and autonomic dysfunction of varying severity.

T   Prolonged benzodiazepine use may lead to withdrawal symptoms if they are abruptly stopped or following the use of flumazenil (benzodiazepine antagonist), manifesting with anxiety, agitation, tremors, headaches, muscle cramps, hyperactive delirium and sometimes seizures.

F   It has been reported that in patients in whom the α2-agonist, dexmedetomidine, has been used as an infusion for up to 7 days, withdrawal symptoms may occur within 24-48 hours of cessation. Symptoms include nausea, vomiting and agitation.

T Opioid and sedative withdrawal is overlooked in critical care and often attributed mistakenly to another cause such as alcohol or illicit drug withdrawal.

F Nicotine replacement therapy may be helpful in reducing nicotine withdrawal symptoms. However, nicotine replacement therapy should be avoided in patients with haemodynamic compromise, a history of severe arrhythmias, myocardial infarction, stroke, uncontrolled hypertension, renal and hepatic impairment. It is not completely safe due to these contraindications.

1. Barr J, Puntillo K, Ely EW, et al. Clinical practice guidelines for the management of pain, agitation, and delirium in adult patients in the intensive care unit. Crit Care Med 2013; 41(1): 263-306.

2. Waldmann C, Soni N, Rhodes A. Oxford Desk Reference Critical Care. Oxford, UK: Oxford University Press, 2008.

3. http://www.evidence.nhs.uk/formulary/bnf/current/4-central-nervous-system/410-drugs-used-in-substance-dependence/4102-nicotine-dependence/nicotine-replacement-therapy?q=Nicotine%20replacement%20therapy.

Answer 31: Necrotising fasciitis: True b & d

F Type I infections are polymicrobial with Type II infections caused by group A *Streptococci*.

T Clindamycin inhibits toxin production and has anaerobic activity.

F Blistering and bulla formation are late features of necrotising fasciitis.

T Known predisposing risk factors include immunosuppression, diabetes and malnutrition.

F Immediate surgical removal is essential to remove the source of infection and toxins, and remove infarcted tissue, followed by planned surgery at regular intervals until the necrotic process stops.

1. Davoudian P, Flint NJ. Necrotizing fasciitis. Contin Educ Anaesth Crit Care Pain 2012; 12(5): 245-50.

Answer 32: Considering inhalational poisoning: All True

T   Carbon monoxide (CO) poisoning may initially present with headache, myalgia, dizziness and/or neuropsychological impairment. This may rapidly progress to confusion, loss of consciousness and death.

T   A cherry red appearance of the skin can occur in CO poisoning but is uncommon.

T   The elimination half-life of CO is over 4 hours in room air. This may be reduced to 80 minutes with 100% FiO_2 and under 30 minutes with hyperbaric O_2 at 3Atm.

T   Hyperbaric O_2 therapy at 3Atm should be considered for patients who are pregnant, comatose and in the presence of a HbCO greater than 40%.

T   Cyanide poisoning can also present with a cherry red skin appearance and a bitter almond odour. Unexplained and persistent lactic acidosis with a raised anion gap despite adequate resuscitation should raise the suspicion of cyanide toxicity. Cyanide blocks and inhibits ATP production and cellular utilisation of oxygen, thus leading to raised lactate from anaerobic metabolism.

1.   www.toxbase.org.

2.   Bishop S, Maguire S. Anaesthesia and intensive care for major burns. *Contin Educ Anaesth Crit Care Pain* 2013; 12(3): 118-22.

3.   Hamele M, Poss WB, Sweney J. Disaster preparedness, pediatric considerations in primary blast injury, chemical and biological terrorism. *World J Crit Care Med* 2014; 3(1): 15-23.

Answer 33: In patients with decompensated chronic liver disease: True c

F   Hypoglycaemia is common and usually responds to intravenous dextrose.

F   Oesophageal varices are not a contraindication to the passage of a fine-bore NG tube, although insertion should be avoided in the days immediately following acute variceal bleeding. Upper GI bleeding is a common cause and consequence of decompensation in chronic liver disease.

T   Patients with chronic liver disease and ascites should be sodium restricted. Diuretic therapy with furosemide and spironolactone should be considered. Hyponatraemia is also common despite total body sodium overload.

F   Hyperaldosteronism often results in chronic liver disease secondary to increased splanchnic blood flow, high cardiac output and low systemic vascular resistance.

F   Up to 50% of renal dysfunction in acute on chronic liver failure is due to: pre-renal failure as a consequence of volume depletion, drug nephrotoxicity, sepsis, intrinsic renal disease and outflow obstruction. HRS is rare and a diagnosis of exclusion in the presence of cirrhosis, ascites and no improvement in renal function after 48 hours with volume expansion, cessation of diuretics and treatment of sepsis.

1.   Waldmann C, Soni N, Rhodes A. *Oxford Desk Reference Critical Care*. Oxford, UK: Oxford University Press, 2008.

2.   EASL. EASL clinical practice guidelines on the management of ascites, spontaneous bacterial peritonitis, and hepatorenal syndrome in cirrhosis. *J Hepatol* 2010; 53: 397-417.

Answer 34: Regarding lumbar puncture (LP) in suspected meningoencephalitis: True b-d

F   CT scanning is not mandatory to determine the safety of performing a LP but should be considered first in critical care patients with: moderate or severe impairment of consciousness (GCS <13, or fall in GCS point >2); focal neurological signs (unequal, dilated or poorly responsive pupils); seizures; hypertension and bradycardia or any other signs suggestive of raised intracranial pressure. A normal head CT does not guarantee that lumbar puncture will be safe in suspected meningoencephalitis.

T   Normal opening pressure is 10-20cmH$_2$O. It is high in bacterial and tuberculous infection. A normal-high value is seen in viral infection and a high very-high value is seen with fungal infection.

T   Peripheral red blood cells (RBCs) in the CSF caused by a traumatic tap, artificially increases the white cell count (WBC) and protein level, thereby confounding diagnosis. Corrective formulae may be used to reduce diagnostic uncertainty. Providing the blood WBC is normal (not too high or low) a correction can be made for traumatic tap, by subtracting one CSF WBC for every 500 to 1000 RBCs in the CSF. Also, the true CSF protein level can be estimated by subtracting 0.1g/dL protein for every 100 red blood cells (or subtracting 10mg/L for every 1000 RBCs/mm³). This approximation will suffice in most cases.

T   CSF lactate may be helpful in determining bacterial meningitis from viral CNS infections, as a CSF lactate less than 2mmol/L is said to rule out bacterial disease.

F   In about 5-10% of adults with proven HSV encephalitis, initial CSF findings are normal with no pleocytosis and a negative HSV polymerase chain reaction (PCR). If the first LP is normal in a patient with suspected HSV encephalitis, a second CSF examination 24-48 hours should be undertaken for HSV PCR before the diagnosis can be safely excluded.

1.   Soloman T, Michael BD, Smith PE, *et al.* Management of suspected viral encephalitis in adults - Association of British Neurologists and British Infection Association National Guidelines. *J Infect* 2012; 64: 347-73.

2.   Longmore M, Wilkinson IB, Davidson EH, *et al. Oxford Handbook of Clinical Medicine.* Oxford, UK: Oxford University Press, 2010.

Answer 35: Regarding microscopic examination of cerebrospinal fluid (CSF): All False

F   In tuberculous meningoencephalitis, CSF cell count is usually only slightly increased and is often less than 500/mm³. Very high counts of up to 100,000/mm³ are associated with bacterial infection. Viral and fungal infections usually have a CSF cell count of 5-1000/mm³. A normal CSF cell count is less than 5/mm³.

F   Bacterial infection is associated with a neutrophilic pleocytosis (differential). A lymphocytic differential is seen normally and in viral tuberculous and fungal infections.

F   Clear coloured CSF is a normal finding. CSF is cloudy in bacterial infection, cloudy-yellow in tuberculous infections and clear-cloudy in fungal infections. 'Gin' clear CSF is said to be associated with viral infections.

F   A normal CSF: plasma glucose ratio is 50-66%. It is often normal in viral infections, low (<40%) in bacterial infections, very low (<30%) in tuberculous infections and low-normal in fungal infections.

F   A normal protein count is <0.45g/L. Bacterial infection has a high protein count >1g/L, viral normal-high 0.5-1g/L, tuberculous high very-high 1.0-5.0g/L, fungal normal-high 0.2-5.0g/L.

1.   Soloman T, Michael BD, Smith PE, *et al.* Management of suspected viral encephalitis in adults - Association of British Neurologists and British Infection Association National Guidelines. *J Infect* 2012; 64: 347-73.

Answer 36: Controversies in the management of septic shock (2012-2014): True a

T   Targeting a mean arterial blood pressure of 80-85mmHg compared with 65-70mmHg during resuscitation of patients in septic shock was found not to improve mortality at either 28 or 90 days. New diagnosis of atrial fibrillation was higher in the high-target mean arterial pressure (MAP) group compared to the normal MAP group. In patients with chronic hypertension, the higher-MAP group needed less renal replacement therapy than the lower-MAP group.

F   The ALBIOS study found in patients with severe sepsis that albumin replacement in addition to crystalloids compared to crystalloids alone did not improve the rate of survival at 28 or 90 days.

F   The IVOIRE study found no evidence that high-volume haemofiltration at 70ml/kg/hr when compared to standard-volume haemofiltration at 35ml/kg/hr for a 96-hour period leads to a reduction in 28-day mortality or improvements in haemodynamic profile or organ function.

F   Drotrecogin alfa (activated) or recombinant activated protein C was found in the PROWESS-SHOCK trial (follow-up to the PROWESS trial which did show a mortality benefit), not to significantly reduce mortality at 28 or 90 days compared to placebo in patients with septic shock. Serious bleeding rates were similar in the two groups.

F   Following on from the Rivers study in 2001, where early goal-directed fluid therapy (EGDT) was found to be of benefit in severe sepsis and septic shock, a number of large studies have been undertaken to verify these findings. The PRoCESS study found that protocol-based EGDT in septic shock resulted in significantly more crystalloid being given (>1.0L difference) compared to both the protocol-based standard therapy and usual care group. Dobutamine use and blood transfusion was higher in the EGDT group compared to usual care. No significant difference was seen in 90-day or 1-year mortality or the need for organ support between the groups. Recently, similar to PRoCESS, the ARISE investigators found that in critically ill patients presenting to the emergency department with early septic shock, EGDT did not reduce all-cause mortality at 90 days. Significantly more fluid and vasopressor use was seen in the EGDT group compared to standard care. The results of a third study into EGDT, the ProMISE study, is currently awaited.

1. Asfar P, Meziani F, Hamel JF, et al. High versus low blood-pressure target in patients with septic shock. New Engl J Med 2014; 370(17): 1583-93.

2. Caironi P, Tognoni G, Masson S, et al. Albumin replacement in patients with severe sepsis or septic shock. New Engl J Med 2014; 370: 1412-21.

3. Joannes-Boyau O, Honore PM, Perez P, et al. High-volume versus standard-volume haemofiltration for septic shock patients with acute kidney injury (IVOIRE Study): a multicentre randomised controlled trial. Intensive Care Med 2013; 39: 1535-46.

4. Ranieri VM, Thompson BT, Barie PS, et al. Drotrecogin alfa (activated) in adults with septic shock. New Engl J Med 2012; 366(22): 2055-64.

5. Rivers E, Nguyen B, Havstad S, et al. Early goal-directed therapy in the treatment of severe sepsis and septic shock. New Engl J Med 2001; 345: 1368-77.

6. The ProCESS investigators. A randomised trial of protocol-based care for early septic shock. New Engl J Med 2014; 370: 1683-93.

7. The ARISE Investigators and the ANZICS Clinical Trials Group. Goal-directed resuscitation for patients with early septic shock. New Engl J Med 2014; 371(16): 1496-506.

Answer 37: Considering mechanisms of antibiotic action: True a, d & e

T   Penicillins act by inhibiting the enzyme transpeptidase that forms the lattice cross-links of bacterial cell walls and exert a bacteriocidal effect. The β-lactam ring of the penicillin molecule confers the anti-transpeptidase activity.

F   Co-trimoxazole and trimethoprim inhibit the conversion of dihydrofolate to tetrahydrofolic acid (a co-enzyme involved in the synthesis of purine bases and thymidine which are needed for DNA and RNA synthesis), by inhibiting dihydrofolate reductase.

F   Metronidazole damages bacterial DNA. It is bactericidal and also has activity against protozoa and amoebic organisms.

T   Vancomycin inhibits bacterial cell wall production and cell synthesis.

T   Rifampicin prevents RNA transcription and protein synthesis. It is bactericidal against mycobacteria, Gram-positive and Gram-negative organisms.

1.   Bromley L. Microbiology for anaesthetists - the pharmacology of antibacterial and antiviral drugs (Part 1). Anaesthesia Tutorial of the Week 190, 2010. www.aagbi.org/education/educational-resources/tutorial-week.

Answer 38: Regarding intravenous anaesthetic agents: True b & d

F   Thiopentone may precipitate an acute porphyric crisis and is absolutely contraindicated in patients with porphyria. Cardiac output, stroke volume and systemic vascular resistance are all reduced following use.

T   Ketamine may be given intramuscularly for induction of anaesthesia if the intravenous route is not available. The dose for intramuscular induction is 4-10mg/kg compared to 2mg/kg for intravenous use.

F   Patients allergic to eggs are usually allergic to egg protein or albumin. Lecithin, a phosphatide, is the egg component found in some propofol preparations. It is unlikely that allergic reactions are due to these components. There is also no evidence that propofol is allergenic in patients who are sensitive to soya beans due to all the protein within the soya bean oil being removed.

T   Etomidate even after one single induction dose (0.3mg/kg intravenous) has the potential for adrenocortical suppression, which has been associated with increased critical care mortality.

F   Thiopentone is highly lipid-soluble and extensively metabolised by oxidative processes in the liver. Less than 1% of the dose of thiopentone is excreted unchanged renally.

1. Pai A, Heining M. Ketamine. *Contin Educ Anaesth Crit Care Pain* 2007; 7(2): 59-63.
2. Peck TE, Hill SA, Williams M. *Pharmacology for Anaesthesia and Intensive Care*, 3rd ed. Cambridge, UK: Cambridge University Press, 2008.

Answer 39: Propofol: True a & e

T   The induction dose of propofol is 1-2mg/kg intravenously. Bolus induction may need to be modified depending on patient condition, as propofol causes systemic vascular resistance to fall with reduced sympathetic activity and myocardial contractility, exacerbating hypotension. Caution is also required in the haemodynamically unstable critical care patient or elderly patient.

F   Metabolic acidosis, atrial fibrillation, ventricular or supraventricular tachycardia, bradycardias and asystole are the most common presenting features of PRIS. The metabolic acidosis is thought to occur due to the renal dysfunction, rhabdomyolysis and lactic acidosis that can occur. Hypertriglyceridaemia, hepatomegaly, hyperkalaemia and lipaemia are often other significant features. Management involves the cessation of propofol and use of alternative sedation (alfentanil/midazolam). Once PRIS occurs it is difficult to treat, often requiring increasing cardiovascular and respiratory support with renal replacement therapy. Prolonged infusion in children on the paediatric intensive care unit was found to be associated with a higher mortality.

F   Propofol has a large volume of distribution of 4L/kg. It is 98% protein bound. Following bolus administration its action is short, due to the rapid decrease in plasma levels as it is distributed to well-perfused tissues.

F   Inadvertent intra-arterial injection of propofol does not appear to cause any adverse effects, although onset of anaesthesia is delayed. Intra-arterial injection of thiopentone is an anaesthetic emergency, as it is associated with tissue ischaemia/necrosis due to precipitation of crystals in blood vessels.

T   Increasing levels of creatine kinase (CK) in the absence of other pathological causes raises the possibility of PRIS and associated propofol-induced cardiac/skeletal necrosis and rhabdomyolysis.

1. Peck TE, Hill SA, Williams M. *Pharmacology for Anaesthesia and Intensive Care*, 3rd ed. Cambridge, UK: Cambridge University Press, 2008.

2.   Loh NHW, Nair P. Propofol infusion syndrome. *Contin Educ Anaesth Crit Care Pain* 2012; 13(6): 200-2.

Answer 40: Regarding the principles of pharmacokinetics: All False

F   Bioavailability is defined as the fraction or proportion of an oral drug dose reaching the systemic circulation, <u>compared</u> with the same dose given intravenously. Bioavailability may be estimated from the ratio of the areas under the concentration-time curves for an identical oral and intravenous drug bolus. Bioavailability = AUCoral/AUCiv.

F   Unlike the rest of the gastrointestinal tract, drugs absorbed from the buccal and rectal mucosa are absorbed directly into the systemic circulation and do not undergo first-pass metabolism by the gut or liver.

F   The intrinsic activity of a drug is its ability to interact with a receptor and produce a response, otherwise known as the efficacy. This is represented by the height of the dose-response curve on a graph of response against drug concentration.

F   Competitive antagonists shift the dose response curve to the right. Non-competitive antagonists do not shift the dose response curve to the right; they shift it down by reducing the maximum obtainable response.

F   The therapeutic index of a drug is the ratio of median lethal dose (LD50) divided by the median effective dose (ED50). A low therapeutic index indicates that drug levels should be monitored, for example, warfarin, as toxic levels may easily be achieved.

1.   Peck TE, Hill SA, Williams M. *Pharmacology for Anaesthesia and Intensive Care*, 3rd ed. Cambridge, UK: Cambridge University Press, 2008.

Answer 41: Regarding drugs used on the intensive care unit: True a, b & d

T   Laudanosine is a product of Hoffman degradation of atracurium which is cleared by hepatic pathways. It has insignificant neuromuscular blocking activity.

T   Clonidine exerts beneficial sedative and antihypertensive effects in ICU patients. It decreases the release of noradrenaline from sympathetic nerve terminals via a negative feedback mechanism involving agonism of presynaptic α2-adrenoceptors in the brainstem.

F   Rifampicin, along with barbiturates, phenytoin, carbamazepine, tobacco and chronic alcohol use, induces cytochrome p450 which can lead to increased metabolism of a number of other drugs by the liver.

T   There are three subgroups of Class I antiarrhythmics: Ia — disopyramide, quinidine, procainamide; Ib — lignocaine, mexiletine; and Ic — flecainide, propafenone.

F   Midazolam's imidazole ring closes at pH values greater than 4, resulting in increased lipid solubility and clinical effects following exposure to physiological pH.

1.   Peck TE, Hill SA, Williams M. *Pharmacology for Anaesthesia and Intensive Care*, 3rd ed. Cambridge, UK: Cambridge University Press, 2008.

Answer 42: Suggested physiological goals for the active management of a heart-beating donor include: True b, d & e

F   Recommended donor cardiovascular goals include: heart rate 60-120 beats/min, systolic blood pressure >100mmHg and mean arterial pressure greater or equal to 70mmHg.

T   Heart-beating donors should have arterial blood gas measurements in the range of: pH 7.35-7.45, $PaCO_2$ 4.7-6kPa and PaO_2 greater than or equal to 10.7kPa.

F   Donors should have a serum sodium between 130-150mmol/L. Cranial diabetes insipidus is a common and potentially avoidable cause of hypernatraemia in this patient group.

T   Donors should have a serum glucose of 4-8mmol/L, along with serum electrolytes — potassium, calcium, magnesium and phosphate — within normal serum ranges.

T   If a pulmonary artery catheter is being used, a cardiac index of at least 2.4L/min/m², systemic vascular resistance of 800-1200 dynes.sec/cm^5 and pulmonary capillary wedge pressure of 6-10mmHg should be targeted.

1. Shemie SD, Ross H, Pagliarello J, *et al*. Organ donor management in Canada: recommendations of the forum on medical management to optimise donor organ potential. *Can Med Assoc J* 2006; 174: S13-20.

2. McKeown DW, Bonser RS, Kellum JA. Management of the heartbeating brain-dead organ donor. *Br J Anaesth* 2012; 108(supp1): i96-107.

Answer 43: Organ donation and consent: True c & d

F   The modified Maastricht classification is used to classify donation after cardiac death patients (DCD). There are five categories (I-V). Most DCD donors come from categories III (anticipated cardiac arrest — controlled) and IV (cardiac arrest in a brain-dead donor — controlled). Categories I (dead on arrival), II (unsuccessful resuscitation) and V (unexpected arrest in ICU patient) describe patients in whom retrieval follows unexpected and irreversible cardiac arrest (uncontrolled DCD).

F   The consent rate in the UK is 63% for DBD and 57% for DCD donors in the period 2007-2009.

T   An advance statement, the organ donor register and exploring any previously held views may help determine consent for donation in a patient who lacks capacity.

T   The Mental Health Act and The Human Tissue Act 2004 provide a structure and statutory framework for seeking consent and actions required by law for donation.

F   When approaching those close to patients about donation, apologetic or negative language should be avoided. A discussion should be had which emphasises that donation is a usual part of end-of-life care, open-ended questions should be used, 'how do you think your relative would feel about organ donation?', and the use of positive language to describe donation should be used.

1. Manara AR, Murphy PG, O'Callaghan G. Donation after circulatory death. *Br J Anaesth* 2012; 108(S1): i108-21.

2. National Institute for Health and Clinical Excellence (NICE). Organ donation for transplantation: improving donor identification and consent rates for deceased organ

donation. NICE Clinical guideline 135, 2011. London, UK: NICE, 2011. http://www.nice.org.uk/cg135.

3. Vincent A, Logan L. Consent for organ donation. *Br J Anaesth* 2012; 108(S1): i80-7.

Answer 44: Absolute contraindications to transoesophageal echo (TOE) include: True d & e

F   Atlantoaxial joint disease is a relative contraindication to TOE as the neck may need to be moved to allow passage of the probe into the oesophagus. TOE may, however, still be used with caution in such patients should image acquisition with transthoracic echo (TTE) be impossible or inadequate.

F   Hiatus hernia is a relative contraindication to TOE and, therefore, TOE may still be used with caution should image acquisition with TTE be impossible or inadequate.

F   Chest irradiation may result in oesophageal stricture and narrowing, making TOE more difficult and potentially hazardous. Prior chest irradiation is a relative contraindication to TOE and may still be used with caution should image acquisition with TTE be impossible or inadequate.

T   A known oesophageal stricture is an absolute contraindication to TOE due to the inability to pass the TOE probe and associated risk of oesophageal perforation.

T   Active upper GI bleeding is an absolute contraindication to TOE. Other absolute contraindications include: recent upper GI surgery, oesophageal tumours, oesophageal diverticula, oesophageal scleroderma and perforated viscus.

1. Waldmann C, Soni N, Rhodes A. *Oxford Desk Reference Critical Care*. Oxford, UK: Oxford University Press, 2008.

Answer 45: Congenital disorders associated with difficult airways in children include: All True

T   Pierre-Robin syndrome is associated with mandibular hypoplasia. Other features that may lead to airway difficulties are micrognathia, glossoptosis (backward displacement of tongue) and a U-shaped cleft palate. Patients may be difficult to bag-mask ventilate and intubate.

T   Treacher-Collins syndrome is associated with bilateral malar and mandibular hypoplasia and obstructive sleep apnoea or airway obstruction whilst awake. Intubation of these patients can be difficult and may be worsened with corrective surgery.

T   Apert syndrome is associated with irregular premature fusion of cranial sutures, midface hypoplasia and hypertelorism, syndactyly, choanal stenosis, progressive calcification of hands, feet and cervical spine. Bag-mask ventilation may be difficult. Intubation is usually straightforward.

T   Down's syndrome is associated with macroglossia, atlanto-axial subluxation and cardiac abnormalities. Children with Down's syndrome may be difficult to hand ventilate due to macroglossia and neck instability. They may require manual in-line stabilisation as a precaution for intubation.

T   Osteopetrosis is associated with increasing bone density, limited mouth opening and neck movement. Obstructive sleep apnoea may be an issue. Patients may prove difficult to bag-mask ventilate and intubate.

1.   Prasad Y. The difficult paediatric airway. Anaesthesia Tutorial of the Week 250, 2012. www.aagbi.org/education/educational-resources/tutorial-week.

Answer 46: Intubation of the critically ill child: True a, b & d

T   Haemodynamic compromise which has failed to respond to initial fluid resuscitation with fluid boluses of up to 60ml/kg is an indication for intubation of a critically ill child.

T   Up to 40% of a sick child's cardiac output may be required to support the work of breathing, and therefore haemodynamic instability may occur on sedating and intubating a critically ill child.

F   In this situation the potential benefits of moving the patient to a place of safety and familiarity such as theatres need to be balanced against the risk of deterioration during transfer. If the patient is deemed too unstable to move, the anaesthetic/critical care team should go to the patient to intubate and stabilise prior to transfer.

T   In extremis, intramuscular ketamine (5-10mg/kg) and suxamethonium (3-4mg/kg) may be used for rapid sequence induction. Suxamethonium can be also given via the intraosseous route (1.5-2mg/kg) and sublingually. Ketamine may be given IO also (2mg/kg).

F   The endotracheal tube internal diameter in mm can be estimated using the formula [age/4]+4. Tube length can be estimated by [age/2]+12 for oral intubation and [age/2]+15 for nasal intubation.

1.   Appelboam R, McCormick B. Intubation of sick children. Anaesthesia Tutorial of the Week 169, 2010. www.aagbi.org/education/educational-resources/tutorial-week.

Answer 47: Regarding disseminated fungal infections: True a & b

T   *Candida* species are the leading fungal pathogens encountered in the hospital setting. *C. albicans* accounts for the majority of infections, but *C. tropicalis*, *C. glabrata* and *C. krusei* together account for about 40% of all *Candida* infections. The overall mortality from candidaemia is 40-68%.

T   Total parenteral nutrition, prolonged ICU stay, the presence of multiple comorbidities, broad-spectrum antibiotic use, acute renal failure with dialysis and the presence of indwelling catheters and inserted devices are all risk factors for the development of fungal infection.

F   A definitive diagnosis of disseminated fungal infection includes: single positive blood culture (a positive fungal blood culture should not be mistaken for a contaminant), fungus cultured on biopsy, burn wound invasion, endophthalmitis, or isolation of fungus from peritoneal fluid or CSF. These criteria are positive in only 30-50% of cases with disseminated fungal infection. Three colonised sites should be regarded as a risk factor rather than a definitive marker of infection.

F   Asymptomatic candiduria does not need to be treated and a change of catheter is usually sufficient to treat the problem. However, drug treatment should be considered in high-risk individuals such as those who are immunocompromised and neutropenic patients.

F   If disseminated fungal infection is suspected, antifungal therapy should not be delayed until blood cultures are positive. Early therapy reduces mortality in disseminated fungal infections. Up to 50% of lethal fungal infections may be culture-negative before death.

1.   Parsons PE, Wiener-Kronish JP. *Critical Care Secrets*, 5th ed. Missouri, USA: Elsevier Mosby, 2013.

Answer 48: Antifungal drugs: True b

F   Amphotericin B, a polyene, binds irreversibly to ergosterol causing cell death through damage to the fungal cell wall.

T   Fluconazole inhibits C-14 α-demethylase which is a fungal enzyme required for the synthesis of ergosterol (the major sterol in the fungal cell membrane). This results in fungal cell death.

F   Caspofungin is an echinocandin. It targets the complex of proteins responsible for synthesis of cell wall polysaccharides. It is used in the treatment of candidaemia.

F   Fluconazole is not nephrotoxic but should be used with caution in patients receiving renal replacement therapy (RRT) due to the unpredictable effects of RRT on drug clearance and thus plasma levels.

F   Fluconazole is not active against *Aspergillus* species, *Candida krusei* and other resistant *Candida* species.

1.   Parsons PE, Wiener-Kronish JP. *Critical Care Secrets*, 5th ed. Missouri, USA: Elsevier Mosby, 2013.

Answer 49: Considering connective tissue disorders and critical care: True b

F   A prolonged Russell viper venom time, prolonged activated partial thromboplastin time (APTT), false-positive test for syphilis (VDRL), positive anti-cardiolipin antibody and positive β2-glycoprotein 1 antibody may all be seen with anti-phospholipid syndrome.

T   DAH may present with haemoptysis and anaemia or catastrophic pulmonary haemorrhage. It may be seen at first presentation of several

453

autoimmune conditions, including: ANCA-associated vasculitis (granulomatosis with polyangiitis [GPA] previously known as Wegener's granulomatosis), systemic lupus erythematosus (SLE), Goodpasture's disease, scleroderma and rheumatoid arthritis.

F   Scleroderma renal crisis is a medical emergency and presents classically with an abrupt onset of hypertension (>150/85mmHg) and acute renal failure. It may precede the diagnosis of systemic sclerosis. Management involves early angiotensin-converting inhibitors (ACEi) and antihypertensives (β-blocker/Ca^{2+}-channel blocker). Renal replacement therapy may be required. Renal function may take up to 3 years to improve.

F   Patients with SLE classically present with a malar-discoid rash, serositis, oral ulcers, photosensitivity, arthritis, neurologic and haematological abnormality, and immunological and renal dysfunction.

F   Anti-Jo-1 is associated with polymyositis. Anti-Scl-70 is associated with diffuse scleroderma. Anti-ribonuclear protein (Anti-RNP) is associated with mixed connective tissue disease (MCTD) and SLE.

1.   Parsons PE, Wiener-Kronish JP. *Critical Care Secrets*, 5th ed. Missouri, USA: Elsevier Mosby, 2013.

Answer 50: The intra-aortic balloon pump (IABP) and clinical practice: True a & e

T   Absolute contraindications to intra-aortic balloon pump use include: severe aortic regurgitation, aortic dissection, previous aortic stenting and end-stage heart failure with no treatment options.

F   The balloon should lie 2-3cm distal to the subclavian artery, approximately at the level of the carina.

F   The IABP-Shock II Trial demonstrated no significant reduction in 30-day mortality with IABP support, in patients with cardiogenic shock following acute myocardial infarction awaiting revascularisation therapy.

F   It is safe to defibrillate whilst an IABP is *in situ*; however, staff need to be clear of the console and its associated connections.

T   Patients with an IABP *in situ* should be positioned no greater than 30° head up, as this can cause migration of the balloon inwards, which can result in aortic arch perforation or subclavian artery occlusion.

1.   Alaour B, English W. Intra-aortic balloon pump counterpulsation. Anaesthesia Tutorial of the Week 220, 2011. www.aagbi.org/education/educational-resources/tutorial-week.

2.   Krishna M, Zacharowski K. Principles of intra-aortic balloon pump counterpulsation. *Contin Educ Anaesth Crit Care Pain* 2009; 9(1): 24-8.

3.   Thiele H, Zeymer U, Neumann FJ, *et al*. Intra-arotic balloon support for myocardial infarction with cardiogenic shock. IABP-SHOCK II Trial Investigators. *N Engl J Med* 2012; 367: 1287-96.

Answer 51: In relation to the human immunodeficiency virus (HIV): True c & d

F   HIV-1 and the less common HIV-2 are RNA retroviruses.

F   25-50% of HIV-infected individuals present to critical care with acute respiratory failure.

T   Surface envelope protein Env binds to the primary receptor CD4 molecule on the host cell. Binding exposes another portion of the Env trimer, which then binds to a co-receptor. This then instigates a series of complex steps, which leads to the fusion of the virus to the host cell membrane allowing fusion.

T   Therapies target the life cycle of the HIV virus. Drugs include: fusion inhibitors, protease enzyme inhibitors and reverse transcriptase (RT) inhibitors.

F   A normal CD4 count is 600-1200 cells/μl. CD4 counts below 350-500 cells/μl may increase the risk of opportunistic infections. Counts <500 cells/μl indicate significant impairment of immune function and the need for anti-retroviral therapy.

1.   Hare CB. Clinical overview of HIV disease, 2006. HIV Insite. UCSF. http://hivinsite.ucsf.edu/InSite?page=kb.

2.   Crothers K, Huang L. Critical care of patients with HIV, 2006. HIV Insite. UCSF. http://hivinsite.ucsf.edu/InSite?page=kb.

Answer 52: Mechanisms of blast injury: True d & e

F   Secondary injury is produced by energised debris and weapon fragments. Tertiary injury is caused by displacement of the victim (e.g. being thrown a distance).

F   The blast wave behaves like an acoustic wave, releasing energy at interfaces between materials of differing acoustic quality. Therefore, air-containing organs are more vulnerable to the damaging effccts of a blast wave than solid organs.

F   Contusions over a certain size, 20mm in the case of colonic contusions, are at a greater risk of late perforation and warrant surgical resection.

T   If a victim has been close enough to the blast to sustain primary injury, overwhelming secondary and tertiary injury are usually also present.

T   *Clostridia* and β-haemolytic *Streptococci* cause the majority of infective complications sustained due to blast injuries in the field, thus making benzylpenicillin an appropriate choice.

1.   Bersten AD, Soni N. *Oh's Intensive Care Manual*, 6th ed. Butterworth Heinemann Elsevier, 2009.

Answer 53: In a patient with carbon monoxide poisoning: True b

F   The precise mechanism of carbon monoxide poisoning is not fully understood but it is thought to exert toxic effects via irreversibly binding to haemoglobin, myoglobin and mitochondrial cytochrome oxidase. It is not directly toxic to the lungs.

T   The oxyhaemoglobin dissociation curve will be shifted to the left.

F   The arterial PO_2 (PaO_2) is unaffected by carbon monoxide toxicity.

F   The elimination time of carbon monoxide is approximately 4 hours in air, which can be reduced to 60-90 minutes with an inspired oxygen concentration of 100%, and reduced even further with the use of hyperbaric oxygen.

F   Pregnancy, unconsciousness, arrhythmias and carboxyhaemoglobin levels greater than 40% are an indication for consideration of hyperbaric oxygen therapy.

1. Yentis SM, Hirsch NP, Smith GB. *Anaesthesia and Intensive Care A-Z. An Encyclopaedia of Principles and Practice*, 3rd ed. Edinburgh, UK: Elsevier Butterworth Heinemann, 2004.

Answer 54: The following physiological changes are seen in pregnancy: d & e

F   Plasma albumin decreases by approximately 5g/L during pregnancy due to the dilutional effects of a 50% increase in plasma volume and also alteration in protein metabolism that frequently occurs during pregnancy.

F   There is a greater fall in diastolic pressure, approximately 10mmHg, compared with systolic pressure which usually falls by 5mmHg.

F   Respiratory alkalosis is normal. Respiratory rate and minute volume are both increased leading to reduced arterial carbon dioxide levels and hence respiratory alkalosis.

T   Basal oxygen consumption is increased by up to 20% in pregnancy due to the additional oxygen demands of the foetus, placenta and uterus, and also increased demand from maternal vital organs. As a result desaturation occurs much faster than in the non-pregnant patient.

T   The uterine vascular bed is responsive to both endogenous and exogenous vasoconstrictors, and thus vasoconstrictors may be used to increase uterine blood flow during pregnancy.

1. Bersten AD, Soni N. *Oh's Intensive Care Manual*, 6th ed. Butterworth Heinemann Elsevier, 2009.

Answer 55: The Confidential Enquiry into Maternal Deaths in the UK 2006-2008 (Centre for Maternal and Child Enquiries: CEMACE): True a & d

T   The overall mortality rate decreased during this period; however, there was an increase in the maternal mortality rate from genital tract sepsis.

F   Substandard care was implicated in 70% of direct deaths and 55% of indirect deaths.

F   Sepsis was the leading cause of direct death during the triennia. The death rate from thrombosis and thromboembolism fell. This may be a reflection of the recent publication of national clinical guidelines and standards on prevention of thromboembolic disease.

T   The death rate from cardiac causes was 2.31 per 100,000 maternities.

F   There were seven deaths directly attributable to anaesthesia: two involved a failure to ventilate the lungs; four involved postoperative complications, including opiate toxicity, pulmonary aspiration, possible incompatible blood transfusion and cardiac arrest after a surgical abortion; and one occurred due to acute haemorrhagic leucoencephalitis.

1.   Centre for Maternal and Child Enquiries (CMACE). Saving mothers' lives: reviewing maternal deaths to make motherhood safer: 2006-08. The Eighth Report of the Confidential Enquiries into Maternal Deaths in the United Kingdom. *Br J Obstet Gynaecol* 2011; 118(Suppl. 1): 1-203.

Answer 56: Obstetric haemorrhage: True c & e

F   Although deaths from major obstetric haemorrhage are reducing in the UK, it is still thought to account for up to 50% of maternal deaths worldwide.

F   Women who have had one or more Caesarean sections and placenta praevia are deemed to be at high risk of developing placenta accreta, as per the UK National Patient Safety Agency guidance.

T   The National Patient Safety Agency has issued a care bundle entitled "Placenta praevia after Caesarean section care bundle: the six elements". This bundle also includes recommendations for consultant supervision, on-site availability of blood and blood products, multidisciplinary pre-operative planning and consent for possible life-saving interventions, e.g. interventional radiology, cell salvage and hysterectomy.

F   PPH is defined as the loss of 500ml or more of blood in the first 24 hours following delivery. It can be minor (500-1000ml) or major (more than 1000ml).

T Factor VIIa may be still used as an adjuvant to standard pharmacological and surgical measures in the management of life-threatening PPH, in consultation with a haematologist. Fibrinogen should be above 1g/L and platelet count greater than 20 x 10^9/L, otherwise Factor VIIa is unlikely to be effective.

1. Centre for Maternal and Child Enquiries (CMACE). Saving mothers' lives: reviewing maternal deaths to make motherhood safer: 2006-08. The Eighth Report of the Confidential Enquiries into Maternal Deaths in the United Kingdom. *Br J Obstet Gynaecol* 2011; 118 (Suppl. 1): 1-203.

2. National Patient Safety Agency. Placenta praevia after Caesarean section care bundle: the six elements. Available at: http://www.nrls.npsa.nhs.uk/resources/type/toolkits/?entryid45=66359.

3. Royal College of Obstetricians and Gynaecologists. Prevention and management of postpartum haemorrhage. Available at: http://www.rcog.org.uk/womens-health/clinical-guidance/prevention-and-management-postpartum-haemorrhage-green-top-52.

Answer 57: Electrocardiography findings in electrolyte disorders include: True a, b & d

T Hyperkalaemia makes the resting membrane potential of cardiac myocytes less negative and as a result, impulse conduction through the myocardium is slowed down. This leads to prolongation of the PR interval.

T Hyperkalaemia reduces the repolarisation time of cardiac myocytes, resulting in a shortened QT interval.

F Prominent U-waves may develop in hypokalaemia. J-waves are seen in hypothermia.

T Hypocalcaemia leads to a reduced influx of calcium ions into the myocyte during the plateau phase of the cardiac action potential, which leads to prolongation of the ST segment and QT interval.

F Bradycadia tends to develop with hypermagnesaemia, in addition to hypotension, and an increased PR interval and QRS duration.

1. Waldmann C, Soni N, Rhodes A. *Oxford Desk Reference Critical Care*. Oxford, UK: Oxford University Press, 2008.

Answer 58: Regarding fluids used for resuscitation: True b & e

F   It is thought that the transvascular exchange of fluid is determined by the endothelial glycocalyx layer, which has been identified on the luminal surface of endothelial cells. The subglycocalyx space is thought to produce a colloid oncotic pressure that is an important determinant of transcapillary flow.

T   The structure and function of the endothelial glycocalyx layer is a key determinant of membrane permeability in pathophysiological states and varies between different organs. The integrity or permeability of this layer varies under different inflammatory and pathological states and affects the distribution of resuscitation fluids.

F   The Fluid Expansion As Supportive Therapy (FEAST) study found that the use of boluses of albumin or saline for resuscitation in febrile children with impaired perfusion in sub-Saharan Africa resulted in similar rates of death at 48 hours. However, comparing bolus fluid resuscitation with no bolus therapy was associated with a significantly increased rate of death at 48 hours. The principal cause of death was cardiovascular collapse.

F   The use of HES is associated with increased rates of renal replacement therapy and adverse events in the critically ill.

T   Albumin use is regarded as the reference colloid solution. It is deemed safe in most critically ill patients and may have a role in early sepsis. However, from the Saline versus Albumin Fluid Evaluation (SAFE) study, albumin was associated with increased mortality in traumatic brain injured patients.

1.   Myburgh JA, Mythen MG. Resuscitation fluids. *New Engl J Med* 2013; 369: 1243-51.

Answer 59: Following liver transplantation: True b & c

F   The risk of intracranial hypertension remains for 48 hours following transplantation, or longer if there is graft dysfunction. Hepatic encephalopathy may develop, where it was not previously present, due to severe graft dysfunction or primary graft non-function.

T   Few studies have looked at the relationship between liver transplantation and the need for post-transplantation renal replacement therapy; however, those who develop severe renal failure necessitating RRT have worse outcomes than those who do not.

T   Reducing AST levels by 50% each day following transplantation is a useful indicator of adequate graft function. Other markers necessary for monitoring of graft function include glucose, bilirubin, alkaline phosphatase, gamma glutamyl transpeptidase, lactate and arterial blood gases.

F   It is characterised by poor graft function from the time of reperfusion and usually results in hyperlactataemia, coagulopathy, metabolic acidosis, hypoglycaemia, hyperkalaemia, rapid elevation in aminotransferase concentrations and a systemic inflammatory response in the first few hours postoperatively.

F   Ultrasound is undertaken routinely in the postoperative period and if there is a rise in transaminase measurements. However, if there is a suspicion of hepatic artery thrombosis or if the vessel is not visualised on ultrasound, CT angiography should be performed.

1.   Afonso AC, Hidalgo R, Zurstrassen MPVC, *et al*. Impact of renal failure on liver transplantation survival. *Transplant Proc* 2008; 40(3): 808-10.

2.   Bersten AD, Soni N. *Oh's Intensive Care Manual*, 6th ed. Butterworth Heinemann Elsevier, 2009.

Answer 60: Regarding heart-lung transplantation: True a & b

T   Indications for heart-lung transplantation include primary pulmonary hypertension, end-stage suppurative pulmonary disease and end-stage bilateral lung disease associated with significant cardiac failure.

T   Denervation occurs below the level of the tracheal anastomosis and the cough reflex below this level is lost, resulting in an abnormal cough.

F   Rejection is more likely to manifest in the lungs before the heart, therefore, frequent monitoring of pulmonary function and possibly transbronchial biopsies will be required.

F   Infection secondary to immunosuppressive therapy is the leading cause of mortality in the first 6 months following heart-lung transplantation.

F   In the early postoperative phase, infiltrates are likely to be a result of the implantation response. Deterioration in PaO_2 and appearance of infiltrates after 48-72 hours should raise the suspicion of rejection rather than the implantation response.

1.   Bersten AD, Soni N. *Oh's Intensive Care Manual*, 6th ed. Butterworth Heinemann Elsevier, 2009.

Answer 61: Following severe crush injuries: True c & d

F   Calcium is sequestered in muscle at the time of muscle necrosis, and is released during muscle recovery, thus hypocalcaemia is usually seen following crush injuries.

F   Creatine kinase levels are the most sensitive indicators of muscle damage following crush injuries, although serum creatinine is also often elevated.

T   Adequate intravenous fluid replacement is the mainstay of treatment of rhabdomyolysis. The addition of mannitol and bicarbonate to fluid loading have no impact on the development of acute kidney injury, need for dialysis or mortality in patients with a creatine kinase level >5000U/L.

T   Fasciotomy of a compartment should be performed once pressures exceed 30mmHg, as irreversible muscle and nerve damage may ensue otherwise.

F   It typically gives a 'snowstorm' appearance; however, radiography may be normal and, therefore, fat embolism cannot be excluded on X-ray findings alone.

1.   Waldmann C, Soni N, Rhodes A. *Oxford Desk Reference Critical Care*. Oxford, UK: Oxford University Press, 2008.

2.   Brown CV, Rhee P, Chan L, Evans K, *et al*. Preventing renal failure in patients with rhabdomyolysis: do bicarbonate and mannitol make a difference? *J Trauma* 2014; 56(6): 1191-6.

3.   Yentis SM, Hirsch NP, Smith GB. *Anaesthesia and Intensive Care A-Z. An Encyclopaedia of Principles and Practice*, 3rd ed. Edinburgh, UK: Elsevier Butterworth Heinemann, 2004.

Answer 62: Regarding the Injury Severity Score (ISS): True b & d

F For the ISS the maximum score is 75, with a total score generated from assessment of six different body regions. Each system is scored 1 to 6, with 6 denoting an injury incompatible with life. The three highest scores are then squared and added together to give the overall score.

T The six body regions included are as follows: head, face, chest, abdomen, extremity and external.

F The squares of the three highest Abbreviated Injury Scale (AIS) scores are added together to gain the ISS. As the highest score for any system in a patient still alive is 5, the maximum score is $5^2 + 5^2 + 5^2 = 75$.

T An AIS score of 6 describes an injury that is incompatible with life and thus the maximum score is assigned to that patient regardless (ISS 75).

F The ISS is a non-linear scoring system and the incidence of scores is unevenly distributed as a result of how the score is calculated. For example, it is very common for a patient to score 9 or 16, uncommon to score 14 or 22 and impossible to score 7 or 15.

1. The Trauma Audit and Research Network. Outcome prediction modelling: the Injury Severity Score. Available at: https://www.tarn.ac.uk.

Answer 63: The following may cause a raised urinary sodium and plasma hyponatraemia: True b, c & e

F Post-TURP syndrome tends to cause a low urinary sodium level and osmolality with plasma hyponatraemia.

T Plasma hyponatraemia with a raised urinary sodium level (>40mmol/L) suggests water retention and/or renal sodium loss. This picture may be seen with hypothyroidism due to a failure to excrete excess plasma water.

T Raised urinary sodium and hyponatraemia occurs with SIADH due to excessive release of ADH from the posterior pituitary, resulting in water retention. This creates a dilutional hyponatraemia and concentrated urinary sodium levels.

F   Psychogenic polydipsia tends to cause a low urine osmolality and sodium level, as the excess water consumed is handled in the usual fashion by the kidneys and excreted as free water, resulting in dilute urine.

T   Cerebral salt wasting causes a raised urinary sodium and plasma hyponatraemia due to a renal sodium transport abnormality, resulting in excess renal sodium loss. In contrast to SIADH, patients tend to be total body sodium depleted and dehydrated.

1.   Waldmann C, Soni N, Rhodes A. *Oxford Desk Reference Critical Care*. Oxford, UK: Oxford University Press, 2008.

Answer 64: Regarding pelvic trauma: True c-e

F   Most pelvic fractures result from motor vehicle accidents.

F   The superior and inferior gluteal arteries may be injured during pelvic trauma causing blood loss and hypovolaemia. They arise from the internal iliac artery.

T   The pelvis is usually damaged in trauma by one of the following three mechanisms of injury: anterior-posterior compression and/or lateral compression resulting in fractures and vertical compression causing instability.

T   The superior gluteal artery is the most commonly injured artery in pelvic trauma and may lead to brisk bleeding and haemodynamic compromise. Other arteries susceptible to damage are the lateral sacral, iliolumbar, obturator, vesical and inferior gluteal arteries.

T   An 'open book' fracture can quadruple the volume of the retroperitoneal space due to the volume of bleeding that is associated with such injuries.

1.   Geeraerts T, Chhor V, Cheisson G, *et al*. Clinical review: initial management of blunt pelvic trauma patients with haemodynamic instability. *Crit Care* 2007; 11(1): 204.

Answer 65: Withdrawal of treatment: True a-d

T   Futility of ongoing treatment should lead to the consideration of withdrawal of treatment. Defining futility is a grey area and therefore seeking wider opinions from colleagues, patients and their families, institutional ethics committees and even courts of law may sometimes be required.

T   When considering the withdrawal of treatment, many factors should be taken into consideration including the burden of ongoing treatment, likely futility of ongoing treatment, patient's previously expressed wishes, wider utilisation of healthcare resources and the patient's best interests.

T   Discussions should involve the patient if at all possible, although this is often not possible in the critically ill, due to the burden of illness or treatment on their capacity and conscious level.

T   In some cases where ethical or legal considerations are present, a court of law may be needed to rule on withdrawal of treatment.

F   Hastening death is viewed in some cultures as euthanasia, which is illegal in UK practice. However, it is paramount to ensure that the patient's best interests are served at all times during the process of dying and thus the judicious use of anxiolytics and analgesics to ensure comfort during death is acceptable.

1.   Waldmann C, Soni N, Rhodes A. *Oxford Desk Reference Critical Care.* Oxford, UK: Oxford University Press, 2008.

2.   International Code of Medical Ethics. Declaration of Geneva. World Medical Association, 1994.

Answer 66: The following are acceptable methods of randomisation of patients for a randomised controlled trial (RCT): True d

F   The only acceptable method of randomisation described is the use of sequentially numbered sealed envelopes that contain computer-generated random numbers that are then used to assign the recruited patients to arms of the study.

F   Toss of a coin is not considered an acceptable means of randomisation for an RCT, as it is potentially open to bias.

F   Any randomisation method that relies upon the date of enrolment is potentially open to bias and therefore not acceptable for randomisation of patients in a RCT.

T   Sequentially numbered sealed envelopes containing a computer-generated number that is used to assign to different groups is an acceptable means of randomisation for a RCT.

F   Sequential allocation of patients at recruitment is potentially open to bias and therefore is not considered to be an acceptable means of randomisation for a RCT.

1.   Stewart LA, Parmar MK Bias in the analysis and reporting of randomized controlled trials. *Int J Technol Assess Health Care* 1996; 12(2): 264-75.

Answer 67: The following may introduce inaccuracy in the recording of oxygen saturations via pulse oximetry: True a-c & e

T   Pulse oximetry readings are calibrated from healthy volunteers, with lower readings being extrapolated from data gathered at higher oxygen saturations. Therefore, saturation readings below 70% are less accurate.

T   Hypothermia results in reduced peripheral perfusion and vasoconstriction, both of which can lead to inaccuracies in the recording of oxygen saturations via pulse oximetry.

T   The irregular nature of atrial fibrillation makes maximum and minimum absorption more difficult to measure and, hence, can make pulse oximetry less accurate.

F   The effect of hyperbilirubinaeamia has been debated in the literature but the consensus view is that it does not affect the accuracy of pulse oximetry readings. Hyperbilirubinaemia may affect the accuracy of results taken from co-oximetry however.

T   Methaemoglobinaemia tends to cause falsely low saturation readings via pulse oximetry, usually around 84%. This is because methaemoglobin has similar absorption at both emitted wavelengths to oxyhaemoglobin and deoxyhaemoglobin.

1.   Waldmann C, Soni N, Rhodes A. *Oxford Desk Reference Critical Care*. Oxford, UK: Oxford University Press, 2008.

Answer 68: Acute severe asthma: True c-e

F   Gas trapping and dynamic hyperinflation with generation of intrinsic positive end-expiratory pressure (PEEPi) is responsible for worsening pathophysiological features in life-threatening asthma. High intrinsic PEEP impairs gas exchange, increases the work of breathing and the risk of barotrauma.

F   Large negative pressures generated by inspiratory effort along with PEEPi can impede right atrial filling and cardiac output.

T   Immediate management of status asthmaticus involves oxygen, salbutamol or terbutaline nebulisers, ipratropium bromide nebulisers and corticosteroids. Magnesium 1.2-2g IV over 20 minutes may provide additional benefit and can be repeated. Hypermagnesaemia is associated with respiratory failure due to muscle weakness, so overuse is not recommended.

T   Ventilatory settings in acute asthma are contentious with some matching PEEP at closing pressure (PEEPc) to PEEPi. However, the initial ventilatory settings should adopt a low rate of ventilation (12-14 breaths/min), protective tidal volume ventilation (4-8ml/kg), sufficient FiO_2 to maintain saturations greater than 92%, relatively long expiratory times (up to I:E 1:4) and little to no PEEP ($<5cmH_2O$).

T   The use of extracorporeal CO_2 removal ($ECCO_2R$) devices and extracorporeal membrane oxygenation (ECMO) have been reported in patients in extremis, although further research is required to determine their precise role in the management of severe refractory asthma.

1.   Stanley D, Tunnicliffe W. Management of life-threatening asthma in adults. *Contin Educ Anaesth Crit Care Pain* 2009; 8(3): 95-9.

2.   http://www.sign.ac.uk/pdf/qrg101.pdf.

3.   Baker A, Richardson D, Craig G. Extracorporeal carbon dioxide removal (ECCO2R) in respiratory failure: an overview, and where next? *J Intensive Care Soc* 2012; 13(3): 232-7.

Answer 69: The following have been demonstrated to reduce the incidence of ventilator-associated pneumonia (VAP): True b-d

F   Prophylactic antibiotics have no role in the prevention of VAP.

T   Head-up tilt has been demonstrated to reduce the incidence of VAP in ventilated patients as micro-aspiration of content from the GI tract is reduced in the upright position.

I   Daily sedation holds have been demonstrated to reduce the length of time that patients spend intubated and ventilated on critical care and is associated with a reduction in VAP incidence.

T   Subglottic irrigation devices reduce the build-up of organisms on the endotracheal tube and thus reduce colonisation and biofilm development. This in turn leads to a reduction in VAP development.

F   Whilst low tidal volume ventilation is undoubtedly of benefit in ventilated patients, it has no specific effect on the incidence of VAP.

1.   Hunter JD. Ventilator-associated pneumonia. *Br Med J* 2012; 344: e3325.

Answer 70: Regarding the Berlin definition for acute respiratory distress syndrome (ARDS): True b & c

F   The timing of ARDS must occur within 1 week of a known clinical insult and new or worsening respiratory symptoms.

T   The definition requires bilateral opacities to be evident on chest imaging — either chest X-ray or CT scan — which is not attributable to effusions, lobar collapse or pulmonary nodules.

T   ARDS exists where respiratory failure cannot be fully explained by cardiac failure or fluid overload. Objective assessment with ultrasound may be required to exclude hydrostatic oedema if no risk factors are present.

F   The Berlin definition classifies ARDS into mild, moderate and severe. This is determined by the PaO_2/FiO_2 ratio: mild: a PaO_2/FiO_2 ratio of less than 300mmHg (39.9kPa) with positive end-expiratory pressure (PEEP) or continuous positive airway pressure (CPAP) >5cmH$_2$O (may be delivered non-invasively); moderate: a PaO_2/FiO_2 ratio of less than 200mmHg (26.6kPa) with PEEP >5cmH$_2$O; severe: a PaO_2/FiO_2 ratio of less than 100mmHg with PEEP >5cmH$_2$O.

F   Severe ARDS is defined as a PaO_2/FiO_2 ratio of less than 100mmHg (13.3kPa) with PEEP >5cmH$_2$O.

1.   The ARDS Definition Task Force. Acute respiratory distress syndrome. The Berlin definition. *JAMA* 2012; 307(23): 2526-33.
2.   Ferguson ND, Fan E, Camporota L, *et al.* The Berlin definition of ARDS: an expanded rationale, justification, and supplementary material. *Intensive Care Med* 2012; 38: 1573-82.

Answer 71: Predictors of successful extubation: True c-e

F   Most patients that fail a spontaneous breathing trial (SBT) will fail within the first 30 minutes, so continuation for 2 hours is unnecessary.

F   A rapid shallow breathing index of <105 predicts successful extubation.

T   Increased age has been identified as an independent risk factor for failed extubation.

T   Upper airway abnormalities increase the risk of a failed extubation. Often such abnormalities are not evident on a SBT, resulting in problems with airway patency on extubation.

T   Several patient-related factors have been demonstrated to be associated with a reduced likelihood of successful extubation. These include: increased age, positive fluid balance prior to extubation, pneumonia as a presenting illness, a prolonged period of invasive ventilation, anaemia and low serum albumin.

1.   Esteban A, Alía I, Gordo F, *et al.* Extubation outcome after spontaneous breathing trials with T-tube or pressure support ventilation. The Spanish Lung Failure Collaborative Group. *Am J Respir Crit Care Med* 1997; 156(2): 459-65.
2.   Yang KL, Tobin MJ. A prospective study of indexes predicting the outcome of trials of weaning from mechanical ventilation. *N Engl J Med* 1991; 324(21): 1445-50.
3.   Frutos-Vivar F, Ferguson ND, Esteban A, *et al.* Risk factors for extubation failure in patients following a successful spontaneous breathing trial. *Chest* 2006; 130(6): 1664-71.
4.   Rothaar RC, Epstein SK. Extubation failure: magnitude of the problem, impact on outcomes, and prevention. *Curr Opin Crit Care* 2003; 9(1): 59-66.

Answer 72: Relating to the control of solutes and water in the kidney: True c & d

F   Approximately 99% of the filtered load of sodium is reabsorbed (27,000mmol/day) throughout the collecting system, with 25% absorbed in the loop of Henle and about 65% reabsorbed in the proximal tubule.

F   Substances reabsorbed in the proximal tubule include: sodium (70% reabsorbed from glomerular filtrate), water (70%), chloride (70%), bicarbonate (90%), urea (50%), glucose (100%), albumin (100%), amino acids, phosphates, sulphates. Substances secreted in the proximal tubule include: organic acids (e.g. penicillins, thiazides), organic bases (e.g. histamine, thiamine), EDTA and hydrogen ions.

T   The relative impermeability to water of the thin and thick limbs of the ascending loop of Henle means urine leaving the loop of Henle is hypotonic, with Na^+ and Cl^- passively diffusing (thin limb) and being actively transported (thick limb) out into the interstitium.

T   Reabsorption of glucose filtered at the glomerulus occurs, within the nephron, in the proximal convoluted tubule. This process, which utilises secondary active transport, can be overwhelmed by excess plasma glucose and, hence, exceed the maximum tubular reabsorption rate and glucose will then be identified in the urine.

F   In their 'natural state' the collecting ducts are not permeable to water, with aquaporins extracting water in the presence of anti-diuretic hormone (ADH).

1.   Gwinnutt M, Gwinnutt J. Renal physiology (Part 2). Anaesthesia Tutorial of the Week 274, 2012. www.aagbi.org/education/educational-resources/tutorial-week.

Answer 73: The following are true in the management of diabetic ketoacidosis (DKA): True a & b

T   Cerebral oedema remains the commonest cause of mortality, especially in adolescents and young children. Acute lung injury and comorbid states such as sepsis are associated with increased mortality in DKA patients.

T   The use of bedside ketone meters is now recommended; however, if blood ketone measurement is not available, venous pH and bicarbonate should be used in conjunction with bedside blood glucose monitoring to assess treatment response.

F   Fluid replacement followed by insulin administration, are the paramount therapeutic interventions. However, even in obese patients, insulin infusions of >15 units per hour are unlikely to be indicated. Fixed rate infusions at 0.1 units/kg are currently recommended.

F   Guideline recommendations are to commence a 10% dextrose infusion when blood glucose falls to less than 14mmol/L. This is to avoid hypoglycaemia and to continue insulin infusions to suppress ketogenesis.

F   Although this remains an area of controversy, excessive bicarbonate may cause a rise in the CO_2 partial pressure in the cerebrospinal fluid and may lead to a paradoxical increase in cerebrospinal fluid acidosis. In addition, the use of bicarbonate in diabetic ketoacidosis may delay the fall in blood lactate: pyruvate ratio and ketones when compared with intravenous 0.9% sodium chloride infusion. There is some evidence to suggest that bicarbonate treatment may be implicated in the development of cerebral oedema in children and young adults.

1.   Savage MW, Dhatariya KK, Kilvert A, *et al.* Joint British Diabetes Societies guideline for the management of diabetic ketoacidosis. *Diabetic Med* 2011; 28(5): 508-15.

2.   Joint British Diabetes Societies Inpatient Care Group. *The Management of Diabetic Ketoacidosis in Adults*, 2nd ed. London, UK: Joint British Diabetes Societies Inpatient Care Group for NHS Diabetes, 2013. http://www.diabetes.org.uk/Documents/About%20Us/What%20we%20say/Management-of-DKA-241013.pdf.

Answer 74: In relation to hyperosmolar hyperglycaemic state (HHS) in adults with diabetes, the following statements are correct: True a & d

T   HHS has a higher mortality than DKA and is associated with vascular complications such as peripheral arterial thrombosis, stroke and myocardial infarction. Levels of dehydration and metabolic disturbance are more severe in HHS with onset over days versus hours in DKA.

F   Characteristic features of HHS include: hypovolaemia, marked hyperglycaemia (>30mmol/L) without significant hyperketonaemia (<3mmol/L) and a raised serum osmolality which is usually >320mOsm/kg. There is also absence of significant acidosis (pH >7.3).

F   Fluid losses are likely to be higher than this with estimated fluid losses being 100-220ml/kg.

T   The rate of fall of plasma sodium should not exceed 10mmol/L in 24 hours; intravenous 0.9% sodium chloride should be used as the principal fluid to restore circulating volume and reverse dehydration. Seek specialist advice.

F   The fall in blood glucose should be no more than 5mmol/L/hr and low-dose IV insulin (0.05 units/kg/hr) should ONLY be commenced if the blood glucose is no longer falling with IV fluids alone OR immediately if there is significant ketonaemia.

1.   Scott A, Claydon A, Kelly T, et al. The management of the hyperosmolar hyperglycaemic state (HHS) in adults with diabetes. Joint British Diabetes Societies Inpatient Care Group, August 2012. http://www.diabetologists-abcd.org.uk/JBDS/JBDS_IP_HHS_Adults.pdf.

Answer 75: The following conditions are currently (2013-14) recommended indications for the institution of therapeutic hypothermia (TH): True a & d

T   This statement is currently true as per recommendations from the American Heart Association (AHA) and the International Liaison Committee on Resuscitation (ILCOR). However, the 2013 Targeted Temperature Management (TTM) trial found that survival and neurological outcomes were not statistically different between patients cooled to 33°C versus those cooled to 36°C. Current ILCOR recommendations are to continue current TTM treatment recommendations pending formal consensus, whilst recognising that some clinicians may use a target temperature of 36°C pending further guidance.

F   Avoidance of hyperthermia would appear prudent in acute ischaemic stroke (AIS), but current recommendations would not recommend TH outside of clinical trials.

F   Induced hypothermia during aneurysm surgery may be a reasonable option in some cases but is not routinely recommended (Class III, Level of Evidence B). Surface cooling to prevent hyperthermia following subarachnoid haemorrhage is often utilised during critical care management.

T   Studies have demonstrated a reduction in poor outcome following TH in perinatal asphyxia with a relative risk reduction of up to 15% and a number needed to treat (NNT) of 9. The National Institute for Health and Care Excellence recommends cooling for neonates with a gestational age of more than 36 weeks who are at risk of hypoxic brain injury at delivery. Treatment should be commenced within 6 hours of the hypoxic insult.

F   Whilst TH has been shown to improve survival in animal studies of sepsis, there is currently no clear human evidence. Also, hypothermia has been identified as an independent risk factor for increased mortality in patients with sepsis.

1.   Raithatha A, Pratt G, Rash A. Developments in the management of acute ischaemic stroke: implications for anaesthetic and critical care management. *Contin Educ Anaesth Crit Care Pain* 2013; 13(3): 80-6.

2.   Raithatha AH, Faulds M, Porter R, Bryden D. Therapeutic hypothermia treatments for the critically ill and injured. *Br J Intensive Care* 2011; Winter: 122-8.

3.   Nielsen N, Wetterslev J. Cronberg, *et al*; TTM investigators. Targeted temperature management at 33°C versus 36°C after cardiac arrest. *N Engl J Med* 2013; 369: 2197-206.

Answer 76: In relation to hyponatraemia, the following statements are true: True b-e

F   Acute 'profound' hyponatraemia can be defined as the biochemical finding of a serum sodium concentration of <125mmol/L, which is documented to exist for <48 hours. 'Profound' has replaced 'severe' in the latest European Society of Intensive Care Medicine (ESICM) guidelines to avoid confusion with severe as a description of symptomology.

T   The serum sodium concentration will rise when correcting for hyperglycaemia. This equates to adding 2.4mmol/L to the measured serum sodium concentration for every 5.5mmol/L incremental rise in serum glucose concentration above a standard value of 5.5mmol/L serum glucose concentration.

T   Beer potomania, primary polydipsia and low solute intake can all be considered in this context.

T   Both the syndrome of inappropriate anti-diuretic hormone secretion (SIADH) and cerebral salt wasting would be consistent.

T   The latest guidelines (Spasovski *et al*, 2014) recommend the use of 150ml of 3% hypertonic saline, or equivalent, over 20 minutes during the first hour of management of hyponatraemia with severe symptoms, regardless of whether hyponatraemia is acute or chronic.

1.   Spasovski G, Vanholder R, Allolio B, *et al* Clinical practice guideline on diagnosis and treatment of hyponatraemia. *Intensive Care Med* 2014; 30: 320-31.

Answer 77: Concerning patient safety initiatives: All False

F   A 2006 prevalence study in England showed that 42.3% of bloodstream infections are likely to be associated with a central line.

F   The head of the bed should be elevated to between 30-45° to reduce passive aspiration of gut organisms into the larynx and trachea.

F   Sedation holds should be done on a daily basis to reduce the amount of sedative drugs given to patients. An assessment of readiness of extubation should be made during the sedation hold.

F   2% chlorhexidine (alcoholic 70%) should be used for skin asepsis prior to central line insertion. The weaker 0.5% solution is used to sterilise skin prior to central neuraxial blockade.

F   TPN should be administered through a separate line or a dedicated lumen on the central line.

1.   http://www.patientsafetyfirst.nhs.uk.
2.   Horner DL, Bellamy MC. Care bundles in intensive care. *Contin Educ Anaesth Crit Care Pain* 2012; 12(4): 199-202.

Answer 78: Transpulmonary pressure (TPP) and ventilator-associated lung injury: True a-d

T   At end-inspiration, the TPP is the principal force maintaining inflation of lung units and thus is an important factor in the genesis of ventilator-induced lung injury (VILI).

T   TPP is calculated from alveolar pressure minus the pleural pressure, and thus alveolar and pleural pressure differences may both play an important role in the pathophysiology of VILI.

T   In a study by Talmor *et al*, where PEEP was set to achieve an end-expiratory pressure of 0-10cmH$_2$O and end-inspiratory TPP was limited to 25cmH$_2$O using oesophageal TPP monitoring, a trend towards reduced 28-day mortality in ARDS was noted.

T   In patients receiving NIV who generate high negative pleural pressures, TPP may be extremely high despite low delivered pressures, thus increasing the risk of barotrauma.

F   Barotrauma occurs due to regional lung over-distension leading to lung damage, air leaks and pneumothoraces. It is not directly caused by high airway pressures. Volutrauma occurs due to high absolute lung ventilatory volumes leading to alveolar rupture and air leaks.

1.   Talmor D, Sarge T, Malhotra A, *et al*. Mechanical ventilation guided by esophageal pressure in acute lung injury. *New Engl J Med* 2008; 359: 2095-104.

2.   Slutsky AS, Ranieri VM. Ventilator-induced lung injury. *New Engl J Med* 2013; 369: 2126-36.

Answer 79: The following statements are true in relation to renal replacement therapy (RRT) and vascular access: True b & e

F   In patients with a high likelihood of needing long-term RRT, subclavian catheters should be avoided due to the risk of thrombosis and stenosis in patients who may later need formation of an arteriovenous fistula for long-term dialysis.

T   Adequately sized catheters are likely to allow good flow rates, which may help prolong filter life.

F   Although earlier studies showed higher rates of CRBSI with femoral routes of access, more recent studies and meta-analysis have shown no difference in rates of CRBSI between different sites.

F   Intermittent haemodialysis may be provided via arteriovenous fistulae to haemodynamically stable patients on critical care.

T   High-access pressure is one of the alarms that may be triggered by a problem with the access catheter.

1.   Waldmann C, Soni N, Rhodes A. *Oxford Desk Reference Critical Care*. Oxford, UK: Oxford University Press, 2008.

2.   Marik PE, Flemmer M, Harrison W. The risk of catheter-related bloodstream infection with femoral venous catheters as compared to subclavian and internal jugular venous catheters: a systematic review of the literature and meta-analysis. *Crit Care Med* 2012; 40(8): 2479-85.

3.   Arulkumaran N, Montero RM, Singer M. Management of the dialysis patient in general intensive care. *Br J Anaesth* 2012; 108(2): 183-92.

Answer 80:   When prescribing continuous renal replacement therapy (CRRT), the following statements are correct: True c

F   There is increasing evidence that HVHF versus standard volume haemofiltration (SVHF) does not confer a survival advantage in patients with acute kidney injury (AKI), including those with septic shock. Recent studies including the RENAL, ATN and IVOIRE trials have not supported the use of HVHF.

F   HVHF does not confer any mortality benefit in non-septic shock patients, and has the additional problems of reduced filter life, a greater risk of cardiovascular instability and an increased need for electrolyte replacement.

T   The filtration ratio is a measure of haemoconcentration in the filter (filtrate removed as a percentage of blood flow). It is how much blood is going into the filter compared with how much ultra-filtrate is taken out. Too high a value is thus associated with clotting in the filter. Different manufacturers have carrying guidance but generally aiming to keep the filtration ratio below 25-30% will prevent clotting in the filter.

F   Replacement fluid can be added pre- or post-filter and in combination. Increasing the pre-dilution will 'thin' the blood by reducing the haematocrit and thus reduce the likelihood of filter clotting. However, increasing pre-dilution will reduce effective solute clearance.

F   Bicarbonate-based replacement solutions are increasingly preferred to lactate-based solutions as they have a more reliable buffering capacity, but as they are more unstable they must be prepared immediately prior to use.

1.   Joannes-Boyau O, Honore PM, Perez P, et al. High-volume versus standard-volume haemofiltration for septic shock patients with acute kidney injury (IVOIRE Study): a multicentre randomised controlled trial. *Intensive Care Med* 2013; 39: 1535-46.

2.   Bellomo R, Cass A, Cole L, et al; RENAL Replacement Therapy Study Investigators. Intensity of continuous renal-replacement therapy in critically ill patients. *N Engl J Med* 2009; 361: 1627-38.

3.   The VA/NIH Acute Renal Failure Trial Network. Intensity of renal support in critically ill patients with acute kidney injury. *N Engl J Med* 2008; 359: 7-20.

4.   Prowle JR, Schneider A, Bellomo R. Clinical review: optimal dose of continuous renal replacement therapy in acute kidney injury. *Crit Care* 2011; 15(2): 207.

Answer 81: Regarding anticoagulation and continuous renal replacement therapy (CRRT): All True

T   This remains the most common practice worldwide with recent survey data suggesting citrate anticoagulation is limited to 0-20% of treatments.

T   This is a grade 1A recommendation of the Kidney Disease Improving Global Outcomes (KDIGO): acute kidney injury (AKI) guideline, with a grade 2C recommendation to use argatroban rather than other agents in HIT patients without severe liver failure undergoing RRT.

T   The depletion of ionized calcium interrupts clotting cascade activation at several stages. Since citrate is a small molecule (molecular weight 258 Da), the calcium-citrate complex is easily removed by diffusion and/or convection and minimal effects on systemic anticoagulation are seen.

T   Citrate anticoagulation requires an exogenous infusion of calcium to replace that lost in the effluent.

T   Citrate accumulation, reduced citrate clearance and lower values of ionised calcium have been demonstrated in patients with acute liver failure or severe liver cirrhosis and thus citrate anticoagulation is contraindicated in severe liver failure.

1.   Kidney Disease Improving Global Outcomes (KDIGO): KDIGO clinical practice guideline for acute kidney injury. *Kidney Int* Suppl 2012; 2: 2.

2.   Oudemans-van Straaten HM, Kellum JA, Bellomo R. Clinical review: anticoagulation for continuous renal replacement therapy - heparin or citrate? *Crit Care* 2011; 15(1): 202.

3.   Morabito S, Pistolesi V, Tritapepe L, *et al*. Regional citrate anticoagulation in cardiac surgery patients at high risk of bleeding: a continuous veno-venous hemofiltration protocol with a low concentration citrate solution. *Crit Care* 2012; 16(3): R111.

Answer 82: Hypernatraemia: True a & b

T   Hypernatremia is most often due to unreplaced water that is lost from the gastrointestinal tract (vomiting or osmotic diarrhoea), skin (sweat), or the urine (diabetes insipidus or an osmotic diuresis due to glycosuria in uncontrolled diabetes mellitus or increased urea excretion resulting from catabolism or recovery from renal failure).

T   In chronic hypernatraemia, aim for a reduction in serum sodium concentration of less than 0.5-0.7mmol/L per hour.

F   Hypovolaemic patients with hypernatraemia should initially be managed with isotonic solutions.

F   Central diabetes insipidus (neurogenic) is caused by a condition of the hypothalamus or pituitary gland in which there is a deficiency in the amount of ADH produced.

F   In patients with central diabetes insipidus, a synthetic analogue of ADH, desmopressin, is the treatment of choice. It is available in oral, intranasal, subcutaneous and intravenous preparations.

1.   Bersten AD, Soni N. *Oh's Intensive Care Manual*, 6th ed. Butterworth Heinemann Elsevier, 2009.

Answer 83: Regarding temporary cardiac pacing: True b & c

F   Sometimes poorly tolerated but sedation/analgesia may help.

T   VVD is a mode which acts on the ventricle only: ventricular pace, ventricular sense and dual ventricular trigger or inhibition.

T   Capture describes the ability of the electrical impulse to initiate myocardial depolarisation.

F   Output should be set at 2-3x the threshold level (<1.0V ventricular wires, <1.5V atrial wires).

F   Sensitivity represents the ability of the pacemaker to detect myocardial activity. The sensitivity dial indicates the minimum voltage that the pacemaker is able to sense. Decreasing the sensitivity dial thus increases pacemaker sensitivity. The dial is set at 2mV if there is no underlying rhythm.

1.   Resuscitation Council (UK). Advanced life support, 6th ed. London: Resuscitation Council (UK), 2011. www.resus.org.uk.

2.   Waldmann C, Soni N, Rhodes A. *Oxford Desk Reference Critical Care.* Oxford, UK: Oxford University Press, 2008.

Answer 84: Anaesthesia and MRI: True c & e

F   Magnetic resonance imaging (MRI) involves interaction of a magnetic field generated by a scanner and magnetic fields generated by nuclei.

F   In a T1-weighted image, fat appears bright (high signal) and water appears dark. In T2-weighted images, fat appears dark and water bright.

T   Standard pulse oximeters have caused patient burns due to induction currents. Fibre-optic probe connections are preferable.

F   Standard infusions pumps become projectiles (due to being highly ferromagnetic) or malfunction when in the MRI environment.

T   Switching of the gradient fields creates loud acoustic noise above 85dB. This can potentially cause hearing loss.

1.   Reddy U, White MJ, Wilson SR. Anaesthesia for magnetic resonance imaging. *Contin Educ Anaesth Crit Care Pain* 2012; 12(3): 140-4.

Answer 85: Concerning intracranial pressure (ICP) monitoring: True a, b & d

T   Although this is a strong statement, it is the current recommendation from the Brain Trauma Foundation (BTF), to use ICP monitoring in all salvageable patients with severe traumatic brain injury and an abnormal CT scan.

T   ICP monitoring should be instituted in salvageable patients with a severe traumatic brain injury and a normal CT scan, if more than two of the following are present: age >40 years, unilateral or bilateral motor posturing or systolic blood pressure <90mmHg.

F   There is level II and III evidence available as described in the BTF guidelines, in relation to the decision making as to whether or not an ICP bolt is inserted in traumatic brain injury.

T   The BTF guidelines recommend the ventricular catheter as the most accurate and reliable method of measuring ICP, as compared to intraparenchymal devices.

F   The BTF guidelines recommend a threshold of 20mmHg, although it is acknowledged that this value is not supported by strong evidence.

1.   Brain Trauma Foundation. Guidelines for the management of severe traumatic brain injury: a joint project of the Brain Trauma Foundation, American Association of Neurological Surgeons (AANS), Congress of Neurological Surgeons (CNS) and AANS/CNS Joint Section on Neurotrauma and Critical Care, 2007. https://www.braintrauma.org.

Answer 86: Regarding acid-base balance: True b-e

F   The use of 0.9% sodium chloride for resuscitation may produce a smaller plasma strong ion difference, leading to an increased $[H]^+$ concentration.

T   In renal tubular acidosis, urinary strong ion difference is high whilst plasma strong ion difference is low. This occurs due to abnormal renal tubular chloride handling.

T   In Type 2 renal tubular acidosis, there is increased proximal tubular chloride resorption. Types 1 and 4 renal tubular acidosis occur due to reduced ammonium production distally and proximally, respectively.

T   Acetazolamide increases the renal excretion ratio of sodium to chloride, increasing serum chloride and reducing serum strong ion difference. This mechanism underlies the correction of metabolic alkalosis.

T   Neurologically, metabolic alkalosis may cause seizures, confusion and drowsiness, as well as cerebral vasospasm.

1.   Burdett E, Roche AM, Mythen MG. Hyperchloraemic acidosis: pathophysiology and clinical impact. *Transfus Altern Transfus Med* 2003; 5(4): 424-30.

2.   Bersten AD, Soni N. *Oh's Intensive Care Manual*, 6th ed. Butterworth Heinemann Elsevier, 2009.

3.   Moviat M, Pickkers P, van der Voort PHJ, van der Hoeven JG. Acetazolamide-mediated decrease in strong ion difference accounts for the correction of metabolic alkalosis in critically il patients. *Crit Care* 2006; 10: R14.

Answer 87: In relation to thyroid function tests, which of the following statements are true?: True b-e

F   In overt hyperthyroidism, free T4 and free T3 levels are usually high, the exception being isolated T3 or isolated T4 toxicosis. For example, in isolated T4 toxicosis, levels of free T4 will be raised, whereas levels of free T3 will be normal.

T   Increased TSH in the presence of normal or low free T4 suggests primary hypothyroidism, i.e. intrinsic thyroid abnormality. In contrast, a decreased TSH in the presence of low free T4 suggests secondary (pituitary origin) hypothyroidism.

T   The euthyroid sick syndrome refers to alterations in serum thyroxine and TSH levels in patients with various non-thyroidal illnesses. It results from alterations in transport and metabolism of peripheral thyroid hormone induced by non-thyroidal illnesses such as infection, malignancy, trauma and starvation. Total T4 levels decrease in moderate to severe illness associated with the euthyroid sick syndrome.

T   See Table 5.1 comparing sick euthyroid syndrome with primary hypothyroidism.

Table 5.1. Thyroid hormone changes in euthyroid sick syndrome and primary hypothyroidism.

Hormone changes	Euthyroid sick syndrome	Primary hypothyroidism
Serum total T3 & T4	Serum T3 decreased proportionately more than T4	Serum T4 decreased proportionately more than T3
TSH	Normal/mild decrease	Increased
Reverse T3	Increased, especially in severe illness	Low
Free T4	Free T4 usually normal	Free T4 reduced

T   Euthyroid hyperthyroxinaemia is characterised by increased T4 with variable T3 and TSH, with increased peripheral conversion of T4 to T3. Euthyroid hyperthyroxinaemia may be caused by drugs (e.g. amiodarone), hyperemesis, acute psychiatric illness and hyponatraemia.

1.   Parsons PE, Wiener-Kronish JP. *Critical Care Secrets*, 5th ed. Missouri, USA: Elsevier Mosby, 2013.

2.   Ligtenberg JJ, Girbes AR, Beentjes JA, *et al.* Hormones in the critically ill patient: to intervene or not to intervene? *Intensive Care Med* 2001; 27(10): 1567-77.

Answer 88: Non-invasive ventilation (NIV): True a-d

T   NIV decreases the work of breathing and may aid weaning from mechanical ventilation.

T   Can reduce the need for intubation and hospital morbidity.

T   Failure of NIV is associated with a higher mortality in respiratory failure.

T   The greatest benefit of NIV use is seen in patients with respiratory failure caused by acute COPD exacerbation or cardiogenic pulmonary oedema.

F   Severe respiratory acidosis (<pH 7.25) is not a contraindication for a short trial of NIV (1-2 hours) in a monitored environment, where prompt intubation and ventilation may be undertaken as rescue, if

NIV fails. Coexistent severe metabolic with respiratory acidosis may suggest a mixed aetiology and other organ dysfunction, resulting in a greater incidence of NIV failure.

1.   Waldmann C, Soni N, Rhodes A. *Oxford Desk Reference Critical Care*. Oxford, UK: Oxford University Press, 2008.

2.   McNeil GBS, Glossop AJ. Clinical applications of non-invasive ventilation in critical care. *Contin Educ Anaesth Crit Care Pain* 2012; 12(1): 33-7.

Answer 89: Rotational thromboelastometry (ROTEM®): True d

F   With ROTEM®, whole blood with activators is incubated in a disposable cuvette (four parallel channels). A pin rotates in either direction while the cuvette remains stationary. Restriction of pin rotation is detected as the clot strength increases, by an optical system and is translated into the ROTEM® tracing. With thromboelastography (TEG), whole blood is added to two disposable heated cups. A pin attached to a torsion wire is immersed in the blood, whilst the cup rotates in either direction. A mechanical-electrical transducer converts pin torsion into a TEG trace.

F   ROTEM® uses tissue factor in the EXTEM cuvette to assess the extrinsic clotting pathway and contact activator in the INTEM cuvette to assess the intrinsic clotting pathway.

F   INTEM assesses the intrinsic clotting pathway.

T   The FIBTEM cuvette is an additional assay that contains the platelet inhibitor cytochalasin D and calcium. The maximum clot firmness (MCF) generated when compared to EXTEM baseline represents the fibrinogen contribution to clot strength.

F   The normal range for clotting time (CT) is: INTEM 137-246s and EXTEM 42-74s. This is the time until initiation of fibrin (period to 2mm amplitude on tracing), similar to the R-time on TEG. The clot formation time (CFT) normal range is: INTEM 40-100s and EXTEM 46-148s, and is similar to the K-time on TEG. It is a measurement of clot kinetics.

1.   Srivastava A, Kelleher A. Point-of-care coagulation testing. *Contin Educ Anaesth Crit Care Pain* 2013; 13(1): 12-6.

Answer 90: Biological weapon poisoning: True a, c & e

T   Ricin is derived from castor oil beans. It is most toxic via inhalation or injection, as it is partially degraded enterally by digestive enzymes. It cannot pass through unbroken skin. 5-10µg/kg is deemed a fatal dose. Management includes decontamination, the use of personal protective equipment (PPE) and general critical care support for multi-organ failure.

F   Anthrax is an infection caused by the Gram-positive bacteria, *Bacillus anthracis*. Spores are 1-5µm in size and can reach the alveolar space. Incubation can take days to weeks, and symptoms are non-specific, including fever, myalgia, headache, cough and sweating. Human to human transmission does not occur, so standard isolation practice is appropriate. Inhalational anthrax has a high fatality rate. Two to four days after initial symptom presentation, severe respiratory failure can occur with evidence of a widened mediastinum, suggestive of mediastinal lymphadenopathy or haemorrhage. Ciprofloxacin and doxycycline are often used in management.

T   VX causes acetylcholine accumulation to occur at muscarinic and nicotinic receptors due to inhibition of acetylcholinesterase (AChE), causing autonomic instability, central excitation/depression, coma and apnoea. Exposure effects include miosis (pupil constriction), salivation, bronchospasm, chest tightness and rhinorrhoea. Systemic absorption rapidly produces systemic features: nausea and vomiting, abdominal pain, fasciculation, weakness, tremor, convulsions, bradycardia or tachycardia, involuntary defecation and urination and cardiovascular collapse. Management includes the use of PPE, and IV atropine boluses (5mg in adult, 50-75µg/kg in a child) repeated every 5 minutes until 'atropinised' and the heart rate is greater than 80/min (this may require >100mg/hr of atropine in some cases). Pralidoxime is a reactivator of phosphorylated AChE and can be given at a dose of 30mg/kg IV over 30 minutes in a critical care setting followed by an infusion of 8mg/kg/hr for 12-24 hours.

F   *Yersinia pestis* is a Gram-negative bacillus known to cause plague. It exists naturally in three forms: septicaemic, bubonic and pneumonic. Pneumonic plague is the most likely to be used in a terrorist attack, causing multi-lobar, haemorrhagic and necrotising bronchopneumonia. Patients develop a cough and fever which then progresses to pneumonia. There is no rapid test for *Yersinia pestis* to confirm plague. Large numbers of people presenting with severe pneumonia, haemoptysis and sepsis may be the first sign of an attack. Streptomycin, gentamicin and doxycycline are used in the management dependent on policy.

T   Smallpox (*Variola major*) is highly contagious and has been eradicated since 1971. However, remaining samples still exist in some countries. The incubation period is 7-19 days following exposure. Initial presentation is non-specific including fever, malaise, vomiting, headache and backache, following which an erythematous macular rash occurs, progressing to papules then pustules in a centrifugal pattern. Death occurs in the second week due to multi-organ failure caused by overwhelming viraemia. Treatment is supportive. Vaccination provides full immunity.

1.   www.toxbase.org.

2.   http://www.hpa.org.uk/webc/HPAwebFile/HPAweb_C/1194947401128.

3.   Geoghegan J, Tong JL. Chemical warfare agents. *Contin Educ Anaesth Crit Care Pain* 2006; 6(6): 230-4.

4.   Hamele M, Poss WB, Sweney J. Disaster preparedness, pediatric considerations in primary blast injury, chemical and biological terrorism. *World J Crit Care Med* 2014; 3(1): 15-23.

Intensive Care Resources

Below is a list of intensive care resources which have proved invaluable not only for revision purposes but also in continuing professional learning and development:

American Board of Internal Medicine
www.abim.org

Anaesthesia Tutorial of the Week. AAGBI
www.aagbi.org

Anaesthesia UK: Critical Care UK
www.frca.co.uk

Continuing Education in Anaesthesia, Critical Care and Pain
www.ceaccp.oxfordjournals.org

Critical Care Reviews
www.criticalcarereviews.com

Crit-IQ
www.crit-iq.com

European Society of Intensive Care Medicine
www.esicm.org

Faculty of Intensive Care Medicine UK (FICM)
www.ficm.ac.uk

Life in the fast lane
www.lifeinthefastlane.com

Indian Society of Critical Care Medicine
www.isccm.org

Intensive Care Monitor
www.intensive-care monitor.com

Intensive Care Society
www.ics.org.uk

Intensive Care Society of Ireland
www.icmed.com

Society of Critical Medicine
www.sccm.org

The American Board of Surgery
www.absurgery.org

The College of Emergency Medicine UK
www.collemergencymed.ac.uk

The College of Intensive Care Medicine Australia and New Zealand.
www.cicm.org.au

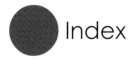 Index

Locators are in the form paper number.question number.